Medical Law & Professional Ethics

Second Edition

Lois Ritter
University of Nevada, Reno
Reno, Nevada

Donald Graham
Attorney
Sacramento, California

Publisher
The Goodheart-Willcox Company, Inc.
Tinley Park, Illinois
www.g-w.com

About the Authors

Lois Ritter, *EdD, MS, MA, MS-HCA, PMP, CHDA, CPHIMS*

Lois Ritter teaches in the Master of Public Health program at the University of Nevada, Reno and is a research consultant. She holds a doctoral degree in education and master's degrees in health science, social and cultural anthropology, and healthcare administration. She has conducted national and statewide research on topics such as telehealth, human trafficking, and substance abuse. She is a published author of several journal articles and textbooks and has presented at international, national, and regional conferences.

Donald Graham, *JD, MA*
Attorney
Sacramento, California

Donald Graham is an attorney and also holds a master's degree in urban studies. He has been licensed for over 20 years in both California and Washington State. His practice involves both civil and criminal justice matters, including personal injury, medical licensing, and Medicaid fraud. Mr. Graham's career has included serving as Deputy Director of the Los Angeles Regional Criminal Justice Planning Board, as an instructor for the Criminal Justice Planning Institute at the University of Southern California, as a consultant to the National Council of Juvenile and Family Court Judges, and as Administrator of the regional Developmental Disabilities Center in Orange County, California. During the past 15 years, he has been periodically involved in assessing programs delivering services for children's mental health, child abuse, and homelessness. Mr. Graham's published works include articles, journals, and a textbook on a variety of related topics.

TOOLS FOR STUDENT AND INSTRUCTOR SUCCESS

Student Tools

Student Text

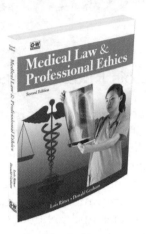

Medical Law & Professional Ethics presents important concepts regarding legal and ethical responsibilities in the healthcare field. It describes various medical laws and explains their impact on people working in this industry. It also addresses the patient-professional relationship, including privacy issues related to the increasingly digital format of healthcare delivery. Plentiful scenarios and case studies apply concepts within the chapter, helping students to apply chapter content in realistic cases.

Study Guide

The supplemental Study Guide that accompanies *Medical Law & Professional Ethics* includes instructor-created questions and activities to help students recall, review, and apply concepts introduced in the book.

Instructor Tools

LMS Integration

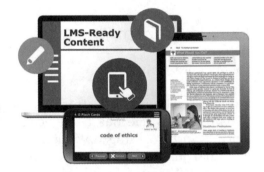

Integrate Goodheart-Willcox content into your Learning Management System for a seamless user experience for both you and your students. LMS-ready content in Common Cartridge® format facilitates single sign-on integration and gives you control of student enrollment and data. With a Common Cartridge integration, you can access the LMS features and tools you are accustomed to using and G-W course resources in one convenient location—your LMS.

G-W Common Cartridge provides a complete learning package for you and your students. The included digital resources help your students remain engaged and learn effectively:

- **eBook content.** G-W Common Cartridge includes the textbook content in an online format. The eBook is interactive, with highlighting, magnification, and note-taking features.
- **Study Guide content.** Students can have access to a digital version of the Study Guide.
- **Drill and Practice.** Learning new vocabulary is critical to student success. These vocabulary activities, which are provided for all key terms in each chapter, provide an active, engaging, and effective way for students to learn the required terminology.

When you incorporate G-W content into your courses via Common Cartridge, you have the flexibility to customize and structure the content to meet the educational needs of your students. You may also choose to add your own content to the course.

For instructors, the Common Cartridge includes the Online Instructor Resources. QTI® question banks are available within the Online Instructor Resources for import into your LMS. These prebuilt assessments help you measure student knowledge and track results in your LMS gradebook. Questions and tests can be customized to meet your assessment needs.

Online Instructor Resources

Instructor Resources provide all the support needed to make preparation and classroom instruction easier than ever. Available in one accessible location, the OIR includes Instructor Resources, Instructor's Presentations for PowerPoint®, and Assessment Software with Question Banks. The OIR is available as a subscription and can be accessed at school, at home, or on the go.

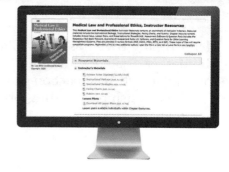

Instructor Resources One resource provides instructors with time-saving preparation tools such as answer keys, lesson plans, pretests, posttests, and other teaching aids.

Instructor's Presentations for PowerPoint® These fully customizable, richly illustrated slides help you teach and visually reinforce the key concepts from each chapter.

Assessment Software with Question Banks Administer and manage assessments to meet your classroom needs. The question banks that accompany this textbook include hundreds of matching, completion, multiple choice, and short answer questions to assess student knowledge of the content in each chapter. Using the assessment software simplifies the process of creating, managing, administering, and grading tests. You can have the software generate a test for you with randomly selected questions. You may also choose specific questions from the question banks and, if you wish, add your own questions to create customized tests to meet your classroom needs.

G-W Integrated Learning Solution

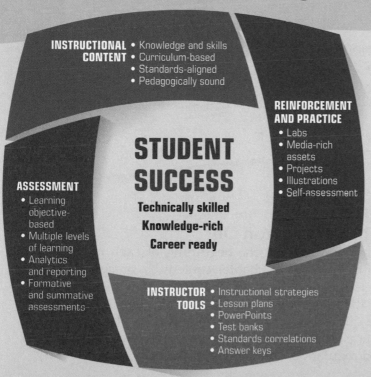

INSTRUCTIONAL CONTENT
- Knowledge and skills
- Curriculum-based
- Standards-aligned
- Pedagogically sound

REINFORCEMENT AND PRACTICE
- Labs
- Media-rich assets
- Projects
- Illustrations
- Self-assessment

STUDENT SUCCESS
Technically skilled
Knowledge-rich
Career ready

ASSESSMENT
- Learning objective-based
- Multiple levels of learning
- Analytics and reporting
- Formative and summative assessments

INSTRUCTOR TOOLS
- Instructional strategies
- Lesson plans
- PowerPoints
- Test banks
- Standards correlations
- Answer keys

The G-W Integrated Learning Solution offers easy-to-use resources that help students and instructors achieve success.

▶ **EXPERT AUTHORS**
▶ **TRUSTED REVIEWERS**
▶ **100 YEARS OF EXPERIENCE**

EMPLOYABILITY SKILLS · TECHNICAL SKILLS · ACADEMIC KNOWLEDGE · INDUSTRY RECOGNIZED STANDARDS

Guided Tour

Medical Law & Professional Ethics will help students understand the legal and ethical responsibilities associated with careers in the healthcare field. The text describes various medical laws and explains their impact on people working in this industry. It also addresses the patient-professional relationship, including privacy issues related to the increasingly digital format of healthcare delivery.

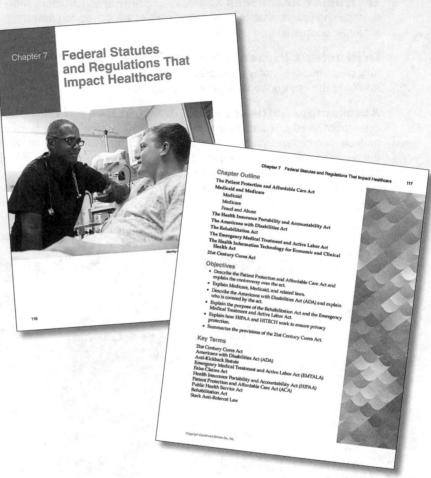

Chapter Orientation

Each chapter begins with an outline and a list of objectives to guide student learning as they read the material presented. Each objective is aligned with the content headings, as well as with the summary at the end of the chapter. This alignment provides a logical flow through each page of the material so that students may build on individual knowledge as they progress through the chapters.

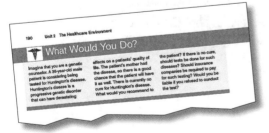

What Would You Do?

These scenarios at the beginning of each chapter help orient students to chapter content by presenting examples of real-life legal issues healthcare workers may face on the job. Considering these examples and answering the question "What would you do?" will pique student interest and increase understanding of how various laws and regulations are applied in the healthcare industry.

Ethical Dilemma Scenarios

Located within each chapter, Ethical Dilemma scenarios describe situations in which, whether or not the legal issue is clear, the ethical implications need to be understood. Reflecting on these situations and thinking about the ethical effects of various actions will deepen student understanding of ethics in healthcare.

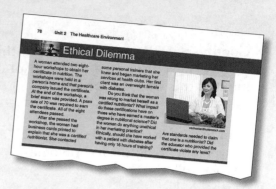

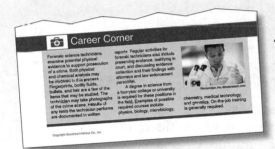

Career Corner

These features provide insight into careers related to the content of each chapter. Reading this information broadens student recognition of the many possible careers within the healthcare industry.

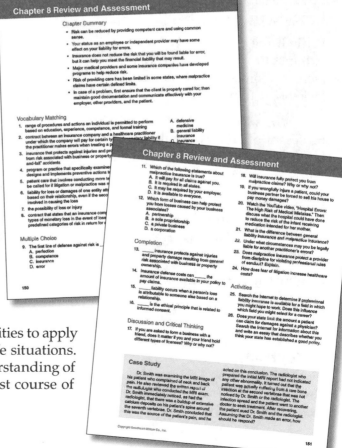

End-of-Chapter Activities

End-of-chapter material provides an opportunity for students to review and apply the concepts presented in the chapter.

- A concise **Chapter Summary** reiterates the chapter objectives and provides a brief review of the content for student reference.
- **Review** questions, including matching, multiple choice, completion, discussion, and critical thinking questions, highlight basic concepts and vocabulary presented in the chapter so students can evaluate their understanding of the material.
- **Application** activities challenge students to apply chapter concepts.
- **Case Studies** provide additional opportunities to apply both legal and ethical principles to real-life situations. Considering these cases adds greater understanding of chapter content as students ponder the best course of action in each case.

Reviewers

Goodheart-Willcox Publisher and the authors would like to thank the following instructors who reviewed selected manuscript chapters and provided valuable input into the development of this textbook program.

Kim Bishop, RHIT, MLT, RMA, AHI(AMT)
Instructor of Medical Technologies
Panola College
Carthage, TX

Marion Bucci
Faculty, Health Care Professions
Montgomery County Community College
Blue Bell, PA

Patty Bucho
Allied Health Instructor
Long Beach City College
Long Beach, CA

Billie Buda
Adjunct Professor RMA (EMT)
Jackson Community College
Jackson, MI

Dr. Donna Burge
Professor of Human Anatomy and Physiology
Lord Fairfax Community College
Warrenton, VA

Imke Casey
Health Information Technology Instructor
Lake-Sumter State College
Leesburg, FL

Debbie Curtin, BS, LVN, CT
Nurse
CIS Healthcare Management
Pasadena, CA

Jessica Ennis
Medical Assisting Program Director
Gwinnett Technical College
Lawrenceville, GA

Sandra Flynn
Instructor
Guilford Technical Community College
Jamestown, NC

Diane Harrison-James
Professor
South Suburban College
South Holland, IL

Angela Hennessy
Instructor, Business Administration
Corning Community College
Corning, NY

Dien Ho
Associate Professor of Philosophy and Health Care Ethics
MCPHS University
Boston, MA

Lisa Huehns
Allied Health Instructor
Lakeshore Technical College
Cleveland, WI

Robert Johnson
Instructor
Ivy Tech Community College
Indianapolis, IN

Patricia Kelly
MLT/PBT Program Director
Mississippi Delta Community College
Drew, MS

Shauna LaMagna
Program Coordinator and Assistant Professor
  of Medical Assisting
Montgomery County Community College
Blue Bell, PA

Christine Malone
Tenured Health Sciences Instructor
Everett Community College
Everett, WA

Patricia Mannie
Dental Hygiene Instructor
St. Cloud Technical and Community College
St. Cloud, MN

Lisa G. Mayer
Assistant Professor, Esquire
Bergen Community College
Paramus, NJ

Tanya Nix
Assistant Professor of Medical Assisting
Northeast Texas Community College
Mt. Pleasant, TX

Patricia Padilla
Adjunct Instructor
Craven Community College
New Bern, NC

Emily Peterson
Faculty; Human, Social, and Behavioral
  Sciences
Washtenaw Community College
Ann Arbor, MI

Linda Pristelski
Health Information Technology Instructor
Northeast Wisconsin Technical College
Green Bay, WI

Nicole Procise
Instructor, Health Care Support
Ivy Tech Community College
Fort Wayne, IN

Alice Pyles
Radiology Program Director
Mississippi Delta Community College
Drew, MS

Michael Randolph
Medical Assistant Instructor
Gateway Technical College
Racine, WI

Pat Reinhart
Faculty, Nursing Assistant/Home Health Aide
Minneapolis Community and Technical
  College
Minneapolis, MN

Marty Richardson
Nursing Professor, Nursing Coordinator
Grayson College
Denison, TX

Carmen Robinson
Adjunct Professor
Contra Costa College
San Pablo, CA

Mary Rost
RN, Advanced Health Careers I Instructor
JP McCaskey High School
Lancaster, PA

Cathy Soto
Faculty, Medical Assisting
El Paso Community College
El Paso, TX

Angelika Stachnik
Clinical Coordinator, Radiography Instructor
Elgin Community College
Elgin, IL

Miasha Torain
Instructor; Administrative and Clinical B.S.,
  CMA (AAMA)
Alamance Community College
Graham, NC

Teresa Wangler
Professor
Oakland Community College
Bloomfield Hills, MI

Brief Contents

Contents

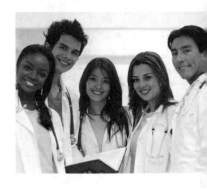

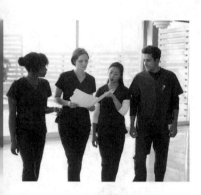

Unit 3
Healthcare, Law, and Ethics across the Lifespan

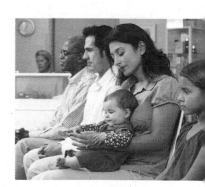

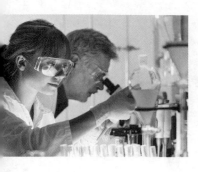

To the Student

We developed this book to provide you with a sense of how the professional rules of ethics and the legal system support efforts to provide good professional care to patients while honoring patient autonomy and protecting their rights. We hope you will enjoy reviewing our description of how professional ethics and law support your participation in the healthcare system while serving people regardless of where they are in their lifespan.

We have limited our discussion to the healthcare and legal systems in the United States. You should be aware that each country has varying rules and there are few, if any, enforceable standards between countries. While there are some efforts to develop international standards, the global system is still unregulated. You must be cautious if you intend to perform any work outside the United States.

While we provide some history, much of this book focuses on the nature and complexity of the current US legal system. Professional associations, the federal government, state governments, and local governments are each involved in the healthcare system. Therefore, if you wish to work in healthcare, you will need to know the framework created for your career by a network of standards, rules, written laws, and evolving case law. We hope to take the mystery and fear out of the complexity of the US system and give you some confidence in how rewarding your career in healthcare can be.

To take the mystery and fear out of reading this book, please take a few minutes to scan through the table of contents to see how the book is organized into major sections that contain several specialized chapters. This structure provides a pathway through this challenging material and may give you a useful framework for addressing real life situations as they arise in your career.

Our book is divided into three major sections, or units. *Foundations of Medical Law and Ethics* includes an introduction to and background on legal and ethical rules. *The Healthcare Environment* describes the framework of certification and licensing and the context of civil laws, criminal laws, and specific healthcare-related statutes. Within this framework are methods for managing risk and the patient-professional relationship. This section also covers health information technology, genetics and drugs, and facilities administration. *Healthcare, Law, and Ethics across the Lifespan* includes a discussion of laws related to minors, adults, and older adults.

Both professional ethics and law change regularly as society changes. However, we hope you find the framework we provide useful in organizing new information on these topics as these standards, rules, and laws evolve over time.

Regardless of which part of the complex healthcare system you select to be part of, you are entering into an important career. We understand the importance of your undertaking and know that you bring your own unique skills and abilities to the system of care. If you can recognize the general framework of professional law and ethics that every competent participant must understand, then you will be an important member of a critical team, prepared to treat patients who put their life in the hands of the healthcare system. Even if you do not continue with a career in healthcare, you will find this book useful to you as a patient and health-care customer.

Lois Ritter
Donald Graham

Unit 1 Foundations of Medical Law and Ethics

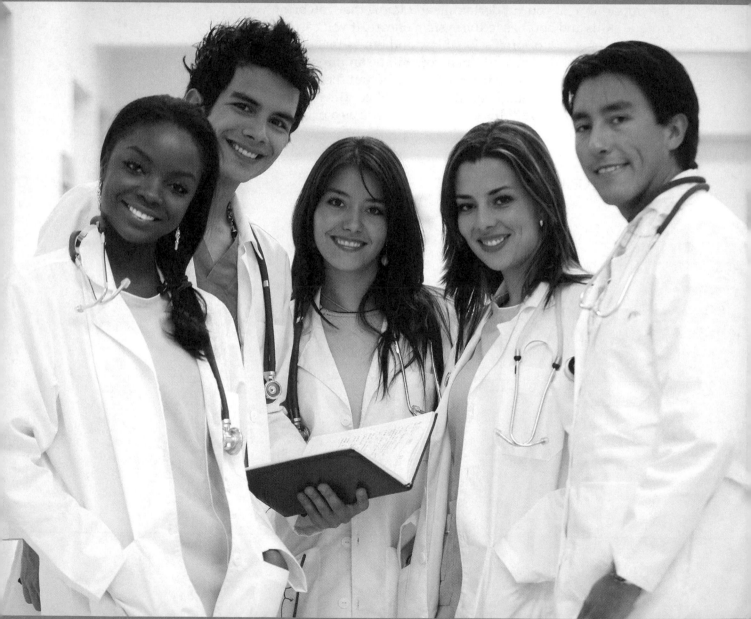

ESB Professional/Shutterstock.com

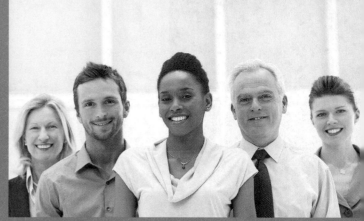
Rido/Shutterstock.com

Chapter 1

Overview of Medical Law and Ethics

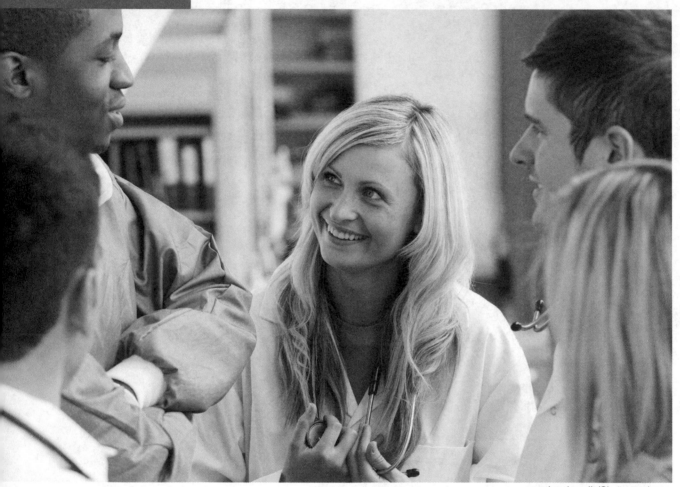

wavebreakmedia/Shutterstock.com

Chapter Outline

The Importance of Studying Medical Law and Ethics
A Brief History of Medical Law
The Relationship between Law and Ethics
The Healthcare Industry
Laws and Ethics Related to Health Careers

Objectives

- Explain the importance of medical law and ethics.
- Describe the history of medical law and ethics.
- Explain how law and ethics are interrelated, yet distinct.
- Explain why and how business is involved in healthcare.
- Summarize the effects of laws and professional ethics on the healthcare industry.

Key Terms

ethics
fee-for-service model
law
morality
philosophy
regulation
rule
value-based healthcare delivery model

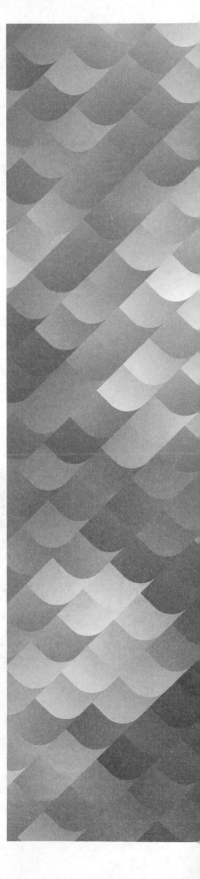

What Would You Do?

Imagine that you are a pediatric nurse practitioner. You strongly believe that children should be immunized.

A parent is not in favor of having her child immunized for religious reasons. Do you try to convince the parent to

have the child immunized? Do you have a legal and ethical responsibility to do so?

People need and want good healthcare. Some people believe that having access to healthcare services is a basic human right. Others disagree, thinking that each individual needs to earn or pay for access to healthcare. Whatever you may believe, everyone desires access to well-trained healthcare providers.

Because good health is a common human interest, societies throughout the world encourage people to learn and practice the specialized skills required to provide quality healthcare. As you consider or pursue a career in healthcare and develop your knowledge and skills, you should be aware of and understand the responsibilities associated with being a healthcare professional. Some healthcare practitioners must be licensed or certified in order to work in their profession. These practitioners are usually rewarded for their education and training with secure and long-term employment. Many healthcare professionals also earn higher-than-average monetary compensation, as well as admiration in their community (Figure 1.1).

This chapter provides a brief history of medical law and ethics and then discusses the relationships between health, laws, ethics, and business.

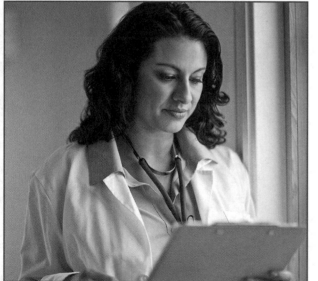

Erickson Stock/Shutterstock.com

Figure 1.1 Physicians must complete many years of schooling before they can practice. All of this preparation leads to a rewarding career and respect from the community.

The Importance of Studying Medical Law and Ethics

There are many reasons for studying medical law and ethics. One reason may be that you are required to study these topics as part of your coursework, which leads to a degree or prepares you for a certain career. Another may be that you are naturally interested in these subjects. Medical law and ethics touch careers, such as being a firefighter or a social policy analyst, that you would not have thought possible. But whether you want to pursue a career in health, law, or anything else, medical law and ethics can provide valuable insights for your personal life as well as your professional life.

Studying law and ethics provides a framework for structuring people's actions and assists with making the right decisions when what is right or wrong is not obvious. There are times when professional ethics and laws may be contradictory to your personal beliefs. For example, you may be personally against using infertility drugs, but as a health-care provider, you may be obligated to prescribe them under your agreement with the medical facility.

Understanding medical law and ethics also can help you avoid litigation and find comfort in the decisions that you make. The right decisions in healthcare are not always obvious. For example, is providing medical treatment for a patient who is in a coma and is brain dead the right way to care for the patient? Is it the legal way?

In addition, people who know and understand medical law and ethical rules can make significant contributions to society. They can assist others with making good decisions, whether those decisions involve individuals, groups, or large populations, directly or indirectly. For example, an administrator of a senior home who follows ethical rules can be a role model for others to treat residents with respect and to follow good clinical practices.

The fields of medicine and law have each developed over thousands of years. Each has its own separate foundation of philosophy, skill, and knowledge. No one really expects a doctor to practice law or a lawyer to practice medicine, although a number of individuals have learned both fields and have become qualified to practice in both professions.

These two fields literally affect every person in every society in one way or another. It is important to know the relationship of these fields to each other whether you end up actually working in these fields, or simply wish to better understand them as a patient or client. Interestingly, both fields struggle equally in attempting to determine what is right or wrong conduct in a certain situation. This chapter explores the complexity of this task.

A Brief History of Medical Law

Throughout the development of civilization, medical law and ethics have been influenced by factors such as social issues, religious authority, and advances in scientific knowledge and technology. Therefore, these topics have evolved to reflect important changes in philosophy and society. Since the earliest recorded history, the practice of medicine has been a special area of reward and discipline (Figure 1.2).

Code of Hammurabi
Financial rewards for good care included the following:
Law 215. *If a physician make a large incision with an operating knife and cure it, or if he opens a tumor (over the eye) with an operating knife, and saves the eye, he shall receive ten shekels in money.*
Law 216. *If the patient be a freed man, he receives five shekels.*
Law 217. *If he be the slave of someone, his owner shall give the physician two shekels.*
These rewards were balanced by the first known written punishments for failing to provide proper care:
Law 218. *If a physician make a large incision with the operating knife, and kill him, or open a tumor with the operating knife, and cut out the eye, his hands shall be cut off.*
Law 219. *If a physician make a large incision in the slave of a freed man, and kill him, he shall replace the slave with another slave.*
Law 220. *If he had opened a tumor with the operating knife and put out his eye, he shall pay half his value.*
Of course, modern discipline is not as harsh as in Hammurabi's time, and incentives to encourage medical practitioners have outweighed the penalties throughout the ages. Yet punishment for not providing proper care is still imposed in the form of malpractice lawsuits and professional censure.

Figure 1.2   Excerpts from the Code of Hammurabi, carved in stone in 1790 BCE.

The first physician on record, dating back to about 2600 BCE, was an Egyptian known by the name Imhotep (Figure 1.3). He established some early techniques for the treatment of wounds, broken bones, and even tumors. Born as a commoner, Imhotep was later worshipped as a god by the Egyptians.

Ancient Egyptian rulers developed a practice to pay members of the upper class who were permitted to practice medicine. Later, in the 6th century BCE, Greek philosophers began exploring the nature of the physical world and morality, laying the foundation for formal medical ethics. Later and most notably, Hippocrates (460–370 BCE)—the "father of modern medicine"—advised medical practitioners to "first, do no harm" (see chapter 2 for further discussion). In the Dark Ages (about 500 to 1000 AD), religious beliefs heavily influenced medical practice, as written knowledge and communication were greatly limited by the effects of war and disease. During the Middle Ages and the Enlightenment (1000 to 1790 AD), major advances in both medicine and law occurred.

Gradually, evolving from mid-15th century English efforts to regulate who could practice medicine, medical practice training and specialized ethical rules were adopted, ending the custom of allowing citizens to simply declare themselves healers and provide creative approaches to curing maladies for a fee. From colonial times in the United States to the present, a large number of laws, rules, ethical guidelines, and career opportunities have evolved.

The Relationship between Healthcare, Law, and Ethics

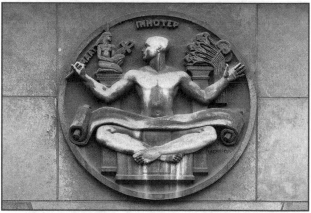

Zvonimir Atletic/Shutterstock.com

Figure 1.3 Ancient Egypt is the origin of many aspects of healthcare, including the first physician on record—Imhotep.

By definition, **law** is a binding system of rules that are recognized by a community and used to regulate the conduct or action of its members. These rules are enforceable by a controlling authority. While a law is recognized as binding, it may not always be clear. This is not surprising when you consider that laws derive from a society's beliefs and that those beliefs and their interpretation and meaning can and do change over time.

As mentioned previously, personal health and safety are important to all members of society. Therefore, a multitude of laws and regulations concerning healthcare have been developed at all levels of government. Like laws, **regulations** are directives made and maintained by an authority. For example, there are state regulations related to health and safety requirements for caregivers. A **rule** is one of a set of explicit or understood regulations or principles governing conduct within a particular activity or sphere. A rule may, for example, deal with the state licensing requirements for child care centers. Legislatures often pass laws that government agencies then turn into more specific regulations and rules.

Healthcare laws regulate governmental operations and private institutional programs while protecting individual rights. Examples include laws guiding the delivery of national healthcare programs such as Medicare, the state licensing of physicians, and the operation of county public health clinics. You will learn more about healthcare law within the framework of our different levels of government in Chapter 3.

The word *ethics* is derived from the Greek word *ethos*, which means "character." The issues of morality and ethical decision-making are strongly related to human conduct. Various theories have been offered throughout the centuries in an attempt to answer the question, "Do morals exist?" For example, a German philosopher of the 19th century, Immanuel Kant (1724–1804), deeply thought about this question (Figure 1.4). For Kant, the source of moral justification is the *categorical imperative*, which means that an act becomes imperative (or commanded) when it should to be applied to everyone. It is *categorical* because it

law
a rule or action that is prescribed by a governmental authority and has a binding legal force

regulation
a rule made and maintained by an authority

rule
an explicit or understood regulation or principle that governs conduct within a specific activity or situation

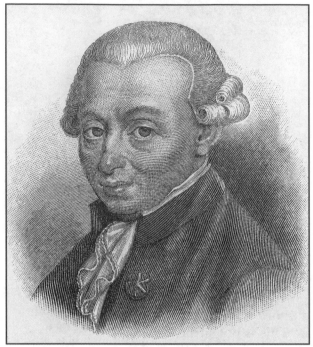

Nicku/Shutterstock.com

Figure 1.4   The writings of Immanuel Kant, as well as other philosophers, helped shape current understanding of ethics.

philosophy
the study of the truths and principles of existence, reality, knowledge, values, or conduct that guide behavior

morality
the quality of practicing the right conduct; defines correct conduct according to an individual's ideals and principles

ethics
a set of principles of right and wrong conduct; a system of values that guides behavior in relationships with people in accordance with social roles

applies to people unconditionally, despite their ability to think of reasons to act otherwise. The professional ethics discussed in the following chapters are essentially categorical imperatives that apply to specific professions.

Medical law evolved from the same general background as all other law. It has a history involving thousands of years of human philosophical, political, moral, and religious discussion about the proper conduct of people and society. **Philosophy** addresses fundamental concepts of consciousness and an individual's ability to actually conduct decision making based on free will as opposed to external predetermination of individual conduct.

Morality is a subset of philosophy that addresses concepts of right and wrong, proper conduct, good and evil, and other concepts intended to provide some guidance to individuals and society. Morality is usually implemented by individual interpretations of concepts of right and wrong, which are often based in philosophical and religious teachings. Of course, your own beliefs of proper conduct and obligation are very important, but they alone cannot guide your work in the healthcare field. You also will be influenced by professional ethics, which differ from morality.

Established by a specific group, **ethics** are externally defined principles that govern the standards of behavior for individuals within that group as to what is good or bad. These principles might include national ethics, professional ethics, social ethics, organizational ethics, or family ethics. Think of it this way: Morals refer to an individual's own principles regarding right and wrong, while ethics involve and adhere to an external system in which those morals are applied. So, while a person's moral code is usually unchanging, the ethics he or she practices can depend on outside systems.

Professional ethics are not laws applied to all citizens, but are rules that dictate whether certain actions by individuals in a designated group are considered ethical behavior or not. For example, the American Bar Association has established a rule that says, "a lawyer shall deposit into a client trust account legal fees and expenses that have been paid in advance, to be withdrawn by the lawyer only as fees are earned or expenses incurred."

Often there is no conflict between a person's individual morality and a group's ethical standards. There are situations, however, in which differences of opinion arise, and it is important to know that you cannot always rely on your own sense of moral or ethical conduct. You never have to give up your own personal moral standards. If you do not want to follow the ethical rules set up by others, you can choose not to work in that particular field.

For instance, repeated major surgeries on a terminally ill patient with little hope of improving might raise your concern as to whether continued surgeries are warranted. Are you serving the patient's best interest by interfering with natural death? What does the patient want? Are these surgeries a waste of medical time and resources needed by others? In this situation, whether you are the surgeon or a participating allied healthcare professional, you would need to make important personal and professional decisions (Figure 1.5).

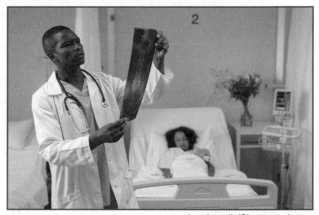

wavebreakmedia/Shutterstock.com

Figure 1.5 Doctors and other healthcare professionals often have to make difficult ethical decisions.

When trying to determine what constitutes ethical conduct in the healthcare field, you might be tempted to simply follow shorthand concepts such as Hippocrates' advice to "do no harm" or the Golden Rule to "do unto others as you would have them do unto you." While these concepts underlie many moral and ethical ideas, you must first look to established laws and ethical rules, which may differ slightly from what we might otherwise consider proper. This practice of knowing and checking laws and ethical standards is fundamental to working in healthcare and can help you avoid inadvertently imposing your own values on others.

Professional associations establish ethical rules to provide guidance to those practicing within a particular healthcare field. In most cases,

Ethical Dilemma

You work in the human resources department for an organization that manufactures an over-the-counter drug. The business is small and owned by a man who has been very good to you over the years. You have been receiving calls about people having adverse reactions to the drug. You approach your boss and inform him of the complaints. He said he will look into it, but he never follows up with you. The calls continue to trickle in, so you approach him again. He informs you that they have identified a bad batch of the drug, that it will cost too much to recall it, and not everyone is becoming ill. The effects are minimal, he says, and the problem has been resolved. He instructs you to take a message if anyone else calls.

What do you do? Is this a legal issue? an ethical issue? Is it part of your job to act on this problem? What if you do? What if you don't act? Where should you look for guidance to help decide?

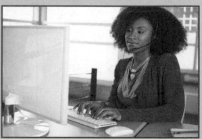

ESB Basic/Shutterstock.com

ethical standards are enforced by suspending the membership of any individuals who fail to conform to the approved standards. Governmental laws and regulations may impose monetary penalties and, in some cases, incarceration for unqualified, unethical, or incompetent actions.

A guideline for easier navigation of these complex topics is the old railroad track warning sign stating, "Stop, Look, and Listen." It is best to wait until you have assessed the patient's current situation, listened to the patient, and followed your training protocols, including relevant professional ethics rules, before jumping into action.

The Healthcare Industry

Of course, patient care is at the heart of healthcare, yet it is part of a complex system of people and resources. Encouragement for effective delivery of healthcare is as old as written law itself, going back as far as 1790 BCE. For example, chiseled in stone is the 3,800-year-old Code of Hammurabi, which contains over 280 laws (Figure 1.6). Several of these laws describe specific rewards for physicians who provided good care, as well as punishments for those who failed to provide proper care. As has been the case since early Egyptian times, payment of money has been an incentive and reward for people providing medical care. The US healthcare system focuses on patient care, but it is a large business sector within the US economy. The 3.6 trillion dollar United States healthcare industry makes up about 17.7 percent of the entire US economy.

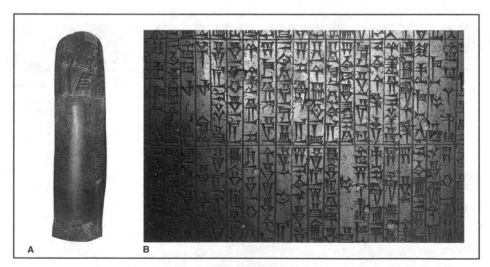

jsp/Shutterstock.com

Figure 1.6   A—the stone on which the Code of Hammurabi is carved; B—close-up of the carved laws

Career Corner

The healthcare field is changing rapidly, which makes it an exciting and diverse area in which to work. How and where care is provided, who provides the healthcare services, and how the care is financed are just a few examples of how the healthcare field is being altered. As a result of these changes, there is a variety of settings where healthcare professionals can work. These settings include:

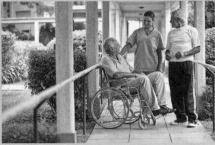
hxdbzxy/Shutterstock.com

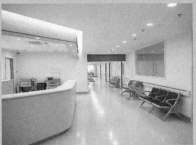
Robert Kneschke/Shutterstock.com

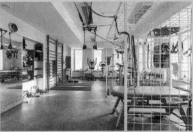
Photographee.eu/Shutterstock.com

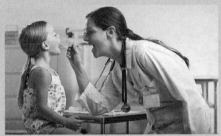
AVAVA/Shutterstock.com

- physical and occupational clinics
- social services agencies
- health insurance companies
- healthcare professional associations
- hospitals
- urgent care centers
- retail health clinics
- nursing and assisted-living homes
- mental health facilities
- public health departments
- rehabilitation centers
- skilled nursing facilities
- academic institutions
- research firms

When people think of healthcare careers, they often think of doctors and nurses, yet there is a wide array of careers in the healthcare sector. For example, a genetic counselor works with families to assess and understand their risk of an inherited medical condition, and then provides education. Genetic counselors have specialized training in medical genetics and counseling. They spend much of their day meeting with patients to help them understand the ways genetics affect their lives and the lives of their unborn offspring.

Many healthcare workers work directly with patients. For example, a home health aide may visit patients at home to assist with activities of daily living. A school counselor may meet with students at a high school.

However, not all healthcare workers engage with patients.

For example, a medical records clerk, transcriptionist, or quality inspector does not engage in direct care. Nevertheless, healthcare is always focused on the hands-on care of individuals and rewards those involved in their care while adhering to legal and ethical guidelines. Not all healthcare workers earn six-figure salaries, but many high-paid and rewarding jobs are available.

As you read this book, you will see various healthcare careers mentioned, but there are many other careers to discover. Use the Internet to find websites with information about healthcare careers. What new careers did you find?

Laws and Ethics Related to Health Careers

The business of healthcare has evolved beyond simply rewarding individual care providers with good compensation and prestige. The healthcare business environment now encourages large-scale commercial activities that increase health system capabilities. In the United States and other Western societies, this has resulted in healthcare becoming "big business."

In many cases, the potential large-scale financial returns are necessary to encourage the development and advancement of medical care. Medical advancements, such as magnetic resonance imaging or new medications, can take many years to develop and many more years to obtain approval from regulatory agencies. Debate continues on how much it actually costs to bring new drugs and technologies to market, but regardless, it is a substantial sum.

The government provides incentives that encourage companies to invest in the development of new medicines and technologies. An example is the government's granting of patents and copyrights, which create short-term monopolies for inventors of medical devices and drugs. By controlling the use of the inventions and rewarding the inventor's efforts, the government seeks to improve healthcare services. Similarly, the government may grant geographic service areas to specific hospitals to provide trauma care or other specialized services in certain locations.

Sometimes large-scale, long-range business opportunities are not sufficient to bring about the needed remedies. In these cases, the government may undertake the development of knowledge and techniques through organizations such as the National Institutes of Health (NIH) or the Centers for Disease Control and Prevention (CDC). An example is research on herbs, such as ginseng, which has been identified as having healing properties. Because it is an herb, it cannot be patented, so private companies would not receive a return on their investment for their research. That is why this type of research is often government funded.

New legal and ethical questions are currently being debated about drug pricing. Traditionally, development and delivery costs were the essential considerations in setting prices, depending on how long it might take to recover a reasonable profit on investment. Recently, this practice has changed to set pricing based on "value" to patients rather than costs to developers.

A **value-based healthcare delivery model** is one in which providers, including hospitals and physicians, are paid based on patient health outcomes. This model is being applied to replace the **fee-for-service model** used in the past, which rewarded providers by volume of hours or other measures of care.

The emerging value-based model may greatly affect how healthcare work is performed and rewarded. Additionally, opportunities for

value-based healthcare delivery model
payment model in which healthcare providers are compensated based on patient health outcomes

fee-for-service model
payment model in which healthcare providers are compensated according to volume of hours or other measures of care

"gaming the system" or exploiting clients is a concern. For example, Turing Pharmaceuticals increased the price of Daraprim®, a medicine used to treat toxoplasmosis (a parasite-borne infection that can be deadly for babies), by 5,000% to $750 per tablet based on value pricing. The concerns relate to whether the drug improves patient health or is just a measure of how much money can be extorted from desperate parents. This type of change raises many legal and ethical concerns that have yet to be resolved but will affect how healthcare is delivered.

Additionally, the business of healthcare involves many businesses outside of the healthcare industry. Hundreds of supporting businesspeople, such as architects, scientific researchers, and accountants, make their living supporting the work of healthcare providers (Figure 1.7). If you decide to work in the healthcare field, these professionals will be dedicating their careers to helping you perform your tasks and having an opportunity for success.

Whatever your role, it is likely that the business forces of profit and loss, risk assessment, and publicity will complicate your view of law, ethics, and healthcare. Your company, for instance, may have its own sets of business ethics, employee policies, continuing education standards, and performance expectations—all of which will affect your day-to-day decision making. Balancing personal financial interests (keeping a job, for example) with efforts to respond to patients' needs, while at the same time trying to comply with all laws, regulations, and ethical rules, creates a complex challenge even for the most well-trained and motivated person. Despite your own personal benevolence or moral commitment to healthcare, business, with objectives that often conflict with those of high-quality care, will always be a part of your daily life in one way or another.

This tension between the delivery of proper care in an efficient manner and the enforcement of proper standards has actually created supporting industries. Such industries (discussed more fully in later chapters) coexist with and heavily influence the healthcare system. For example, insurance industry practices and professional legal activities create both tensions and safeguards for the healthcare business. Insurance companies provide ways to finance unpredictable and sometimes costly medical treatment, for instance. Similarly, the legal profession—including insurance industry attorneys, corporate business attorneys, and attorneys representing patients—challenges and defends business and professional conduct, and thereby helps frame the boundaries of healthcare business and practice.

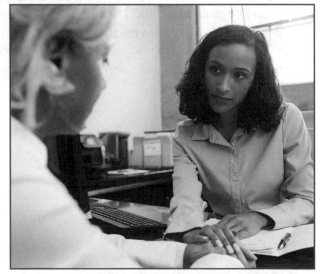

Monkey Business Images/Shutterstock.com

Figure 1.7 In addition to physicians and nurses, the field of healthcare is supported by various business people.

Chapter Summary

- Medical law and ethics are important to society because everyone receives healthcare and depends on providers to act properly.
- Medical law and ethics have existed since the earliest known writings and have evolved as societies have developed over the centuries.
- Laws are imposed by governments to protect society, and ethics are generally created by members of the medical profession to ensure agreed-upon conduct by the providers.
- Business is involved in healthcare as a means to allocate scarce resources and to reward providers for the careful application of their skills for the benefit of patients.
- Overall, laws and ethics shape the limits of provider behavior and ensure quality care for the public and adequate compensation for providers.

Vocabulary Matching

1. the study of the truths and principles of existence, reality, knowledge, values, or conduct that guides behavior
2. rule or action prescribed by a governmental authority that has a binding legal force
3. rule made and maintained by an authority
4. set of principles of right and wrong conduct; a system of values that guides behavior in relationships with people in accordance with social roles
5. explicit or understood regulation or principle that governs conduct within a specific activity or situation
6. the quality of practicing the right conduct; defines correct conduct according to an individual's ideals and principles
7. healthcare providers are compensated according to volume of hours or other measures of care
8. healthcare providers are compensated based on patient health outcomes

A. ethics
B. fee-for-service model
C. law
D. morality
E. philosophy
F. regulation
G. rule
H. value-based healthcare delivery model

Multiple Choice

9. _____ is the name of the first physician on record.
   A. Hippocrates
   B. Imhotep
   C. Plato
   D. Aristotle

10. Which of the following concepts is *not* included in either medicine or law?
    A. skill
    B. creativity
    C. philosophy
    D. knowledge

11. The first known written laws related to medicine were created by the _____.
    A. Egyptians
    B. English
    C. Germans
    D. Greeks

12. Which of the following businesspeople are *not* described in your textbook as being involved in healthcare?
    A. researchers
    B. architects
    C. management coordinators
    D. accountants

13. The term _____ refers to an individual's internal beliefs about what is right or wrong, while the term _____ is related to an external social system that defines what is right or wrong.
    A. ethics, morality
    B. morality, ethics
    C. philosophy, morality
    D. morality, principles

14. Who is known for creating the ethical guidance to "First, do no harm"?
    A. Immanuel Kant
    B. Imhotep
    C. Hippocrates
    D. Hammurabi

Completion

15. The Greek term _____ translates into the term *character*.

16. The Code of _____ includes laws that describe rewards for physicians who provided good care.

17. A(n) _____ has a binding force because it is created by a governing authority.

18. A subset of philosophy that addresses "right and wrong" is _____.

Discussion and Critical Thinking

19. Describe an existing law or rule that could encourage good healthcare.

20. Describe an existing law that will be recognized as a good law 200 years from now.

21. Should you always act on your good intentions? Why?

22. Explain why using caution in the field of healthcare is a good idea.

23. At the beginning of this chapter, there is an example of legal and ethical situations that occur in the healthcare field. What legal or ethical situations have you or your friends and family experienced? How were the situations resolved?

24. How are morals different from professional ethics?

25. Why must laws and ethical rules be considered in light of personal moral convictions?

26. Why might rules related to medicine be among those seen in the earliest written laws?

27. Why does society allow some health-related industries to become "big business"?

28. Explain why the government may decide to become involved in medical research.

Activities

29. Review several current newspaper articles related to medical malpractice cases. Write a two-page paper summarizing three articles that you found. Discuss the key issues involved in the lawsuits you read about, the decision made by the court, and the laws that were related to the legal outcomes. Do you agree with the court's decision? Describe what the healthcare professional should have done differently.

30. Write a one-page paper that describes the health career that most interests you. What courses on law and ethics are required for this field? What are the professional codes that guide these health professionals? What are some of the ethical challenges that they face?

Case Study

Dr. Raven is an experienced orthopedic surgeon with a successful practice. You have worked with him as an operating room (OR) technician for years. Recently, however, he has arrived in the OR with bloodshot eyes and a disheveled appearance. Today you noticed his hands were shaking, and you smelled alcohol when he greeted you. When you asked Dr. Raven if he felt okay, he said he felt fine and appeared annoyed with your question. He is scheduled to perform several surgeries today. You are a single father and really need your job, so you are afraid of reporting this issue to anyone.

- Is it ethical for Dr. Raven to go ahead with the planned procedures? Why or why not?

- Should you report Dr. Raven? Should you do this even if it means losing your job and being unable to provide housing and food for your children? How will you balance your ethical responsibilities as a professional with those as a father?

Chapter 2

Professional Ethics

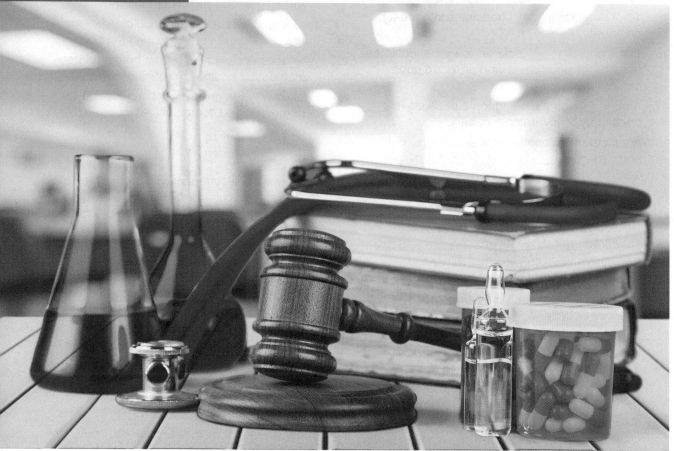

Billion Photos/Shutterstock.com

Chapter Outline

An Introduction to Professional Ethics
    History of Medical Ethics
    Modern Codes of Professional Ethics
The Impact of Politics on Professional Ethics
Ethical Principles
Professional Codes of Ethics and State Laws
Ethical Rights of Patients and Providers
Ethical Decision Making
Bioethics
    Policy Response to Changing Standards of Care
    Medical Ethics Committees

Objectives

- Discuss the history and evolution of medical codes of ethics.
- Explain the impact of politics on professional ethics.
- Describe ethical principles commonly used to guide professional care.
- Explain the relationship between professional codes of ethics and state laws.
- Explain how defined sets of ethical rights help both patients and providers.
- Describe methods of ensuring that decisions are made according to acknowledged ethical standards.
- Identify two types of responses that have evolved to manage difficult bioethical questions.

Key Terms

autonomy
beneficence
bioethics
Common Rule
Hippocratic Oath
Institutional Review Boards
justice
medical ethics committees
non-malfeasance
profession

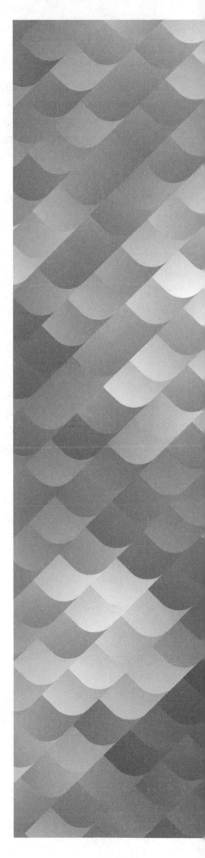

What Would You Do?

After a serious fall that caused him to black out, an 18-year-old skateboarder is brought to the emergency room by his friends. He has a gash on his head and displays all the symptoms of a concussion. After getting stitches, he says he feels better and wants to leave without having a brain CT scan. Should the physician try to convince him to stay and have the test? Would doing so violate the patient's ethical rights? Would the physician be doing harm by letting the skateboarder leave, since his suspected concussion may be affecting his thinking and judgment?

If you decide to pursue a career in healthcare, you will be expected to perform your work according to specific ethical guidelines and standards of care for your chosen field. How do you know where to start? What are the behavioral expectations and guidelines for that profession?

Perhaps the best way to begin is to research the specific code of professional ethics that applies to your intended specialty. Then, broaden your search to determine if potential employers have set certain standards for their employees. Taken together, these codes and standards for behavior will usually include guidelines for honesty, respect, integrity, competence, justice, and professional behavior.

Credentials (licensure and certification) often include a code of ethics that you must follow. Requirements for credentials generally vary among states and different specialties. Even if you select a healthcare career that does not require a specific credential, you will probably work for a person or organization that follows a formal code of ethics. You also may be subject to ethical rules based on your membership in professional organizations. If your intended healthcare specialty does not currently have a code of ethics, one may be developed over the course of your career.

This chapter provides an overview of the changing environment of ethical rules, presents examples of different types of ethical guidelines, and describes the basic ethical principles used in the healthcare field.

An Introduction to Professional Ethics

Professional ethics, as explained in Chapter 1, are defined principles established by a specific group. These principles govern the standards of behavior for individuals within that group. Originally, codes of ethics, or sets of rules, applied only to the "learned professions," which included theology, medicine, and law (Figure 2.1). However, the number of professions regulated by codes of ethics has expanded, particularly in the last 100 years. Generally, these ethical codes address rules within various specialties and define standards for conduct within the scope of practice for each specialty.

The term *profession* derives from a Latin term meaning "to swear (an oath)." The modern definition of **profession** refers to paid work that requires specialized knowledge and skill, and which unqualified people are not allowed to perform. Although the meaning of the term *profession* has changed over the years, certain professions retain the original meaning in their adherence to codes of ethics.

History of Medical Ethics

During the classical Greek era (5th century BC), Hippocrates believed that disease could be studied and cured. He advised medical practitioners, however, to "first do no harm" in recognition that preparation and caution were required for this work. This belief became the basis for the **Hippocratic Oath**, which has provided basic ethical guidance for the medical profession since at least the classical Greek era (Figure 2.2).

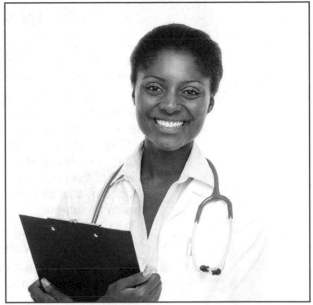

Aila Images/Shutterstock.com

Figure 2.1 Physicians, nurses, and other healthcare professionals have codes of ethics that guide their conduct in the workplace.

This idea still holds true today throughout the various medical fields. In fact, many contemporary medical practitioners take an oath based on Hippocrates' advice. Essentially, if you plan to act in any healthcare situation, you must be sure that you will not engage in actions that make the situation worse than it is already. You must be prepared both technically and emotionally to follow through and finish the work in as positive a manner as possible. You must act in the same way as any person with sufficient skills and learn to handle the situation without imposing additional difficulties on the patient.

If you are not confident that you have the skills and knowledge to improve a patient's position, you do not have an obligation to perform. In fact, you may be held accountable if you act while knowing that you are not competent to do so. In addition, if you try to improve a patient's condition, you have an obligation to continue until such care is adequately provided and no additional harm has been inflicted. You cannot begin to provide care and then stop, leaving the patient in a worse position than before you started. In some situations, if you realize you cannot adequately help the patient yourself, your obligation may be to seek help from others who are more prepared.

During the Middle Ages, the Hippocratic Oath was just one of several different perspectives on medical practice. For instance, both Indian

profession
a calling that requires specialized training and membership in a group that establishes and enforces codes of conduct or codes of ethics, including requirements for continuing education and payment of periodic membership fees

Hippocratic Oath
an oath attributed to the ancient Greek known as Hippocrates that requires a new physician to swear upon a number of healing gods that he will uphold professional ethical standards; strongly binds the student to his teacher and the greater community of physicians

The Classical Oath of Hippocrates

I swear by Apollo the physician, and Aesculapius, and Hygeia, and Panacea, and all the gods and goddesses as my witness, that, according to my ability and judgment, I will keep this Oath and this contract:

To hold him who taught me this art equally dear to me as my parents, to be a partner in life with him, and to fulfill his needs when required; to look upon his offspring as equals to my own siblings, and to teach them this art, if they shall wish to learn it, without fee or contract; and that by the set of rules, lectures, and every other mode of instruction, I will impart a knowledge of the art to my own sons, and those of my teachers, and to students bound by this contract and having sworn this Oath to the law of medicine, but to no others.

I will use those dietary regimens which will benefit my patients according to my greatest ability and judgment, and I will do no harm or injustice to them.

I will not give a lethal drug to anyone if I am asked, nor will I advise such a plan; and similarly I will not give a woman a pessary to cause an abortion.

In purity and according to divine law will I carry out my life and art.

I will not use a knife, even upon those suffering from stones, but I will leave this to those who are trained in this craft.

Into whatever homes I go, I will enter them for the benefit of the sick, avoiding any voluntary act of impropriety or corruption, including the seduction of women or men, whether they are free men or slaves.

Whatever I see or hear in the lives of my patients, whether in connection with my professional practice or not, which ought not to be spoken of outside, I will keep secret, as considering all such things to be private.

So long as I maintain this Oath faithfully and without corruption, may it be granted to me to partake of life fully and the practice of my art, gaining the respect of all men for all time. However, should I transgress this Oath or violate it, may the opposite be my fate.

Goodheart-Willcox Publisher; translated by Michael North, National Library of Medicine, 2002

Figure 2.2 The principles put forth in the classic Hippocratic Oath have formed a basis for medical codes of ethics for centuries.

and Chinese medical writings called for physicians to practice with humility, compassion, and concern for the patient's well-being.

The first known book on medical ethics, *Adab al-Tabib* (*Conduct of a Physician*), was written in the 9th century AD by Ishaq bin Ali Rahawi. This book became increasingly recognized during the late Middle Ages. Rahawi's work, along with later works by Jewish scholar Maimonides (1138–1204 AD) and by Catholic philosophical leader Thomas Aquinas (1225–1274 AD), served as the basis for a discussion of medical ethics throughout Europe during the Middle Ages.

In 1803, English physician Thomas Percival published his famous *Medical Ethics*, a code of professional conduct for physicians and surgeons (Figure 2.3). In 1847, the American Medical Association (AMA) established the first national code of medical ethics, including some provisions taken directly from Percival's work.

Modern Codes of Professional Ethics

Since the 19th century, more health professions have emerged and numerous ethical codes have been developed. The original rules in these codes are continuously reviewed and interpreted by the organizations that developed them. As science and social values evolve, additional rules are developed in response to changing circumstances.

The AMA's Code of Medical Ethics, for example, has been modified several times since its adoption. These revisions have resulted in the AMA's current code, which is essentially a one-page document of principles, with about 500 additional pages of annotated decisions and interpretations of the code (Figure 2.4). Individual practitioners must know the basic content of the applicable code. They must also remain aware of new interpretations and understand how to apply the latest changes to their daily practice. Codes of professional ethics have been developed for a large number of healthcare practitioners ranging from physicians and nurses to clinical laboratory scientists and medical assistants.

Modern versions of the Hippocratic Oath have been developed and are used to initiate new physicians at a number of universities in the United States (Figure 2.5). Marked differences between the original and modern versions reflect the evolving roles of medicine and its relationship to natural death. For example, Hippocrates could not have anticipated the invention of mechanical life support systems or the role of physicians in decisions to continue or suspend such treatment.

Recently, the number of healthcare professions has increased, creating many new types of practitioners. As a result, there has been an increase in the number of professional groups that need ethical standards to help guide their practice. All professions have one or more governing bodies whose function is to define, promote, oversee, support, and regulate the conduct of its members. In fact, the regulation and enforcement of ethics distinguishes a profession from other occupations. The nature and role of professional organizations is discussed in more detail in Chapter 4.

Ethical rules provide guidance, and practitioners are duty bound by oaths or codes of ethics they have sworn to uphold. They are also bound to work within restraints established by their colleagues and the law via

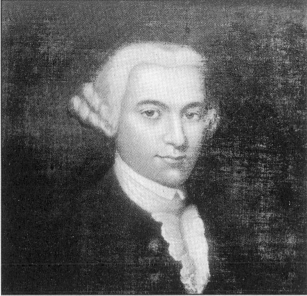

Wellcome Collection

Figure 2.3 Thomas Percival, an English physician, wrote one of the first guides for medical ethics, even inspiring the AMA's national code of ethics many years later.

The AMA Professional Code of Ethics

Preamble

The medical profession has long subscribed to a body of ethical statements developed primarily for the benefit of the patient. As a member of this profession, a physician must recognize responsibility to patients first and foremost, as well as to society, to other health professionals, and to self. The following Principles adopted by the American Medical Association are not laws, but standards of conduct, which define the essentials of honorable behavior for the physician.

Principles of Medical Ethics

I. A physician shall be dedicated to providing competent medical care, with compassion and respect for human dignity and rights.

II. A physician shall uphold the standards of professionalism, be honest in all professional interactions, and strive to report physicians deficient in character or competence, or engaging in fraud or deception, to appropriate entities.

III. A physician shall respect the law and also recognize a responsibility to seek changes in those requirements which are contrary to the best interests of the patient.

IV. A physician shall respect the rights of patients, colleagues, and other health professionals, and shall safeguard patient confidences and privacy within the constraints of the law.

V. A physician shall continue to study, apply, and advance scientific knowledge, maintain a commitment to medical education, make relevant information available to patients, colleagues, and the public, obtain consultation, and use the talents of other health professionals when indicated.

VI. A physician shall, in the provision of appropriate patient care, except in emergencies, be free to choose whom to serve, with whom to associate, and the environment in which to provide medical care.

VII. A physician shall recognize a responsibility to participate in activities contributing to the improvement of the community and the betterment of public health.

VIII. A physician shall, while caring for a patient, regard responsibility to the patient as paramount.

IX. A physician shall support access to medical care for all people.

Copyright 1995–2019 American Medical Association. All Rights Reserved.

Figure 2.4   The articles listed on the first page of the AMA's Professional Code of Ethics.

their professional association. However, every patient is different and new situations constantly arise and present challenging situations. Practitioners are therefore required to use their own independent professional skill and judgment, even while employed by others. The review and enforcement of individual professional decisions by professional associations leads to the continuous evolution and clarification of ethical codes.

Hippocratic Oath: Modern Version
I swear to fulfill, to the best of my ability and judgment, this covenant:

I will respect the hard-won scientific gains of those physicians in whose steps I walk, and gladly share such knowledge as is mine with those who are to follow.

I will apply, for the benefit of the sick, all measures [that] are required, avoiding those twin traps of overtreatment and therapeutic nihilism.

I will remember that there is art to medicine as well as science, and that warmth, sympathy, and understanding may outweigh the surgeon's knife or the chemist's drug.

I will not be ashamed to say "I know not," nor will I fail to call in my colleagues when the skills of another are needed for a patient's recovery.

I will respect the privacy of my patients, for their problems are not disclosed to me that the world may know. Most especially must I tread with care in matters of life and death. If it is given me to save a life, all thanks. But it may also be within my power to take a life; this awesome responsibility must be faced with great humbleness and awareness of my own frailty. Above all, I must not play at God.

I will remember that I do not treat a fever chart, a cancerous growth, but a sick human being, whose illness may affect the person's family and economic stability. My responsibility includes these related problems, if I am to care adequately for the sick.

I will prevent disease whenever I can, for prevention is preferable to cure.

I will remember that I remain a member of society, with special obligations to all my fellow human beings, those sound of mind and body as well as the infirm.

If I do not violate this oath, may I enjoy life and art, respected while I live and remembered with affection thereafter. May I always act so as to preserve the finest traditions of my calling and may I long experience the joy of healing those who seek my help.

Goodheart-Willcox Publisher; source: Louis C. Lasagna, MD.

Figure 2.5 The modern version of the Hippocratic Oath reflects changes in both societal values and technology.

The Impact of Politics on Professional Ethics

In addition to professional associations, various external factors have greatly influenced the changes made to codes of medical ethics. As noted in Chapter 1, healthcare and related ethical codes fall within the domains of philosophy, religion, morality, and politics. None of these domains are static or fixed. As medical practices and new professions evolve, definitions and interpretations of ethical standards of practice will transform. Some changes occur due to a new understanding of human conduct. For example, the atrocities of World War II increased social understanding of the extremes of scientific experimentation.

Nazi Germany's social and political denigration of certain types of people, such as the mentally disabled, religious minorities (Jewish people), and ethnic groups (the Romani people, known as *Gypsies*) led to a reassessment and rededication of many in the healthcare field to ethical conduct. One example was the World Medical Association's adoption of The Nuremberg Code, which addressed the concept of informed consent. This concept developed as a result of the discovery of forced experimentation on prisoners. Later declarations have included the following:

- Declaration of Geneva (1948)—addressed confidentiality and non-discrimination
- Declaration of Sydney (1968)—defined death in light of developments in artificial life support (Figure 2.6)
- Declaration of Oslo (1970)—attempted to reconcile therapeutic abortion with the Hippocratic Oath
- Declarations of Tokyo (1975) and Hawaii (1977)—prohibited physicians' participation in torture and the cruel and unusual punishment of prisoners

These ethical rules were developed partially in response to laws of humanity that were established by the United Nations in response to traumatic world events during World War II.

In 1974, given the variety of healthcare-related disciplines and related ethical codes, the US Department of Health Education and Welfare (now the US Department of Health and Human Services) created a National Commission for the Protection of Human Subjects of Biomedical and Behavioral Research. In 1979, the Commission released The Belmont Report, which defined fundamental ethical principles in healthcare for the United States.

In 2001, immediately after the terrorist attacks on the World Trade Center and the Pentagon, the AMA developed its Declaration of Professional Responsibility. This document called on physicians to "reaffirm [their] historical commitment to combat natural and man-made assaults on the health and well being of humankind." The declaration contains nine tenets, which include respecting human life and dignity, condemning crimes against humanity, treating the sick without prejudice, protecting privacy and confidentiality, and working with colleagues toward advances in medicine and public health.

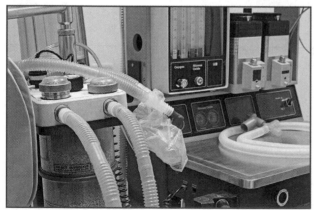

Paul Vinten/Shutterstock.com

Figure 2.6 Artificial life support, such as the ventilator shown here that can help a person breathe, changed the way that those in the field of healthcare thought about death.

Ethical Principles

After thousands of years of development and debate about philosophical, religious, political, and economic principles, and the publication of hundreds of books on medical ethics, a consensus has evolved on the general values that serve as the basis for professional medical ethics. This does not mean there is universal agreement. For example, people continue to debate whether decisions should be based on the rights of the individual, the overall good to society, the happiness of the individual, or the inherent goodness or evil of certain acts. This is, in part, why the study of historically recognized philosophers such as Confucius, Plato, Aristotle, Hobbes, Kant, Mills, and others is included in many college courses.

Despite continued debate, the following principles commonly guide medical professionals in providing patient care:

1. The concept of **autonomy** means that a person has a certain amount of "self-rule." A patient has the right to refuse or choose treatment. This idea is based on respect for the individual's ownership of and right to rule his or her own body. A patient's mental capacity and freedom from duress to make an informed and free decision must be considered in certain cases. The concept of respect for persons is derived from this principle.

    autonomy
    an individual's right to self-determination that is free from undue interference from others

    In respect for a patient's autonomy, a healthcare provider must obtain permission before administering treatment. For example, if a physician thinks that a blood transfusion will help a patient, he or she must first fully explain the pros and cons of the procedure and then obtain the patient's permission before performing that procedure (Figure 2.7). This is known as *informed consent* (see Chapter 9 for further discussion of informed consent).

    Not all patients will give consent, though. For example, Jehovah's Witnesses believe that it is wrong to accept a blood transfusion, even in a life-threatening situation. Therefore, a Jehovah's Witness patient may refuse the procedure. If that happens, the physician must respect the patient's autonomous choice and still carry out his or her ethical responsibility to the patient. In this case, informed by community practice and legal provisions for the free exercise of one's religion, the physician gives greater priority to the principle of patient autonomy than to other values.

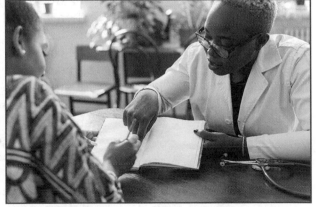

Donenko Oleksii/Shutterstock.com

Figure 2.7 Informed consent is important because it means that patients are fully aware of the procedures that they are agreeing to or refusing.

If the patient is a child, the parents typically have the authority to make these kinds of healthcare decisions. In such a case, if the parents were refusing the life-saving blood transfusion on religious grounds, the healthcare providers might challenge the parents' decision. There is legal precedence for overriding the parents' wishes by appealing to the Juvenile Court Judge who is authorized by the state to protect the lives of its citizens, particularly minors. The court might determine that the child, if making his or her own autonomous decision, would prefer the transfusion to reliance on divine action. The court could override the autonomy of the child's parents as the surrogate decision makers and act in their place. Chapter 13 includes further discussion of the rights of minors related to healthcare.

beneficence
the act of performing goodness, kindness, or charity, including all actions intended to benefit others based on a moral obligation to do so

2. **Beneficence** is the principle that directs a medical practitioner to act in the best interest of the patient and provide skilled assistance to others. This concept means that a practitioner should always act to improve the patient's condition. This often requires practitioners to balance risks and benefits of different treatments, favoring what is in the best interest of the patient.

   For example, if a 98-year-old woman fell and fractured her hip, a physician would need to consider what is best for her (Figure 2.8). It might be normal to recommend surgery for this injury. However, due to the patient's advanced age and the possible impact on her cardiovascular system from surgery, another course of treatment, such as a long period of self-healing with rest and pain medication, might be the best option.

non-malfeasance
the principle that requires a practitioner to do no harm to a patient by not performing up to professional standards, such as through ineffective, careless, or intentional wrongful acts

3. The concept of **non-malfeasance** dictates that a medical practitioner must do no harm to a patient. Harm might occur when a practitioner fails to meet professional standards through ineffective, careless, or intentional wrongful acts. The concept of non-malfeasance is linked to beneficence but focuses on the practitioner's own readiness and personal intent.

   For example, a healthcare practitioner should not undertake an action without having the minimum skill and knowledge that other practitioners performing a similar treatment under similar conditions would have. If a certain dosage of radiation has been proven to help a cancer patient, tripling the dosage may be considered malfeasance if the practitioner is careless of the probable consequences. Well-intended harmful acts are not proper if they would not be undertaken by others with proper skill and training.

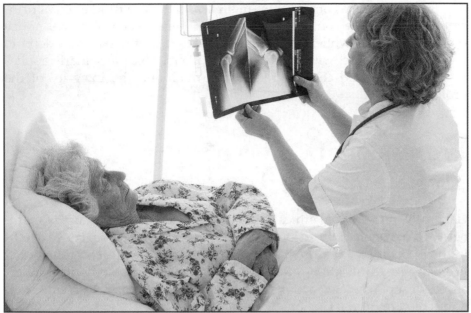

JPC-PROD/Shutterstock.com

Figure 2.8 Sometimes physicians need to make ethical judgments regarding treatment for some older patients, or other patients who may not benefit from surgery.

4. The principle of **justice** concerns the allocation of scarce health resources and decisions involving who gets what treatment (fairness and equality). For example, organ transplantation is an area in which issues of justice commonly arise, especially when there are long waiting lists for organs. Should a newly available donated heart be used to save the life of a 72-year-old man or a 23-year-old woman? Who decides? What criteria are used to make the decision?

    Patients are often placed on the United Network for Organ Sharing (UNOS) list, which is operated under contract from the federal government. UNOS applies the same criteria to all potential transplant recipients. Factors affecting ranking may include tissue match, blood type, length of time on the waiting list, immune status, and the distance between the potential recipient and the donor. For transplants involving the heart, liver, lungs, or intestines, the potential recipient's degree of medical urgency is also considered.

justice
the principle that requires giving others what is due to them, including the fair distribution of benefits, risks, and costs

The values of autonomy, beneficence, non-malfeasance, and justice are embedded in various ways throughout the entire field of professional ethics. Some lists of ethical principles include additional values, such as honesty, truthfulness, and dignity. It is possible, however, to consider these values subsets of respecting patient autonomy.

Similarly, some consider non-malfeasance to be a fundamental principle, but it can be considered a subset of beneficence. You will notice that ethical rules, while fundamentally focused on the patient, extend to professional conduct with colleagues and others. This particularly applies to truthfulness and conduct required to maintain the integrity of the profession.

Professional Codes of Ethics and State Laws

Generally, professional ethics apply only to the ethical conduct of members of a particular profession. However, many professional codes of ethics have been included in state law as a means to enforce professional licensing or certification. In addition, these codes are sometimes referenced in separate legal actions and litigation in attempts to define standards of care in court actions.

For example, the well-publicized case of Terri Schiavo involved administrative hearings, civil litigation, state and federal legislation, and Supreme Court review. Terri Schiavo had been in a "vegetative state" from 1990 to 2005, during which time her husband/conservator wanted to end artificial life support for her (Figure 2.9). The main issues involved in this case were patient ethics and consent. The court had to determine whether statements Terri made earlier in her life about not wanting drawn-out artificial life support should be honored (as requested by her husband) or not (as requested by her parents).

This case involved extraordinary publicity, appeals up through the federal courts, denial of review by the Supreme Court, a special act of Congress to keep Terri at least temporarily alive, and special legislation in Florida that was overturned by the Florida Supreme Court. Ultimately, the original Florida District Court finding in favor of the husband's arguments indicating the patient's previously expressed opinions was allowed to prevail and life support was removed.

Another example involving patient autonomy was the infamous Jack Kevorkian, a Michigan physician who advocated for and practiced assisted suicide. After five trials involving three acquittals and one mistrial between 1994 and 1999, he was convicted of second-degree murder and sent to prison, where he served eight years of a 10- to 25-year sentence.

Although his license had been revoked eight years earlier, Kevorkian claimed he was simply implementing his patient's wishes. However, he

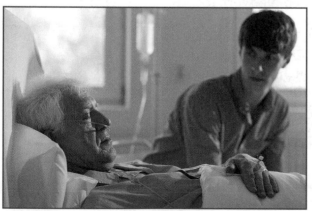
Photographee.eu/Shutterstock.com

Figure 2.9   When a patient is in a vegetative state, the topic of artificial life support may cause ethical issues such as patient autonomy and consent.

was found to have violated the ethical requirement to avoid harming the patient and, of course, breaking a criminal law against voluntarily taking the life of another person. The Kavorkian case led to much public attention to the topics of assisted suicide and right-to-death policies that continues to be debated across the country.

Ethical Rights of Patients and Providers

Sometimes a patient is unable to articulate his or her own informed opinion about a course of treatment. To address this situation, many institutions have published their own set of rights for patients to guide conservators, guardians, or others holding power of attorney for healthcare (see Chapter 5). These patient rights provide additional benefits, such as communicating to the public that the organization recognizes a patient's rights and is committed to patients involved in and directing their care.

These guidelines also provide a means to communicate a provider's rights to candor and respect from the patient. Patient rights can help clarify the roles of patient and provider as they work together to enable quality care, minimize misunderstandings, and reduce the likelihood of costly litigation.

Ethical Decision Making

Medical ethical standards are intended to guide individuals, and, as you have read repeatedly, they are always changing. Medical care provided with these standards in mind often requires moment-to-moment decisions and actions. Ethical missteps in actual practice can occur before you even recognize the existence of an ethical question. Missteps are judged after the fact, when it is too late to correct a violation.

Enforcement of ethical standards by licensing authorities and employers is intended to punish violators but also provide guidance to avoid future problems. When an ethical error occurs, licenses may be suspended or revoked, and a person can even be fired. Licensing authorities always test your knowledge of the rules before allowing you to engage in care, but applying the rules during a busy day can be challenging. You will obtain some understanding of this when you first apply for admission to a health profession or when you undergo orientation. You will want to internalize ethical rules so they are second nature. For example, you might automatically ask yourself if a patient provided informed consent for what you are about to do.

In addition to passing initial entry tests, health professionals must maintain awareness of long-standing rules and the possibility of new rules or new interpretations of existing rules. Many professions require members to engage in a certain amount of continuing education in both the latest practice techniques and ethics rules because both change over time. Generally, you should recognize that, by joining a profession, you will be undertaking a commitment to some level of lifelong learning to keep up with the changing field.

Ethical decision making can be more difficult than you might think. For instance, suppose that you are a primary care provider talking to a married couple. You find yourself in a conversation that involves sensitive, personal information about the husband, who is your patient. He is describing symptoms that indicate a sexually transmitted infection (STI), and recent tests confirmed this diagnosis. You have not received permission from the patient during previous visits or the current discussion to disclose this diagnosis to anyone, including his spouse. This may be particularly true because the patient did not know about his condition when he allowed his wife to sit in on the conversation.

Eventually the patient's spouse should be informed of the diagnosis, in the interest of her own health. At this point, however, your understanding is that the patient would prefer the issue to remain confidential (Figure 2.10). You should consider whether it would be ethical to temporarily refrain from disclosing your diagnosis to the patient until you are able to talk to him in private.

During an emergency, decisions need to be made immediately (see Chapter 9 for further discussion). In other situations, there is time to review formal written opinions from authoritative bodies, such as

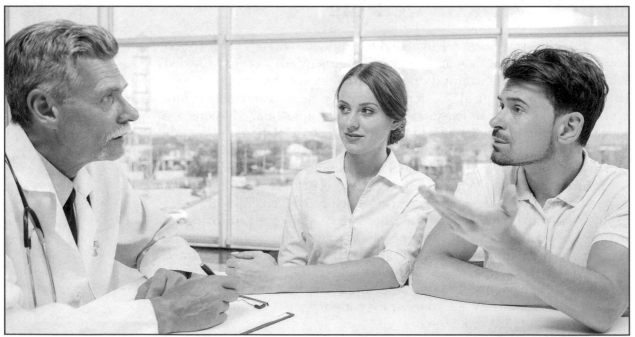

VGstockstudio/Shutterstock.com

Figure 2.10   Even in the case of a married couple, physicians must keep each individual patient's medical information confidential until consent to reveal that information is given.

professional associations. At other times, it may be appropriate to formally seek advice from supervisors, professional colleagues, or **medical ethics committees**.

Generally, if you believe you can legally act, you should first consider if the patient is able to understand and decide issues and can provide autonomous guidance on preferred methods of care (or refusal of care, as the case may be). Next, consider what is in the best interest of the patient (under the principle of beneficence) and whether you can act without harming the patient. Finally, consider whether serving this patient means that you are providing just and equitable care or denying care to others by expending your time or available resources in this manner.

medical ethics committee
a group of knowledgeable healthcare-related experts who are convened to provide advice and assistance in resolving unusual, complicated ethical problems that involve issues affecting the care and treatment of patients

 ## Ethical Dilemma

Imagine that you are a dentist. Consider a situation in which the principle of beneficence calls upon you to assist a patient who is in so much pain that he wishes to have a tooth immediately extracted. Upon examination, you cannot find anything particularly wrong with the tooth and suspect the pain is caused by a nerve issue unrelated to the tooth itself. You believe that the patient should be referred to a specialist for additional assessment. Is it honoring the patient's autonomy to extract the tooth as requested? Might it be malfeasance to honor the patient's wish when not medically indicated? What if you pulled the tooth and the pain continued?

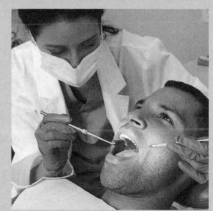

Monkey Business Images/Shutterstock.com

There are several ethical decision frameworks you can use. One example is the five-step decision model described below, which was adapted from the Josephson Institute's approach to ethical decision making:

1. **Determine the facts.** Examine the facts and separate them from assumptions and opinions.

2. **Define and examine the ethical issue.** Define the precise ethical issue and examine which ethical principles and values are involved. Review the ethical guidelines of your profession and organization.

3. **Identify alternatives and their consequences.** Carefully consider the benefits, burdens, and risks to each stakeholder involved in each alternative. Eliminate any impractical, illegal, and improper alternatives.

4. **Evaluate the alternatives.** Compare the alternatives you identified and evaluate the consequences for each. Seek assistance from an ethical committee if needed and available.

5. **Make a decision.** Maximize the benefits to society and minimize the costs and risks. How would you feel if your decision was in the newspaper the next day for your colleagues and family to see?

For the situation presented in the "Ethical Dilemma" in this section, the five-step model could be applied as follows:

- **Determine the facts.** Review the health risks of extracting a healthy tooth and ignoring another probable source of pain. Review the research and clinical guidelines.

- **Define and examine the ethical issue.** The issue is that ethics exist. Consider if other ethical issues exist, such as the right to life and do no harm. Should you honor the patient's autonomy and extract the tooth in the absence of scientific evidence, perhaps violating your duty to act with beneficence? Do other ethical questions exist, such as whether you will do the patient harm by extracting a healthy tooth and potentially misaligning the patient's bite pattern or requiring unnecessary expense to place a bridge or other device?

- **Identify alternatives and their consequences.** Review the legal parameters and previous cases as well as their related outcomes. Review all options, including various alternatives to surgical approaches.

- **Evaluate the alternatives.** Through medical literature, assess the likelihood that pain would continue if the tooth were pulled. Identify methods that could reduce any risks of continued suffering. Discuss the options with experts in this area. Consult with an ethics committee.

- **Make a decision.** Select the option that will create the greatest benefit to society through equitable allocation of health resources, and which will minimize the harm done to the individual. Are you wasting time and resources by performing an unnecessary procedure?

Bioethics

bioethics
the study of the ethical and moral implications of new biological discoveries and biomedical advances

Bioethics is the study of the ethical and moral implications of new biological discoveries and biomedical advances. The field of bioethics involves a broad range of issues related to the application of scientific advances to medical care that often present the dilemma of whether "we can" means "we should." Bioethical dilemmas often go beyond the scope of individual practice and can affect society in general.

For instance, if animals can be cloned, should humans be cloned to serve as spare parts for patients or as surrogate soldiers to prevent injury to draftees? Autonomy and beneficence might lead to a "yes" decision. However, justice, autonomy, and beneficence might be in conflict on an individual level if the clone is identical to the original person or if wars are encouraged by the availability of greater numbers of disposable soldiers.

Does exploring this type of issue reflect a violation of non-malfeasance because the practice does not exist at this point and negative consequences have not been fully determined? It may soon be possible to extend human life indefinitely. Would you be assisting suicide if a patient refuses inexpensive and routine life-extending treatment? Would it be malfeasance if the practice will undoubtedly lead to world hunger due to overpopulation? Two basic responses have evolved to address such difficult issues both at the societal level and for individual practitioners.

Policy Response to Changing Standards of Care

Some bioethical issues are beyond the scope of one practitioner acting alone. Certain issues, such as cloning, are addressed by the general population, who adopt political solutions through the passage of legislation. For example, a number of states have banned human cloning. Somewhat related is the severe restriction the federal government has placed on stem cell research (Figure 2.11). Such large-scale issues may not be encountered during your individual daily practice, but they certainly influence the nature of the healthcare field in general.

Medical Ethics Committees

Medical ethics committees assist practitioners as they attempt to resolve ethical dilemmas. These committees are generally advisory in nature and are established to provide assistance rather than authoritative directives. They are different from the boards or committees that establish ethical rules for specific areas of practice. Those rules are established by professional associations, the government, and employers to encourage thorough consideration of complex clinical issues and to promote good decision making.

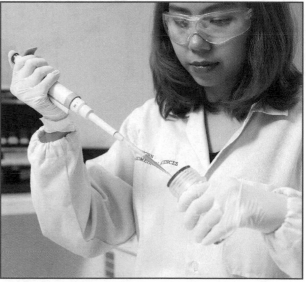

Apple's Eyes Studio/Shutterstock.com

Figure 2.11   Stem cell research is an area in which legislators have responded to a technological advance that could affect healthcare.

Employers may have policies and procedures that outline when medical ethics committees should be used by employees. Practitioners may also be permitted to voluntarily request guidance from such committees on an as-needed basis.

One example of this is the Kaiser Permanente Ethics Committee (Figure 2.12). This committee allows for the identification and discussion of healthcare-related ethical and social questions. When ethical questions are raised, this committee convenes to discuss the situation.

These committees are different from **Institutional Review Boards** (IRBs). IRBs are independent ethics committees that supervise research. IRBs were developed, and are now required, for many forms of research that involve human subjects. This is because while scientific research has produced substantial social benefits, it also has revealed some troubling ethical situations. IRBs exist to protect patients' rights to safety and privacy.

Federal regulations require that research projects involving human subjects be reviewed by an IRB. The IRB must approve the project or determine it to be exempt prior to the start of any research activities.

Institutional Review Boards
groups of experts convened to review proposed research activities at an institution with the focus of protecting the rights and welfare of human subjects recruited to participate in those research activities

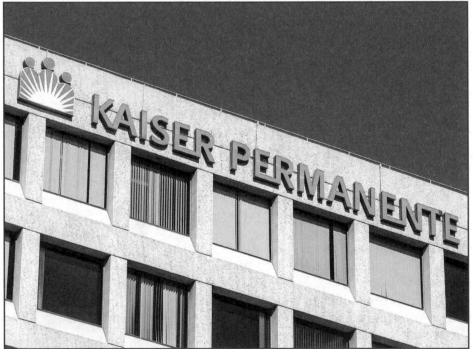

Sundry Photography/Shutterstock.com

Figure 2.12   The Kaiser Permanente Ethics Committee is a group that discusses healthcare-related ethical questions.

Institutions that receive federal support are required to provide a written assurance to the Office for Human Research Protections that describes how the institution will protect the rights and welfare of human subjects.

These assurances also include an agreement to follow the **Common Rule**. In 1991, many federal agencies adopted Subpart A of 45 CFR Part 46, at which time the term "Common Rule" came into use. HHS adopted requirements to provide additional protections for fetuses, neonates, pregnant women, prisoners, and children. The three sets of regulations are the Common Rule, FDA, and VA. These regulations outline the authority and responsibilities of IRBs. The Common Rule has the most detail. Special or additional requirements are outlined in the VA regulations.

Common Rule
the common name for 45 CFR Part 46, Subpart A, which outlines the authority of IRBs and helps protect fetuses, neonates, and pregnant women, prisoners, and children involved in research studies

 ## Career Corner

Bioethicists are concerned with the ethical questions that stem from the collaboration of areas such as life sciences, biotechnology, medicine, politics, law, and philosophy. An understanding of bioethics can be useful when reflecting upon the implications and outcomes of medical procedures, treatment decisions, biomedical and behavioral research, and health policies.

Bioethicists work in a variety of settings, such as healthcare facilities (hospitals, clinics, and skilled nursing facilities), pharmaceutical and biotechnology companies, academic centers, research and compliance boards, and policy organizations.

Bioethicists may consider and advise organizations

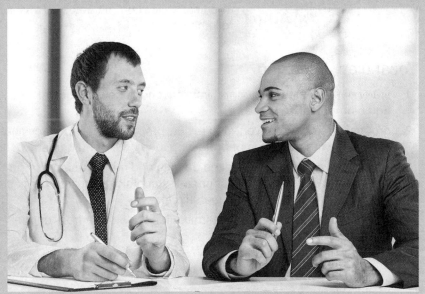
Billion Photos/Shutterstock.com

and individuals on critical social and individual concerns such as informed consent, cultural diversity, and emerging reproductive technologies.

Use the Internet to search for information on academic programs and jobs in bioethics. What types of courses are included in these programs? What are the job requirements?

Chapter Summary

- Medical law and ethics are important to society because everyone receives healthcare and depends on providers to act properly.
- Although basic concepts of medical ethics developed over centuries, formal codes of ethics have evolved during the past few hundred years.
- Codes of ethics are constantly evolving in response to politics and scientific developments.
- The basic concepts of ethics, beneficence, non-malfeasance, and justice provide a framework for dealing with most ethical issues.
- Many professional codes of ethics have been included in state laws as a means to enforce licensing or certification.
- Sets of patient rights developed by institutions help patients and providers work together to enable quality care, minimize misunderstandings, and reduce litigation.
- Ethical decision frameworks, such as the Josephson Institute's decision model, are available to help people make ethical decisions.
- Bioethical issues have required political solutions at the state level; medical ethics committees also assist practitioners with ethical dilemmas.

Vocabulary Matching

1. study of the ethical and moral implications of new biological discoveries and biomedical advances
2. groups of experts convened to review proposed research activities at an institution with the focus of protecting the rights of human subjects
3. calling that requires specialized training and membership in a group that establishes codes of conduct or codes of ethics, requires continuing education, and collects membership fees
4. an individual's right to self-determination that is free from undue interference from others
5. group of healthcare-related experts that provides advice and assistance in resolving complex ethical problems involving patient care and treatment
6. oath attributed to the ancient Greeks that requires a new physician to swear that he will uphold professional ethical standards
7. act of goodness, kindness, or charity, including actions intended to benefit others based on a moral obligation to do so
8. outlines the authority of IRBs and helps protect fetuses, neonates, pregnant women, prisoners, and children involved in research studies
9. principle that requires giving others what is due to them, including the fair distribution of benefits, risks, and costs
10. principle that requires a practitioner to do no harm to a patient by not performing up to professional standards

A. autonomy
B. beneficence
C. bioethics
D. Common Rule
E. Hippocratic Oath
F. Institutional Review Boards
G. justice
H. medical ethics committee
I. non-malfeasance
J. profession

Chapter 2 Review and Assessment

Multiple Choice

11. The four ethical principles include all of the following *except* _____.
    A. equity
    B. autonomy
    C. non-malfeasance
    D. justice

12. A(n) _____ is an ethics committee that reviews research on human subjects.
    A. Research Ethics Committee
    B. Human Subject Ethics Committee
    C. Institutional Review Board
    D. Research Review Board

Completion

13. The regulation for IRBs that has the most detail is the _____.

14. _____ is the organization that created the first formal code of medical ethics.

15. The first step in making an ethical decision is to determine the _____.

Discussion and Critical Thinking

16. Identify two principles included in the AMA Principles of Medical Ethics that involve each of the following ethical concepts:
    autonomy
    beneficence
    non-malfeasance
    justice

17. Compare and contrast the classic Hippocratic Oath with the AMA Code of Ethics.

18. Compare and contrast the original and modern versions of the Hippocratic Oath and explain the differences.

Activities

19. Search the Internet for information about the Stanford Prison study. Write a one-page paper that discusses the following questions:
    A. What ethical violations occurred in this study?
    B. Were the consequences of the experiment foreseeable? Why or why not?
    C. What would you have changed about how the experiment was conducted?

20. Watch the nine-part series, "Miss Evers' Boys," on YouTube. Write a one-page paper that addresses the following issues:

    • What components of the Hippocratic Oath did the physician and nurse violate?

    • What should the physician have done differently?

    • What should the nurse have done differently?

    • What professional codes of ethics did they violate?

Case Study

A 35-year-old female was in a car accident and is now in the intensive care unit. She has multiple injuries and fractures, and her condition continues to worsen. The patient is heavily sedated and on life support. When the accident occurred, her parents were notified. They have been by her bedside since then. The patient's parents informed the hospital staff that she is one month from her divorce being final. Her husband has been physically and verbally abusive throughout their four-year marriage. The husband has not been notified about her accident. However, the patient's soon-to-be ex-husband is her legal next of kin.

• Should the husband be notified?

• Should the husband be responsible for treatment decisions that the patient is now unable to make?

• Do you need more facts? What ethical concepts are presented here?

• Is a choice really available?

Chapter 3

The Source of Law and Regulations

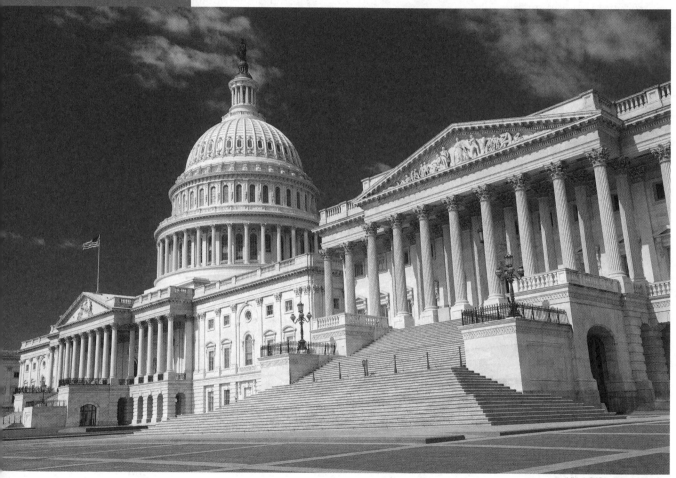

Vlad G/Shutterstock.com

Chapter Outline

The Federal Government

The Constitution of the United States

The Preamble of the Constitution

The Articles of the Constitution

The Amendments of the Constitution

The Constitution and the Hierarchy of Law

The Federal Government's Authority to Regulate Healthcare

State Governments

Local Governments

Objectives

- Describe the purpose of the US Constitution and the role of the federal government in healthcare regulation.
- Explain the differences between the powers of the federal government and the individual state governments, and the effects of these differences on healthcare.
- Identify the roles of local governments in healthcare provisions and regulation.

Key Terms

amendments

articles

Bill of Rights

Cabinet

case law

checks and balances

Commerce Clause

common law

Due Process Clause

Equal Protection Clause

executive branch

full faith and credit

government of limited power

Health Information Technology for Economic and Clinical Health (HITECH) Act

judicial branch

legislative branch

police power

separation of powers

statutes

statutory law

Supremacy Clause

United States Constitution

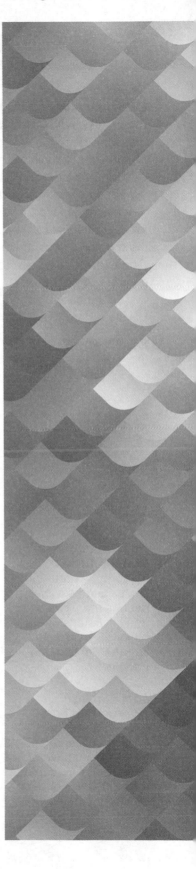

What Would You Do?

As part of the Affordable Care Act's reform to the American healthcare system, the Democratic Obama Administration included a provision that required all health insurance plans to provide many preventive healthcare services for no additional cost beyond the monthly insurance premium. One of these services was birth control.

In January 2012, the US Department of Health and Human Services, following the general model of more than 10 states, issued regulations requiring that preventive services be covered by all insurance plans except those provided directly to religion-based organizations. Almost immediately, there was an outcry by the Catholic Church and Republican Party.

Rather than indignation based on morals or ethics, opposition was raised on the constitutional grounds of the importance of separation of church and state and freedom of religion. Birth control is not against medical ethics, but it is morally objectionable to some. This issue was resolved by changing rules for organizations raising religion-based objections. However, if you, as a healthcare provider, were asked to vote on the issue in Congress, what would you do? How would you vote and why?

United States Constitution
the formal charter of the United States, which defines the powers and limitations of the national government and the rights of the people

common law
rules derived from English law (French law in Louisiana) and tradition that have often been formally adopted into state laws or used to determine decisions in American courts

To understand the relationship between the healthcare system and the legal system in the United States, you must understand that laws and ethical rules have been established to encourage and protect delivery of the best healthcare possible. This may not always work out in practice. However, the fundamental principle is to ensure maximum competence and professional independence for practitioners to whom citizens, including the policymakers themselves, entrust their health and lives.

In the United States, society's rules and regulations are derived from a complex variety of sources. The **United States Constitution** is "the supreme law of the land," which defines and limits the powers of the federal government (Figure 3.1). While the federal government has a pervasive influence on healthcare, it plays a relatively minimal role in actually providing care to patients. The authority and power to train, license, and set standards for actual medical care is retained by the states.

Local governments, through their city planning, business licensing, and other practices, also affect the healthcare provider. In addition, professional associations establish their own independent rules and sanctions, which have a significant impact on members' daily practical decisions. Finally, **common law**, derived from individual case law from England and predating US laws, serves as the basis for bringing challenges to healthcare providers, such as medical malpractice suits that are often based on common law principles.

What is the source of all this governmental authority? Such power derives from a democratic concept that individuals have voluntarily empowered the governing entities to act on behalf of the individual.

For example, the Declaration of Independence suggests that there are Laws of Nature and of Nature's God in which all men are created equal and "endowed by their creator with certain unalienable rights." This chapter explores the nature and roles of the various levels of government authority and their influences on healthcare.

The Federal Government

The United States federal government has a limited role in providing direct patient care other than military and Indian Health Services. Nevertheless, the federal government has tremendous influence and impact on those who practice direct care throughout all of the states. The Patient Protection and Affordable Care Act (ACA), for instance, has affected all healthcare insurance and was intended to standardize and improve access to basic healthcare services for all US citizens.

The Constitution of the United States

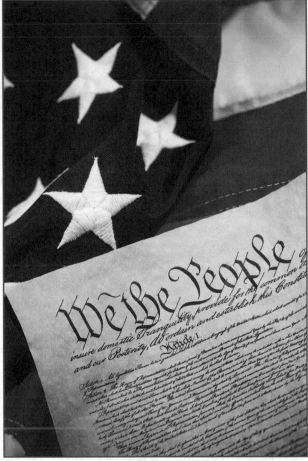

Sean Locke Photography/Shutterstock.com

Figure 3.1 The Constitution contains laws that govern the nation and even apply to healthcare.

The United States' founders' initial draft of the Constitution was intended to establish a permanent governmental structure and address problems that arise from having distinctly separate governing systems: a national government and individual state governments. Thus, the US Constitution created a federal **government of limited power**. Such governments derive the authority to act specifically from the Constitution.

Any power that is not delegated to the federal government in the Constitution is reserved to the states or the people (US Constitution, Amendment X). The Constitution does not limit the rights of the individual citizen; it limits the authority of government. For the federal government to act in any area, it must have Constitutional authority to do so.

government of limited power
a government that can only exert authority it has been given by its constitution

articles
sections of the US Constitution

amendments
additions to the US Constitution that address topics not covered in the original Constitution

The Preamble of the Constitution

The Constitution begins with the Preamble, which is followed by sections called **articles** and **amendments**. Though brief, the Preamble sets forth the purpose of establishing the government (Figure 3.2).

> *We the People of the United States, in Order to form a more perfect Union, establish Justice, insure domestic Tranquility, provide for the common defence, promote the general Welfare, and secure the Blessings of Liberty to ourselves and our Posterity, do ordain and establish this Constitution for the United States of America.*

Figure 3.2   The Preamble to the Constitution indirectly references healthcare in its call to "promote the general welfare."

separation of powers
a purposeful structuring of the government to avoid one person or group of people wielding uncontrolled centralized power

checks and balances
the limitations of each branch of government and the coordination among the branches required to operate the government

legislative branch
the portion of the government made up of lawmakers elected by the people; includes the House of Representatives and the Senate

statutory law
the body of law established by legislatures, as opposed to common law that has been developed over time by case law

Health Information Technology for Economic and Clinical Health (HITECH) Act
a federal law established to promote the adoption of health information technology while protecting patient privacy

Healthcare itself is not specifically mentioned in the Preamble but can be found in the constitutional purpose to promote the general welfare and secure liberty. The provision to "promote the general welfare" has served as justification for extensive government programs such as Medicare, Medicaid, food and drug regulation, and nationally sponsored medical research and disease control.

How do such federal laws, programs, and rules come into being? The carefully designed system of procedures that contributes to their creation is addressed in several articles of the Constitution.

The Articles of the Constitution

The articles of the Constitution are sections of the document that establish and describe the authority and limitations of the three branches of government—legislative, executive, and judicial (Figure 3.3). The three branches were set up by the Constitution to ensure that no one area of federal government became dominant. This **separation of powers** established a system of **checks and balances** in which each branch of government has the ability to perform specific, separate functions that can be limited by one of the other two branches.

Article I of the Constitution created the **legislative branch** and gave certain powers to Congress. Congress is composed of the House of Representatives and the Senate. The most important powers given to Congress are its authority for making federal **statutory law** (written law) and its power to approve federal taxes and expenditures. This permits citizens of the country, who elect the members of Congress, to maintain control over lawmaking and the cost of government.

One example of a statutory law made by Congress that impacts health is the **Health Information Technology for Economic and Clinical Health (HITECH) Act**. The HITECH Act was enacted as part of the American Recovery and Reinvestment Act of 2009 and was signed into law on February 17, 2009. Its purpose was to promote the greater adoption of health information technology while protecting patient privacy detailed in other federal laws, such as the Health Insurance Portability and Accountability Act (HIPAA). It made incentives available for medical facilities to implement and utilize electronic health records (EHR) systems. If a medical facility does not use EHRs, it may face penalties.

Summary of Articles in the US Constitution	
Article Number	**Summary**
I	establishes the first of the three branches of the government, the Legislature
II	establishes the second of the three branches of government, the Executive
III	establishes the third of the three branches of government, the Judiciary
IV	concerns the states; four sections: (1) mandates that all states will honor the laws of all other states, (2) guarantees that citizens of one state be treated equally and fairly like all citizens of another, (3) concerns the admittance of new states and the control of federal lands, and (4) ensures representative democracy
V	details the method of amending, or changing, the Constitution
VI	concerns the United States itself: (1) guarantees that the United States under the Constitution would assume all debts and contracts entered into by the United States, (2) sets the Constitution and all laws and treaties of the United States to be the supreme law of the country, and (3) requires all officers of the United States and of the states to swear an oath of allegiance to the United States and the Constitution when taking office
VII	details the method for ratification, or acceptance, of the Constitution

Goodheart-Willcox Publisher

Figure 3.3   A brief description of the Articles of the US Constitution.

Section 8 of Article I of the Constitution enumerates the powers of Congress. These powers include the authority to levy taxes, regulate commerce, provide for the general welfare, declare war, make rules for government, and establish all laws necessary and proper to carry out its powers.

In addition to specific legislation, such as the ACA, much of the federal government's ability to influence healthcare is based on the implied powers derived from the **Commerce Clause**. This clause asserts that Congress is to regulate commerce between the states. Almost anything that crosses state lines can be regulated by Congress. In addition, under the ACA, the Congressional power to levy taxes was used to require individual citizens to enroll in health insurance programs or pay taxes to the federal Internal Revenue Service. This tax is no longer in effect.

States can accordingly proclaim sovereignty over their traditional control of health and safety, because the US Constitution does not list such powers for the federal government. At the same time, however, program advocates can use this section to argue for more federal services or more federal protection for individual autonomy and privacy. Balancing priorities and issues of morality, people negotiate social values, ethics, and medical science in Congress to establish federal programs that affect healthcare.

Commerce Clause
a clause in the US Constitution that grants Congress extensive power to regulate the economy, particularly the flow of items and information between the states

executive branch
the portion of the government that is empowered to implement the laws established by the legislative branch

Article II of the Constitution created the **executive branch** of government, which is headed by the President (Figure 3.4). The duty of the executive branch is to administer and enforce the laws of the United States as enacted by Congress. The President has influence over Congress through the authority to approve or reject (veto) acts of Congress. While Congress has the sole power to declare war, the executive branch has the sole authority to manage foreign affairs on behalf of the country.

The creation of regulations by administrative agencies within the executive branch is important to the relationship between government and healthcare. For instance, routine, daily healthcare practices can be heavily influenced by reimbursement and service coding requirements established to administer federal programs such as Medicare and Medicaid.

Fifteen executive departments carry out the day-to-day administration of the federal government. The heads of these departments, known as *secretaries*, are appointed by the President and confirmed by the Senate. They serve on an advisory panel called the **Cabinet** and report to the President. Cabinet members are often the President's closest confidants. Department heads of other executive agencies are not included in the Cabinet but still fall under the authority of the President.

Cabinet
the advisory body to the President of the United States, which is made up of the heads of various federal agencies

Healthcare can be affected by any number of these executive branch agencies, often in ways that may be lesser known. For example, the US Patent Office has a significant role in determining who can receive rights and privileges under patent laws that govern new drugs and medical appliances.

The connection between other departments and health is more apparent. The Department of Health and Human Services is the principal

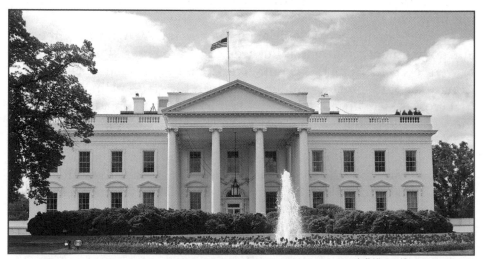

Jeff Kinsey/Shutterstock.com

Figure 3.4   The White House, which is where the President lives, is also the seat of the government's executive branch.

agency for protecting the health of all Americans. It performs a wide variety of tasks and services affecting research, public health, food and drug safety, grants and other funding, data collection, regulations, and health insurance.

Article III of the Constitution established the third branch of government, the **judicial branch**, also known as the *judiciary.* The judiciary interprets the laws of the United States, acts as the final mediator of disputes, and ensures that actions by the other two branches of the federal government, and actions by state and local governments, do not violate the Constitution.

The judicial branch has played a major role in defining fundamental rights to privacy and autonomy that are central to patient rights but are not specifically described in the Constitution. For instance, the Supreme Court has been involved in several high-profile cases to determine if care can be withheld from a person whose life is sustained only by life support, a form of medical technology. Figure 3.5 shows a summary of the structure and roles of the three branches.

Article IV of the Constitution addresses relations between and among the states. It ensures that citizens of the states are entitled to all privileges and immunities afforded to those of each of the states. This article also ensures that laws enacted in one state are given **full faith and credit** (equal recognition) in each of the other states. For example, this clause has been used to ensure that contracts and driver's licenses from one state are recognized in all other states. The fundamental purpose of this Article is to encourage commerce between the states and protect the rights of individual citizens as they move from state to state.

However, Article IV does not force state regulators of medical providers to recognize licensing from other states. While healthcare providers and individual patients can move between states, professional licensing and rights to practice are not required by the Constitution to be recognized across state lines. This can have a significant effect on availability of services and standards of practice.

For example, you can receive advice from your physician who is licensed in your state over the telephone, but a physician practicing from any other state cannot have the same conversation with you. In some instances, such as nursing, interstate compact agreements among the states have created reciprocity rights that allow recognition of out-of-state licenses.

The Amendments of the Constitution

The body of the Constitution itself is amazingly brief, but it has been expanded by the addition of amendments to address issues that have arisen over time. Within four years of the Constitution being ratified, the first 10 amendments were passed. Collectively, these first 10 amendments are referred to as the **Bill of Rights** and are designed to protect people from government infringement on their fundamental rights (Figure 3.6).

judicial branch
the portion of the government made up of judges and courts that resolve issues involving the application of laws

full faith and credit
the Constitution's requirement that each state recognize the equal powers of each state to establish its own law; has been used to ensure that barriers to commerce and rights of citizenship do not interfere with the nation functioning as a single entity

Bill of Rights
the first ten amendments to the US Constitution, which protect the individual rights of citizens

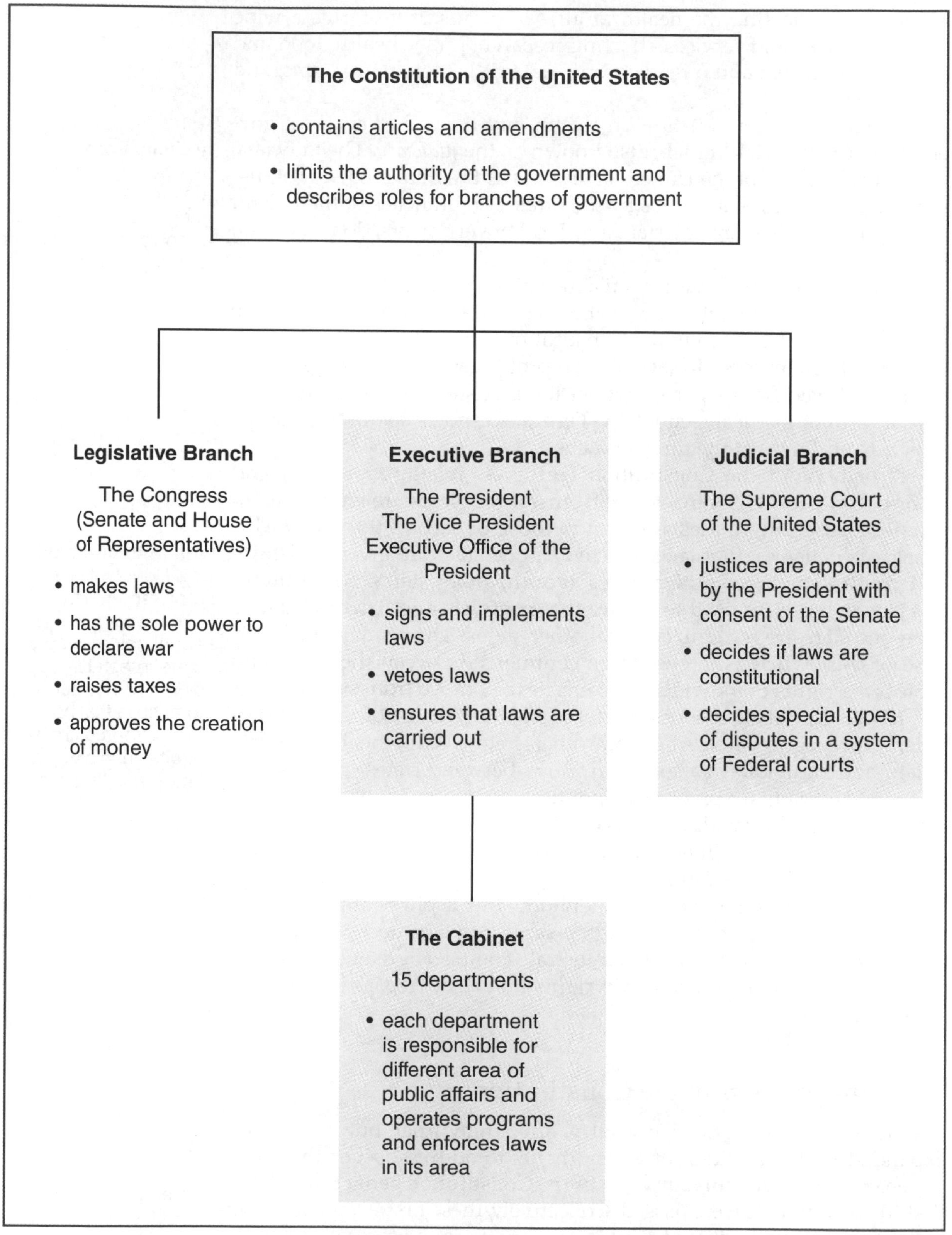

The Constitution of the United States

- contains articles and amendments

- limits the authority of the government and describes roles for branches of government

Legislative Branch

The Congress
(Senate and House
of Representatives)

- makes laws

- has the sole power to declare war

- raises taxes

- approves the creation of money

Executive Branch

The President
The Vice President
Executive Office of the President

- signs and implements laws

- vetoes laws

- ensures that laws are carried out

Judicial Branch

The Supreme Court
of the United States

- justices are appointed by the President with consent of the Senate

- decides if laws are constitutional

- decides special types of disputes in a system of Federal courts

The Cabinet

15 departments

- each department is responsible for different area of public affairs and operates programs and enforces laws in its area

Goodheart-Willcox Publisher

Figure 3.5   The structure of the federal government.

The Bill of Rights

Amendment	Topic	Text
I	religion and freedom of speech	Congress shall make no law respecting an establishment of religion, or prohibiting the free exercise thereof; or abridging the freedom of speech, or of the press; or the right of the people peaceably to assemble, and to petition the Government for a redress of grievances.
II	military	A well-regulated Militia, being necessary to the security of a free State, the right of the people to keep and bear Arms, shall not be infringed.
III	confinement	No Soldier shall, in time of peace be quartered in any house, without the consent of the Owner, nor in time of war, but in a manner to be prescribed by law.
IV	privacy	The right of the people to be secure in their persons, houses, papers, and effects, against unreasonable searches and seizures, shall not be violated, and no Warrants shall issue, but upon probable cause, supported by Oath or affirmation, and particularly describing the place to be searched, and the persons or things to be seized.
V	fair trial	No person shall be held to answer for a capital, or otherwise Infamous crime, unless on a presentment or indictment of a Grand Jury, except in cases arising in the land or naval forces, or in the Militia, when in actual service in time of War or public danger; nor shall any person be subject for the same offense to be twice put in jeopardy of life or limb; nor shall be compelled in any criminal case to be a witness against himself, nor be deprived of life, liberty, or property, without due process of law; nor shall private property be taken for public use, without just compensation.
VI	criminal trial	In all criminal prosecutions, the accused shall enjoy the right to a speedy and public trial, by an impartial jury of the State and district wherein the crime shall have been committed, which district shall have been previously ascertained by law, and to be informed of the nature and cause of the accusation; to be confronted with the witnesses.
VII	trial by jury	In Suits at common law, where the value in controversy shall exceed twenty dollars, the right of trial by jury shall be preserved, and no fact tried by a jury, shall be otherwise re-examined in any Court of the United States, than according to the rules of the common law.
VIII	bail and cruel punishment	Excessive bail shall not be required, nor excessive fines imposed, nor cruel and unusual punishments inflicted.
IX	equal rights	The enumeration in the Constitution, of certain rights, shall not be construed to deny or disparage others retained by the people.
X	federal and state power	The powers not delegated to the United States by the Constitution, nor prohibited by it to the States, are reserved to the States respectively or to the people.

Source: The US National Archives & Records Administration

Figure 3.6 Summary of the Bill of Rights.

For example, the government must respect any objections that you may have to certain types of medical care based on your religious beliefs. The government can only override such objections when it can prove that there is a compelling public interest clearly outweighing the constitutional right of the individual. An example includes requiring children to be immunized before enrolling in school to protect all other children from illness. Even in this situation, however, some states have "opt-out" policies that allow people to forego immunizations based on religious objections.

Ethical Dilemma

Vaccinations are beneficial for individuals and communities. When the majority of a population is vaccinated against a pathogen, the entire community is protected from the pathogen. This is known as *herd immunity*. Herd immunity makes it more difficult for a pathogen to spread. This is the primary rationale for making some vaccinations mandatory in the United States.

All states require children attending public school or state-licensed day care to receive certain vaccinations. These requirements are state specific and therefore vary depending on where you live. The term *mandate* is somewhat misleading when applied to vaccination, however. The last time the United States had a true mandate, requiring vaccination without exception, was during World War I. Today, many states have procedures that allow parents and legal guardians to exempt their children from state vaccination requirements because of religious or personal beliefs, but this is changing due to new epidemics.

Do you think that vaccination exemptions should

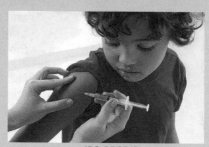

JPC-PROD/Shutterstock.com

exist? Should an individual's preference take priority over the health of the community? Should the government be able to require that all children be vaccinated, or is that a violation of their constitutional rights?

Amendment XIV to the Constitution addresses the civil rights of citizens and contains two important clauses—the Due Process Clause and the Equal Protection Clause.

Due Process Clause
a clause in the Fourteenth Amendment that has been interpreted to mean that citizens cannot be deprived of life or liberty without notice and a right to be heard

The **Due Process Clause** states that a citizen shall not be deprived of life, liberty, or property without due process of law. This clause requires that laws and rules made by the government be reasonable and clear, and that fair procedures must be followed when the rules are enforced. Generally, this means you must be given notice and an opportunity to present information on your own behalf when government action will adversely affect you.

The **Equal Protection Clause** states that no person is to be denied equal protection of the laws. Similar persons must be treated in a similar manner, and the government must have at least a rational reason to treat an individual differently. This clause, along with the Due Process Clause, has been interpreted by the courts to mean that a citizen's fundamental rights may not be infringed upon unless the government meets higher standards, it has a compelling interest in the area, and its actions are necessary.

Due process may affect your healthcare if, for example, your medical care was being provided under a program, such as Medicaid, and you were required to prove you had a low income to qualify for payment of your bills. Before you can be dropped from a program, you are entitled to "notice and a fair hearing." The ACA specifically includes requirements that the healthcare exchange provide due process procedures to applicants. In addition, the process you follow must be essentially the same as any other person, without differentiation based on race, religion, or other conditions that are protected under the law.

The Constitution and the Hierarchy of Law

The application of the Constitution to any particular situation requires an analysis of where the government's power to act originated. Because the United States is a country comprised of 1 national government, 50 state governments, and several territorial governments, a determination of which laws take precedence when conflict between state and federal laws occur is necessary.

The **Supremacy Clause** of the Constitution (Article 6, clause 2) asserts that federal law takes precedence over any conflicting state law. When a variance in the laws applicable to a situation occurs, federal law prevails. Therefore, when a state legalizes the use of medical marijuana within its borders, it has no effect on federal laws against marijuana use. People may still be prosecuted within that state for violating federal law.

However, the discussion of our system of laws does not end here. Our system of government and law is controlled by a distinct hierarchy, the first tier of which is constitutional law (Figure 3.7). For powers delegated to the federal government, the US Constitution is superior to all other law in the country and is often referred to as the *supreme law of the land*. All other laws must be formed within constitutional requirements and comply with constitutional concepts. Laws must not violate any terms of the Constitution or exceed the constitutional authority granted to the government to act.

Other powers not delegated to the federal government are retained by the states, each of which is governed by its own individual constitution. These constitutions are not uniform, and their jurisdictions have

Equal Protection Clause
a clause in the Fourteenth Amendment that is intended to end all remaining discrimination resulting from slavery and requires state laws to protect each citizen equally

Supremacy Clause
a clause in Article VI of the US Constitution that establishes that all federal laws and all treaties made under the authority of the United States are the "supreme law of the land"

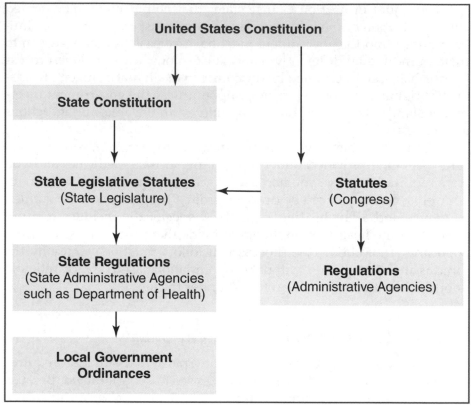

Goodheart-Willcox Publisher

Figure 3.7 The hierarchy of law.

evolved from different historical foundations. For instance, the northeastern states are founded on English common law and have significantly different perspectives on marriage than far western states such as California, Oregon, Washington, Arizona, New Mexico, and Texas, which are influenced by Spanish law. Louisiana's constitution is based largely on civil law derived from France.

statutes
laws established by a legislative body

case law
law that is made by courts as they resolve issues presented to them

The second tier of the hierarchy of law consists of **statutes**, laws, and legislation. A statute is a formal enactment of Congress or a legislature that governs a nation, state, county, or city. The term *statute* is often used to distinguish laws passed by a legislature from **case law** (judicial decisions and interpretations made by judges while deciding on the legal issues before them) and regulations. Statutes include the general and permanent laws of the state, incorporating all new laws, amendments, or repeals of old law. Statutes are superior to all other law except the articles and amendments of the Constitution.

Many governmental agencies, after being authorized by legislation, are permitted to establish regulations, such as those that protect the public's health. For example, a state health or agricultural agency may be legislatively empowered to protect migrant workers by adopting rules to establish minimum health and safety requirements for agricultural labor. Congress or state legislatures must have authority from their Constitution to act in the area being legislated. If the Constitution does not provide such authority, the statute is unconstitutional.

The third level of authority in the hierarchy of law is administrative agency regulations and local governments. Regulations are administrative rules that create or restrict rights and allocate responsibilities to implement programs established by legislation. Regulation can take many forms.

For example, the Occupational Safety and Health Administration (OSHA) regulates health and safety standards in the workplace. Administrative agencies are empowered to write, disseminate, and enforce regulations that implement statutes. Regulations must be consistent with both the legislative objectives that they were designed to achieve and the Constitution.

Local governments, including counties and cities, are authorized to create their own rules (ordinances) if they are not in conflict with federal and state constitutions and laws. Speed limits, zoning regulations, and local parks are examples of topics usually regulated by local ordinances. Counties and cities also may establish their own public hospitals and clinics, as well as paramedic and ambulance services that directly affect healthcare and the work of healthcare providers.

Career Corner

Businesses need sound management to keep them functioning efficiently and effectively. The business of healthcare is no different. Healthcare administrators, also known as *human service administrators*, are professionals who plan, direct, coordinate, and supervise the delivery of healthcare. These professionals have an educational background in the traditional management disciplines taught in a healthcare context as well as coursework in policy and public health. Such programs are available at both the undergraduate and graduate level.

A health policy and administration degree can lead to employment in private or public healthcare organizations, educational institutions, and nonprofit social services organizations. Examples of such employers include county health departments, federal health agencies, pharmaceutical companies, health insurance providers, consulting firms, medical clinics, and medical device and supply companies.

Many graduates get involved in healthcare policy by engaging in careers with local, state, or federal agencies or health-related national

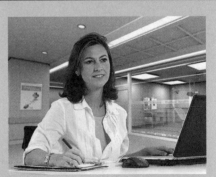
Franck Boston/Shutterstock.com

associations. After reading this chapter, would you be interested in a healthcare administration career? Are you interested in health policy? What types of policies are of interest to you?

The Federal Government's Authority to Regulate Healthcare

Government involvement in healthcare occurs in many ways (Figure 3.8). The question of whether the federal government has the right to legislate or regulate healthcare in a particular manner is raised often. Frequently, the issue involves the Constitution's authorization of government activity in a specific area.

From a literal reading of the Constitution, there is no passage that directly states that the government may legislate in the area of healthcare. However, the fact that the document does not specifically state that government has the power to legislate in an area does not necessarily mean that it is prohibited from doing so. Constitutional interpretation looks to the intent of the document to determine the constitutionality of any governmental action.

The Constitution contains language that many people believe indicates the government's authority to regulate healthcare, with some of the language more obvious than other language. The Preamble of the Constitution states that the government was created, in part, to promote the general welfare. Article 1, Section 8 states that Congress is empowered to provide for the general welfare. These two provisions have long been interpreted to mean that government has an essential duty, and

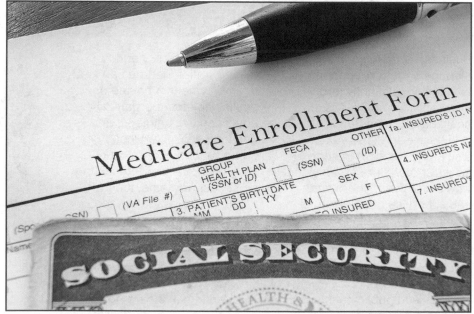

zimmytws/Shutterstock.com

Figure 3.8 The government facilitates several healthcare programs, including Medicare and Medicaid.

accompanying authority, to provide for the safety and welfare of the country and its citizens through healthcare.

This interpretation is implemented through the government's **police power**, which means its obligation to protect public safety and welfare. The authority of the police power is not limited to the federal government but is inherent in the various states' authorities as well. Therefore, when a state creates licensing laws for hospitals or healthcare providers, or enacts public health laws related to contagious diseases, it is exercising its police power.

The ability of Congress to regulate commerce (Article 1, Section 8 of the US Constitution) is closely aligned to the police power. The courts have repeatedly held that Congress has the authority to regulate transactions that are involved in, or impact, interstate commerce. Healthcare makes up 17.7 percent of the US economy and is involved in interstate commerce in many ways, from using the US mail for billing to buying pharmaceuticals from companies across the country.

In the rare instance when the Congressional power under the Commerce Clause is not sufficient to manage all aspects of healthcare, the power to tax has been used. When the individual mandate requiring individual citizens to buy health insurance under the ACA was challenged in the Supreme Court, it was decided that this feature of the ACA was constitutional. The Supreme Court found that while the Commerce Clause did not involve the power to compel individuals to act, the taxing power was available to Congress to shape individual action. In 2017, Congress reduced the unpopular tax to zero starting in 2019.

police power
the basic right of state and local governments to make laws and regulations for the benefit of their communities

State Governments

State government structures generally parallel the structure of the federal government, including their own elected legislatures. Because states have all remaining power not granted to the federal government or prohibited by it, the states are deeply involved in healthcare regulation. Not only do the states regulate healthcare delivery, they often provide direct services such as operating state mental health hospitals. Ever expanding on their inherent power, states have recently been authorized by federal law (by way of the ACA and the Commerce Clause) to establish healthcare exchanges to improve access to health insurance (Figure 3.9).

Individual practitioners, healthcare businesses and organizations, and insurance companies comprise the healthcare field. In addition to these components, state and local governments can operate a full range of healthcare services directly as part of the government, particularly for homeless or mentally ill individuals. Each state is actively participating in healthcare regulation.

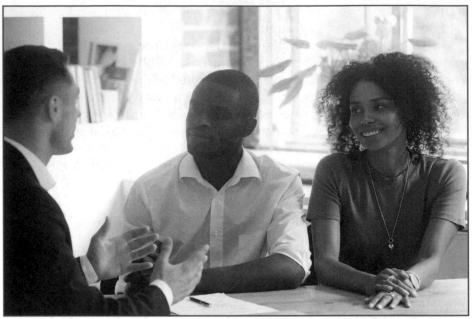

fizkes/Shutterstock.com

Figure 3.9   Healthcare exchanges may help you enroll in a health insurance plan.

Likewise, it is the state court system that is involved in the vast major-ity of lawsuits involving malpractice, battery, assault, wrongful death, and other claims against practitioners. County health departments make a direct and valuable contribution to the health of the community.

Oregon's Death with Dignity Act is an example of the state gov-ernment's role in healthcare. This law allows terminally ill residents of the state to end their lives through the voluntary self-administration of lethal medications. These medications are openly prescribed by a doctor for the purpose of ending one's life. The act requires that the Oregon Health Authority collect information about the patients and physicians who participate and publish an annual statistical report.

Other examples of the state governments' roles in healthcare include licensing and regulation of clinicians; overseeing and engaging in public health activities (health surveillance, sanitation, disease control); financ-ing and delivering individual health services, including Medicaid and mental health programs; and direct healthcare delivery through county and other public hospitals and health departments.

Local Governments

Local governments carry out some of the most important roles in healthcare delivery. They provide a variety of organizational models and services and are involved in healthcare far beyond their role as employers providing employee benefits. Local governments are enmeshed in many facets of health services, including public schools, homeless shelters, food establishments, county hospitals, and transportation. They provide both indirect and direct services. For example, consider emergency medical services. When a person needs emergency medical treatment, many different local organizations may be involved. In almost all cases, a local fire and rescue unit, emergency medical unit, general hospital, and/or contracted provider act during this first medical intervention. Depending on the situation, police presence and even helicopter medical rescue may also be required (Figure 3.10). All of these services are controlled by the local government.

Local governments are heavily involved in public health. This includes the development of laws, such as smoking regulations, and communicable disease surveillance and control. For example, local governments have the authority to quarantine a person who has a communicable disease if the person is not adhering to treatment.

The roles of local governments concerning non-communicable diseases include education, policy development and regulation, data collection and analysis, and supportive services, such as providing free cholesterol level checks or depression screenings. Transportation safety, such as zoning laws and speed bumps, as well as food safety, such as inspecting restaurants, fall under their purview as well. Additional examples of the health-related responsibilities of local governments include environment health management, housing inspections, noise pollution and vector control, water safety, and public awareness and education campaigns.

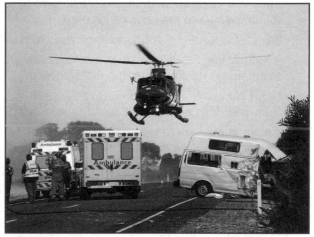

Hypervision Creative/Shutterstock.com

Figure 3.10   Many different local agencies may participate in providing emergency medical assistance to individuals.

Chapter Summary

- The articles of the US Constitution define the three branches of government (legislative, executive, and judiciary) and describe the division of powers among the federal and state governments; the federal government has the power to create statutory laws, including laws that affect healthcare.

- State governments have all remaining power not granted to the federal government or prohibited by it, according to the US Constitution; the state court system is involved in the majority of lawsuits involving malpractice, battery, assault, wrongful death, and other claims against healthcare practitioners.

- Local governments provide actual services to area residents, including emergency health care, public health issues, and public education about healthcare and healthcare resources.

Vocabulary Matching

1. basic right of state and local governments to make laws and regulations for the benefit of their communities

2. law that is made by courts as they resolve issues presented to them

3. a federal law established to promote the adoption of health information technology while protecting patient privacy

4. purposeful structuring of the government to prevent one person or group from wielding uncontrolled centralized power

5. clause in the US Constitution that has been interpreted to mean that citizens cannot be deprived of life or liberty without notice and a right to be heard

6. additions to the US Constitution that address topics not covered in the original Constitution

7. rules derived from English law (French law in Louisiana) and tradition that have been formally adopted into state laws or used to determine decisions in American courts

8. laws established by a legislative body

9. the first ten amendments to the US Constitution, which protect the individual rights of citizens

10. clause in the Fourteenth Amendment intended to end all remaining discrimination resulting from slavery and requires state laws to protect each citizen equally

11. clause in the US Constitution that grants Congress extensive power to regulate the economy, particularly the flow of items and information between the states

12. clause in Article VI of the US Constitution that establishes that all federal laws and all treaties made under the authority of the United States are the "supreme law of the land"

A. amendments
B. Bill of Rights
C. case law
D. Commerce Clause
E. common law
F. Due Process Clause
G. Equal Protection Clause
H. HITECH Act
I. police power
J. separation of powers
K. statutes
L. Supremacy Clause

Multiple Choice

13. The _____ government has the power to license healthcare professionals.
    A. federal
    B. state
    C. local
    D. Both state and local

14. The Health Information Technology for Economic and Clinical Health (HITECH) Act is an example of a health law made by the _____.
    A. judicial branch
    B. Congress
    C. Senate
    D. Supreme Court

Completion

15. The Constitution includes _____ articles.

16. The three branches of the federal government are the judicial, executive, and _____ branches.

17. The _____ branch of government has the authority to create the billing codes needed to administer the Medicare program.

10. The Bill of Rights contains _____ amendments.

19. _____ is composed of the House of Representatives and the Senate.

Discussion and Critical Thinking

20. Do the levels of government and separation of powers in the US democracy inherently lead to a highly complex regulatory environment for healthcare? If so, is this a positive or negative outcome?

21. How do the amendments to the US Constitution help you as a patient?

22. If you were a healthcare practitioner, would you appreciate the special protections given to your patient, or would you be upset with the levels of rules and regulations governing your practice? Address aspects of both options in your answer.

23. Review the Constitution. Where in the document is the right to privacy mentioned?

24. All states allow drivers licensed in another state to drive on their highways. Why are healthcare-related licenses not honored in the same way? Would the reason also have to do with why the federal government does not issue either type of license? Explain.

25. What sections of the US Constitution allow the federal government to legislate and operate programs that affect healthcare?

26. If the US Constitution is the supreme law of the land, why are states so involved in regulating and providing healthcare?

27. Where does the fundamental authority to create healthcare laws come from at the federal and state levels of government?

Activities

28. Reread the scenario presented at the beginning of the chapter. Write a one-page paper that describes your decision in this situation and the reasons supporting your decision.

29. Review two federal laws, two state laws, and two local laws related to healthcare. Write a two-page paper that explains the laws. Include reasons for why you support or do not support each law.

Case Study

A mother refuses to allow a doctor to provide a legally required immunization for her child. The outcome of this case depends on whether the state can display a compelling public interest in preventing the spread of communicable disease. Typically, the decision of the legislature in making laws regarding required immunizations have been upheld. In some states and in some cases, objections based on religious or philosophical grounds have been allowed. Can the child's mother prevail if she objects based on the pain it will cause the child? Can she prevail if her objection is based on religious beliefs?

Unit 2 The Healthcare Environment

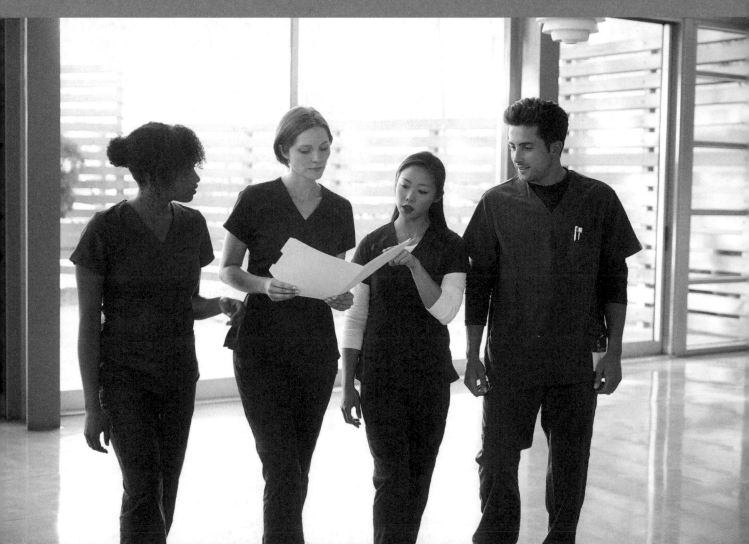

Monkey Business Images/Shutterstock.com

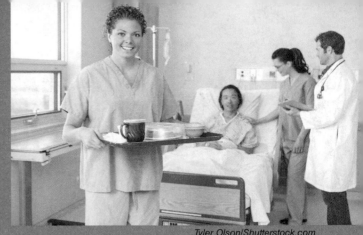
Tyler Olson/Shutterstock.com

Chapter 4

Certification and Licensing of Healthcare Professionals

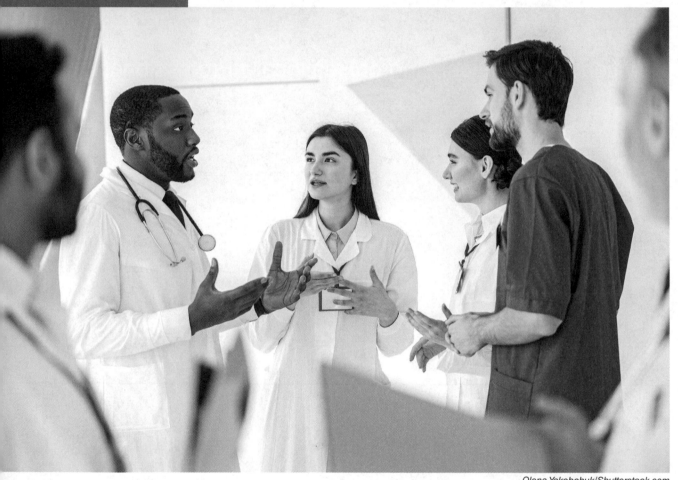

Olena Yakobchuk/Shutterstock.com

Chapter Outline

Healthcare Professions

Licensing and Certification

Licensing

Continuing Education

Codes of Ethics

Suspension and Revocation of Licensure

Certification

Professional Organizations

Objectives

- Identify at least six examples of healthcare professions.
- Describe the benefits of earning a license or certification and the process of obtaining and maintaining it.
- Explain how the rights of professionals and the safety of the public are protected through the licensing and certification of healthcare professionals.

Key Terms

accreditation

allied health professionals

certification

code of ethics

license

professional organization

revocation

suspension

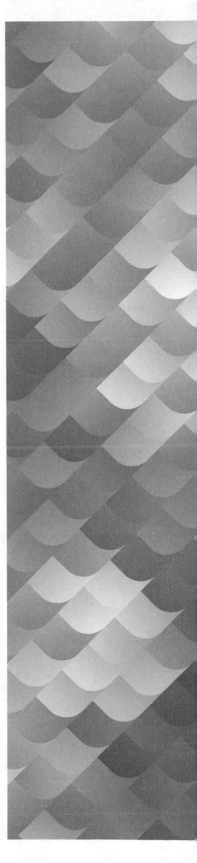

What Would You Do?

Sally just moved to Alabama. She needs to find a new primary care physician and a new acupuncturist. She's worried because she received excellent care from her providers for 20 years before she moved. How can she find potential providers in her new area? How can she be sure that they are qualified and will provide good care?

certification
a document that formally recognizes the recipient as having successfully achieved a specific level of training or demonstrated a specific level of competence

license
a legally authorized permit to work in a given field

Healthcare professionals have special rights and privileges as well as important roles and responsibilities. In some cases, these responsibilities are changing, causing the legal requirements for these professions to change as well. These changes are due, in part, to shortages of healthcare providers and emerging technological advances. As a result of these changes, some health professions have experienced alterations in their **certification** or **license** requirements. Certifications indicate competency in a particular area. Licenses are legally authorized permits to work in a given field.

What types of healthcare jobs require a certification or license? This depends on the specialty involved in a given job. Generally, the level of training and certification or licensure required for a health profession is established by professional associations and may be recognized in state law. Specific employers and programs, such as Medicare, may establish their own additional standards. For instance, the Kaiser Permanente School of Allied Health Sciences awards a certificate for IV and Blood Withdrawal Therapy (phlebotomy) as part of its continuing education program in compliance with the California Health and Safety Code (Figure 4.1).

This chapter discusses some of the evolving healthcare professions and laws related to them. The chapter also provides an overview of licensing and other certifications, the role of professional organizations, and the importance of maintaining good professional conduct. It is through the membership and status associated with a profession that many workers in the healthcare field enjoy special standing in the community.

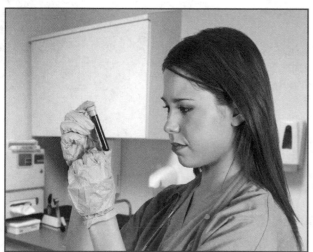

Rob Byron/Shutterstock.com

Figure 4.1   Some healthcare workers, such as phlebotomists, need licenses from specific agencies or organizations.

Healthcare Professions

When people think of working in healthcare, they often think of doctors and nurses. However, there are hundreds of specialized jobs in the field, all with different levels of training and practice requirements. For example, educational requirements can range from a 40-hour certification to six or more years of schooling, residencies, and internships. Jobs that involve direct patient care range from working with newborns to the very elderly, or working with individuals, families, or large groups. There also are many jobs, such as health policy analyst, that involve minimal patient contact.

Without a doubt, you can find a career in healthcare that fits the amount of time you wish to attend school and that matches your personality and interests. This section describes laws and ethics related to a few healthcare careers that are changing (Figure 4.2). Note that there are many other careers in the healthcare field that are not described here.

Selected Healthcare Professions	
Healthcare Profession	**Description**
Community health workers	Community health workers (CHWs) provide outreach, education, referral, follow-up, case management, advocacy, and home visitation services to community members. While no federal requirement for training exists, the health and human services agencies in some states require CHWs to obtain state-level certification. To earn this certification, individuals must pass an approved training program. These programs include specific skills and competencies that students must demonstrate to pass the program. Credentialing and certification programs are often administered by the local health department or another agency at the state level. In addition, academic institutions offer courses, certificates, or degrees in the CHW field.
Pharmacists	According to the Wise Law Group, LLC, "Three common types of state laws regarding pharmacists regulate (1) what the requirements are to be a pharmacist, (2) what a pharmacist may and must do as part of his or her practice and (3) state laws about the supervision of non-professional pharmacy personnel and the limits of their practice."
	Most, but not all, states have laws that require pharmacists to complete an accredited program in pharmacological science and procedures. Sometimes these state laws identify specific courses to be included in a pharmacist's education. Some state laws require pharmacists to pass a competency test for licensure. Some require that pharmacists complete continuing education courses to remain up-to-date in the field. Required classes and tests may be different in each state.
	In most states, pharmacists are not allowed to prescribe medications. As a result, pharmacy practice is limited to preparing, dispensing, and teaching people about medications. Many states have laws that require pharmacists to educate patients about their medications, including instructions for taking them, side effects that may occur, and potential interactions with other drugs. Some states have enacted laws that require pharmacists to monitor the sale of certain over-the-counter medications, such as Sudafed, that are used to make the drug methamphetamine (meth).

Figure 4.2

(Continued)

Selected Healthcare Professions (*Continued*)	
Naturopaths	Naturopaths practice naturopathic medicine, also known as *naturopathy*. Naturopathy is a system of medicine based on the healing power of nature. According to the University of Maryland Medical Center, "Naturopathy is a holistic system, meaning that naturopathic doctors (NDs) or naturopathic medical doctors (NMDs) strive to find the cause of disease by understanding the body, mind, and spirit of the person. Most naturopathic doctors use a variety of therapies and techniques (such as nutrition, behavior change, herbal medicine, homeopathy, and acupuncture)." In Washington, as well as other states, NDs can perform minor office procedures appropriate to a primary care setting, administer vaccinations, and prescribe most standard drugs.
	As of early 2019, 22 states, the District of Columbia, and the United States territories of Puerto Rico and the Virgin Islands had licensing laws for NDs. In these areas, naturopathic doctors must meet certain requirements to receive a license. These requirements include graduating from an accredited four-year residential naturopathic medical school and passing an extensive postdoctoral board examination known as the *NPLEX*. Some states mandate that licensed naturopathic physicians must complete continuing education requirements annually. Naturopathic doctors have a specific scope of practice defined by their state's law.
Home Health and Personal Care Aides	Home health and personal care aides assist individuals who have a disability, chronic illness, or cognitive impairment. These professionals also assist older adults. Home health and personal care aides help clients with activities of daily living, such as bathing and dressing, and they provide services such as light housekeeping or cooking. In some states, home health aides are permitted to give a client medication or check the client's vital signs under the direction of a nurse or other healthcare practitioner.
	Home health and personal care aides are not required to obtain any formal education. However, home health aides working in certified home health or hospice agencies are required to go through formal training and pass a standardized test.
	In some states, the only requirement for employment for these professionals is on-the-job training, which is generally provided by employers. Other states require formal training, which can be obtained through community colleges, vocational schools, elder care programs, and home health care agencies. Background checks on prospective aides are required in some states.
	Home health aides who work for agencies that receive reimbursement from Medicare or Medicaid must obtain a minimum level of training and pass a competency evaluation or receive state certification. Training topics include personal hygiene, reading and recording vital signs, infection control, and basic nutrition. Aides may take a competency exam to become certified without going through any training. These are the minimum requirements by law, but additional requirements for certification differ in each state.
	Aides can be certified by the National Association for Home Care & Hospice (NAHC). Certification is not always required, but many employers prefer to hire certified aides. Certification requires education, experience, paying an exam fee, and passing a written exam.

(Continued)

Selected Healthcare Professions (*Continued*)	
Nurse Aides	The Omnibus Budget Reconciliation Act of 1987 required states to initiate and maintain Nurse Aide Training and Competency Evaluation Programs and Nurse Aide Registries. This requirement was intended to improve the quality of care in long-term healthcare facilities and define training and evaluation standards for nurse aides. This act requires that states review, approve, deny, or suspend training programs as outlined in the Federal Code of Regulations (CFR Title 42, volume 3, part 483). States are also is required to certify and list all individuals who complete a state-approved training program and competency evaluation. In addition, states must list and maintain a registry of all nurse aides who are found to have abused or neglected elderly or vulnerable individuals or misappropriated their property.
Midwives	A licensed direct-entry midwife (LDM) oversees the labor process and childbirth; advises and educates parents about the progress of childbirth; and provides prenatal, intrapartum, and postpartum care. LDMs work in patients' homes, birthing centers, clinics, and midwifery schools as teachers. Midwives are educated through self-study, apprenticeship, midwifery school, or a college-based program. Licensure laws that apply to midwives vary by state. For example, Florida requires licensure, but other states do not have this requirement. However, having a license affects reimbursement. In Oregon, licensure is voluntary, and unlicensed midwives may practice. State law allows only licensed midwives to receive reimbursement under the Oregon Health Plan. LDMs are legally authorized to administer certain drugs and devices in Oregon, including anti hemorrhagics, oxygen, catheters, and sutures.

Goodheart-Willcox Publisher

Licensing and Certification

Depending on the state you live in, you may be required to obtain certification or licensure to pursue your chosen healthcare profession. Each process is described in this section.

Licensing

Many jobs in the healthcare field require licenses (physicians, nurses, pharmacists, and occupational therapists, for example). Licenses are essentially permits issued by state governments or other organizations in accordance with legislation that describes standards for licensing. Licenses are issued when an individual has demonstrated competence in skill, learning, and ethics to meet specific, officially recognized standards. These standards are established to maintain a general level of professional practice in the field and to protect current and potential patients or clients.

A license is intended to protect both the profession and patients from people who have not formally met the minimum standards and have not been issued documentation showing their right to practice. Licenses are usually only valid within a particular state, but some specialties have developed agreements called *interstate compacts*. These agreements allow different states to recognize other states' licenses.

Career Corner

An example of a healthcare profession that may or may not require certification is medical interpreting. The National Board for Certification of Medical Interpreters provides a national certification for medical interpreters, but it is important to research the legal requirements of the state where you will practice. Even if your state does not currently require certification, obtaining a national certification now may help ensure that you meet future employment requirements.

For some professions, the certification process can be complex. For example, different pathways to eligibility for certification are available for diagnostic medical sonographers through the American Registry for Diagnostic Medical Sonography (ARDMS). If a student attends a program in an academic institution that is not accredited, he or she may be able to take the ARDMS certification exam after completing a year of full-time clinical experience. However, most graduates of non-accredited programs are unable to fulfill this clinical experience because they cannot obtain a job without certification.

Non-accredited programs often tell potential students that they will be "ARDMS eligible" upon completion, and that may technically be true. However, caution is important when selecting a program. Students should find out if their academic institution is accredited prior to enrollment. Can you think of any healthcare professions

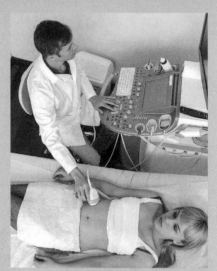
Med Photo Studio/Shutterstock.com

that do not have high enough standards when it comes to licensing? Are there any professions that should have licenses but do not?

Having a license provides some advantages for job applicants. Only people with the appropriate license may apply for certain jobs, and all others are excluded. In addition, a license affords you a certain status with your prospective employer, because you enter into employment already recognized as having a certain proven competence.

One of the rights you have as a licensed professional is for the government to protect the integrity of your profession by prosecuting impostors or those people who attempt to practice without a license. The government will use its police power to protect the public, and your profession, from unqualified people performing tasks that they are not qualified to perform. In doing so, the government effectively protects the "monopoly" that license holders have on their practice. Both criminal penalties (jail or prison time) and civil penalties (monetary fines) can be imposed on people who practice without a valid license. Laws forbidding unauthorized practice can also be applied against anyone who assists someone else to practice without a license.

A licensed healthcare professional receives governmental protection, economic advantage, and prestige from being licensed. However, he or she also carries a responsibility to the licensing authority to ensure that any work authorized by him or her is implemented in a proper manner.

Many healthcare tasks are performed by people who do not require licensure, such as medical assistants, nursing assistants, and occupational therapy aides. Much of that work is performed under the direct supervision or at the direction of licensed individuals or organizations (Figure 4.3). Therefore, a licensed nurse may be responsible for directing tasks performed by a nursing aide, whose job does not require licensure.

Perhaps the greatest right of a licensed healthcare worker is identification as a professional. There is more to licensure than simply paying fees and following administrative procedures. Licenses in the healthcare field are given based on educational requirements and competence demonstrated through internships and examinations. Obtaining licensure shows that you have achieved a level of recognized intellectual and personal achievement.

Your individual license is issued to you with a unique number. It cannot be inherited, loaned to you by a friend, or issued to you by your employer. In addition, if you are laid off by your employer, you still retain your license and identity as a licensed individual.

As long as the licensing authority has not revoked your license for improper conduct, failure to meet continuing education requirements, or negligence in paying your state licensing fee, you remain licensed. Retaining your license provides you with the basis for well-deserved personal satisfaction and ongoing recognition by others of your status, whether you are employed or not.

Typically, obtaining a license entails extensive education and training. These requirements are established by the licensing authority as a prerequisite to even taking a test. The tests generally have a written component, which is sometimes combined with a skills test. A written test or examination will usually include an ethics component as well as clinical competencies. You also will be required to pay a fee.

The entire licensing process creates a significant challenge and requires a commitment of time, money, and effort. For example, you must first obtain basic training and education in the desired field or specialty. Then, typically, you must prepare for the actual exam, which includes applying for the exam, paying the

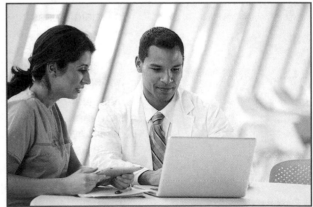

Monkey Business Images/Shutterstock.com

Figure 4.3 Certain healthcare workers, such as this nursing aide, do not require licensure, but must be supervised.

administrative fee for the exam, and taking an optional and often expensive test preparation course. Of course, there is the time and expense of actually taking the exam, as well as ongoing periodic registration fees and continuing education requirements that must be met to maintain the license.

Maintaining a license is a healthcare professional's responsibility (Figure 4.4). If your license is not renewed within the appropriate timeframe, your right to practice is suspended. You may be faced with prosecution for practicing without a license, professional discipline in your workplace, and an increased risk of malpractice claims.

Example of Licensure Requirements

Registered Dental Hygienist

- Dental hygienists are licensed by each state to provide dental hygiene care and patient education.

- To be eligible for state licensure, almost all states require that dental hygienists be graduates of a dental hygiene education program that is accredited by the Commission on Dental Education.

- Almost all states require candidates for licensure to obtain a passing score on the National Board Dental Hygiene Examination (a comprehensive written examination).

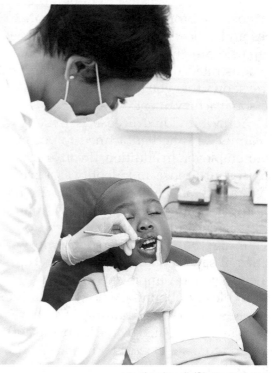

wavebreakmedia/Shutterstock.com

- Most states also require candidates to pass a state-authorized licensure examination. The state or regional examination tests candidates' clinical dental hygiene skills as well as their knowledge of dental hygiene and related subjects.

- Upon receipt of their license, dental hygienists may use the acronym "RDH" after their names to signify recognition by the state that they are a registered dental hygienist.

(Continued)

Figure 4.4   Healthcare fields and occupations have different licensure requirements.

Example of Licensure Requirements (*Continued*)

Mental Health Counselor

- Mental health counselor education requirements vary by state.
- Although some states allow professionals with a bachelor's degree to work in psychology, clinical mental health counseling typically requires a master's degree because these clinical professionals work directly with patients to provide a form of healthcare.

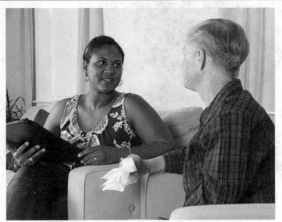

Rob Marmion/Shutterstock.com

- Successful completion of a Council for Accreditation of Counseling and Related Educational Programs certified graduate program qualifies people to sit for the licensing exam. After passing this exam, graduates can practice as a mental health counselor.

Goodheart-Willcox Publisher

Continuing Education

Once a license or certificate is issued, it usually has to be renewed periodically. To do so, a healthcare professional must fulfill a continuing education requirement established by the issuing authority in addition to paying fees or taxes. These requirements encourage providers to keep up to date with new, important knowledge for their practice, thus ensuring that the quality of the profession is upheld. The requirements also help protect the public by preventing incompetence. Of course, they also allow a particular specialty to demonstrate a reputable and responsible appearance to the public.

A specified number of approved continuing education credits must be earned and reported to the licensing authority within certain time limits, often annually. Approved courses are those that have been certified by the licensing authority as meeting certain standards related to format and content. Formats include in-person lectures, audio recordings, and web-based courses (Figure 4.5). The content must be relevant to the specialty in question. Continuing education often requires some additional ethics training as well.

Many commercial entities provide continuing education courses in addition to educational institutions. Some commercial organizations that are approved to deliver continuing medical education (CME) offer the courses at no charge as part of a marketing program or if they received grant money

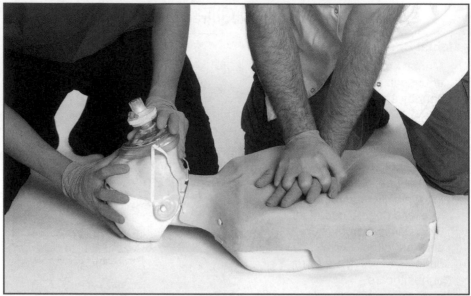

Pakula Piotr/Shutterstock.com

Figure 4.5   The American Heart Association (AHA) frequently updates guidelines for CPR and other rescue techniques, so continuing education classes in CPR are required at intervals for many professionals who work directly with patients.

to provide the training. However, most courses require a fee, which can vary from a few dollars to several hundred dollars. Sometimes an employer will pay for these courses, but you may have to pay this cost on your own.

Codes of Ethics

code of ethics
a set of rules established to guide the conduct of members of a profession

Professional ethics are governed by rules known as **codes of ethics**, which are established by the various specialties. These codes generally provide guidelines for conduct between the professional and the patient.

Information privacy is one example of this. Licensed healthcare providers are granted the special legal privilege to keep the confidences and personal information of their patients private. All licensed and unlicensed healthcare workers are legally required to protect patient health information under the Health Insurance Portability and Accountability Act (HIPAA). However, within the judicial process, there is a recognized need for patients to be able to share highly personal information and confidences with their licensed healthcare providers so that the providers may deliver proper care. Patients may refuse to allow their providers to testify in court about personal medical matters. This is based on the provider-patient privilege. The provider has a right to refrain from disclosing patient secrets without the patient's consent, even in serious criminal cases.

Codes of ethics may also include guidelines for how professionals within a specialty should conduct themselves when working with each other. Health professionals who have been sanctioned for misconduct are required to self-report this information to the appropriate authorities. Failure to do so is a breach of professional ethics, but some individuals disregard this requirement.

To improve public safety, national databases have been established to track disciplinary actions. The National Practitioner Data Bank (NPDB) lists all actions that revoke, suspend, or restrict a license for reasons related to the practitioner's professional competence. Professional associations report all professional review actions that adversely affect a person's membership. Hospital administrators report disciplinary actions that negatively affect a provider's clinical privileges for more than 30 days. They are required to check the NPDB when appointing or reappointing medical, dental, and allied health staff.

Malpractice insurance carriers report all settlements against physicians, dentists, and other licensed healthcare providers. The information can be accessed through state licensing boards, hospitals and other healthcare entities, professional associations, certain federal agencies, and plaintiffs and their attorneys in a malpractice suit. The general public may find information about professionals from organizations such as The Medical Board of California, which will verify professional licenses and provide access to certain public documents, such as lists of disciplinary actions and license revocations that may affect employment.

Healthcare facilities and other organizations that deliver services are also subject to their own specific requirements for obtaining and maintaining certifications and licenses. Those requirements are generally imposed by state regulatory organizations, such as the California Department of Public Health, which monitors facility compliance.

Suspension and Revocation of Licensure

As previously noted, licensing is a function of state police powers that are exercised primarily to protect the public. To this end, certain requirements must be fulfilled to maintain a license. In addition, most licensing depends on maintaining proper, moral, and legal conduct. Licensing organizations usually have a broad range of discretion on determining such violations.

Courts have determined that the US Constitution requires "due process" to be provided before a license may be revoked or suspended. This necessitates a sufficient description of the types of prohibited conduct, giving the accused persons notice of their alleged violations and an opportunity to be heard to oppose any adverse action. Examples of misconduct that may lead to adverse action include drug violations, improper use of credentials after your name, and criminal activity. Finally, performing work beyond the scope of your license can result in suspension or revocation.

suspension
a temporary negation of the rights and privileges granted by a license

revocation
an official government act that permanently takes away all rights afforded by a license

Suspension means the right to practice under the license is taken away for a period of time, and reinstatement may or may not be subject to other conditions, such as additional training. **Revocation** means all rights afforded by the license are permanently taken away. This also can include a broad range of conditions for any future reinstatement. These conditions might include taking additional education courses and passing additional exams. However, revocation proceedings may not always provide a means to reinstate the license. Therefore, the administrative enforcement of licensing standards is generally subject to judicial review in state courts.

While the court may recognize that the licensing agency has much discretion in its decision making, it will determine if there was proper notice, an opportunity to be heard, and sufficient evidence. This is usually based on a preponderance of the evidence, meaning that the evidence shows that the allegations are more likely than not to be true. By the time the matter reaches the court, the burden will be on the health practitioner to prove the licensing agency made an error.

Revocation and suspension hearings are separate from any related civil or criminal prosecutions that might occur in parallel. For example, the State of California waited to begin license revocation proceedings against Dr. Conrad Murray, the physician accused of wrongdoing related to the death of Michael Jackson, until one day after he appeared in court to answer for manslaughter charges.

Positive attributes associated with licensure and certification include self-respect, recognized achievement, better pay, protection from unwarranted competition, and a certain amount of autonomy for your own professional decision making. Your good standing also reflects your adherence to proper professional ethics. While there are numerous benefits to obtaining licensure and certification, there also are increased expectations of your abilities. The more training and official recognition you acquire, the greater rewards you may attain. You also may find, however, that you have greater responsibilities to properly apply your skills and knowledge, including supervising others.

Certification

allied health professionals
healthcare workers who deliver services involving the identification, evaluation, and prevention of diseases and disorders; dietary and nutrition services; and rehabilitation and health systems management

Certification is not mandatory. It is a voluntary process in which an individual, institution, or educational program is evaluated and recognized as meeting certain predetermined standards. Certifications can be issued by governments but are usually made by nongovernmental agencies, such as private companies, professional associations, or medical schools. A certification can indicate a range of accomplishments, from completing a specific course to having demonstrated years of successful practice. The purpose of certification is to recognize people who have formally met training and experience requirements.

Certifications can be issued to both medical professionals and **allied health professionals**. Allied health professions have greatly increased in number over the past 50 years as more and more roles that support traditional, physician-centered care have developed their own associations, standards, and testing procedures (Figure 4.6).

According to the Association of Schools of Allied Health Professions, "Allied health professionals are involved with the delivery of health or related services pertaining to the identification, evaluation, and prevention of diseases and disorders; dietary and nutrition services; rehabilitation and health systems management, among others."

There is some disagreement in the field as to how *allied health professional* is defined. Some view the term narrowly, including about 30 licensed categories. Others take a broader view to include over 200 positions that require licensure or that entail working under the supervision of someone who is licensed.

Figure 4.7 includes examples of allied health positions. Each job classification has its own set of qualifications. Because of the variation in topics, levels of training, and certifying organizations, you must be careful in verifying how any one certification will be recognized as credible or reputable. While it is true that anyone who has been issued a certificate

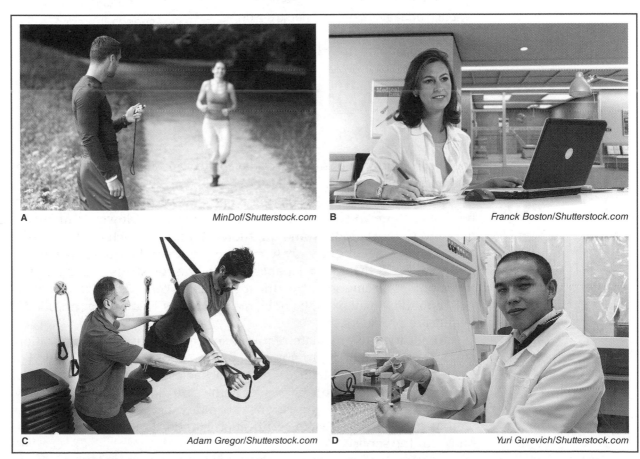

A — *MinDof/Shutterstock.com*
B — *Franck Boston/Shutterstock.com*
C — *Adam Gregor/Shutterstock.com*
D — *Yuri Gurevich/Shutterstock.com*

Figure 4.6 Allied health professionals include: A—athletic trainers; B—hospital administrators; C—physical therapists; D—public health employees.

A Partial List of Allied Health Positions		
anesthesiologist assistant	home care aide	orthoptist
art therapist	kinesiotherapist	orthotist and prosthetist
athletic trainer	magnetic resonance technologist	paramedic
audiologist	medical assistant	physical therapist
community health worker	medical coder	physician assistant
cytotechnologist	medical dosimetrist	polysomnographic technologist
dance/movement therapist	medical interpreter	radiologic technologist
dental hygienist	medical laboratory scientist	radiologist assistant
dietetic technician	medical laboratory technologist	radiology administrator
emergency medical technician	medical librarian	recreational therapist
exercise physiologist	medical technologist	registered dietitian
genetic counselor	nuclear medicine technologist	respiratory therapist
health educator	nurse's aide	sonographer
health information specialist	occupational therapist	speech therapist
	ophthalmic assistant	surgical technologist

Goodheart-Willcox Publisher

Figure 4.7

could claim he or she is certified, the context and nature of the certification must be examined.

For example, after completing a one-day training course, you may be able to claim you are a certified personal trainer. However, many clients and organizations would question the value of such a claim. Other certifications may require greater training but still be questionable. For example, Reiki therapy, a Japanese technique for stress reduction and relaxation, is an emerging treatment practice. A certification in this alternative therapy may or may not be recognized as valuable by traditional healthcare providers.

In addition to any state requirements for obtaining a certification, employers or funding programs may impose other requirements. For example, the federal Medicare program has established its own set of minimum training requirements for home care aides across the country. Anyone training to become a home care aide must comply with these as well as the individual state certification standards if Medicare will be billed for the service.

Certification of people already licensed as healthcare professionals is generally related to specialties (sports medicine, pediatric dermatology, or geriatric medicine, for example) or special competencies. Often, these certifications may only be obtained after the practitioner has been licensed and practicing for some time.

For example, the American Board of Neurological Surgery (ABNS) states that specialty training required prior to certification for residents who began their training on or after July 1, 2019 includes 84 months of neurosurgical residency training in Accreditation Council for Graduate Medical Education (ACGME) accredited programs under the direction of a neurosurgical Program Director. This must consist of the following:

- 54 months of core clinical neurosurgery, including
  - 12 months as chief resident during the last two years of training (postgraduate year 6 or 7);
  - 3 months of basic neuroscience (neurology, neuro-otology, neuroradiology, neuropathology) taken in the first 18 months of training;
  - 3 months of critical care relevant to neurosurgery patients taken in the first 18 months of residency;
  - 6 months of structured education in general patient care (trauma, general surgery, orthopedic surgery, otolaryngology, plastic surgery); and

    21 months spent in one program.
- 30 months of electives, such as neuropathology, neuroradiology, and research; more neurosurgery, possibly in areas of special interest such as complex spine surgery, endovascular, or pediatric neurosurgery; and/or clinical and non-clinical neurosciences.
- Outside rotations of 6 to 12 months at a program accredited by the ACGME may be counted toward the core 54 months of neurosurgery training. The program director must request credit from the ABNS prior to the rotation.

Board certifications generally require continuing education and testing and may involve surveys to determine client satisfaction with the level of care.

Ethical issues may arise in the complex realm of health-related certifications. You must be accurate when claiming certification in recognized skills, because recognized certifications can bring additional prestige and income. Claiming certification in questionable practice areas or certification by unrecognized organizations may not be illegal, but doing so can raise ethical issues.

Ethical Dilemma

A woman attended two eight-hour workshops to obtain her certificate in nutrition. The workshops were held in a person's home and that person's company issued the certificate. At the end of the workshop, a brief exam was provided. A pass rate of 70 was required to earn the certificate. All of the eight attendees passed.

After she passed the workshop, the woman had business cards printed to explain that she was a *certified nutritionist*. She contacted some personal trainers that she knew and began marketing her services at health clubs. Her first client was an overweight female with diabetes.

Do you think that the woman was wrong to market herself as a *certified nutritionist*? What impact do these certifications have on those who have earned a master's degree in nutritional science? Did the woman do anything unethical in her marketing practice? Ethically, should she have worked with a patient with diabetes after having only 16 hours of training?

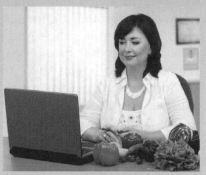

verbaska/Shutterstock.com

Are standards needed to claim that one is a nutritionist? Did the educator who provided the certificate violate any laws?

Professional Organizations

professional organization
a group that consists of individuals who are subject to specific standards regarding training and experience as well as ethical rules

A **professional organization**, or *professional association*, is established to represent the interests of a particular profession. Membership may require possession of a state-issued license. Some specialty associations are organized to enhance the interests of professionals in a particular practice, in a certain geographic area, or according to another characteristic. Many professional organizations also provide accreditation to academic programs and offer certifications.

For example, the Commission on Accreditation for Health Informatics and Information Management Education (CAHIIM) is an independent **accreditation** agency for health informatics programs at colleges and universities. The American Health Information Management Association (AHIMA) offers several certification exams for health informatics and medical coding professionals, but people must have graduated from a CAHIIM-accredited school to qualify for the exam.

accreditation
the process for authorizing or approving a facility, program, or person that conforms to formal standards

The Healthcare Information Management Systems Society (HIMSS), like AHIMA, is a professional organization for health informatics professionals (Figure 4.8). HIMSS also offers certifications, but their requirements are different from AHIMA's.

Major associations establish and maintain standards that protect patients and regulate conduct of professionals in the field. These organizations operate testing and admission processes; conduct, certify, and coordinate continuing education programs; establish, interpret, and enforce ethics rules; and develop advocacy positions on various public policy issues that might affect the profession as a whole.

Associations provide their expert insight in public policy discussions of issues that may affect their members. For example, the American Nurses Association (ANA), acting similarly to a labor union, regularly advocates improving the wages and working conditions of nurses. As stated on their website:

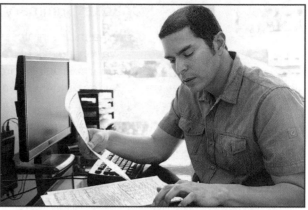

Monkey Business Images/Shutterstock.com

Figure 4.8 Health informatics workers may join the American Health Information Management Association (AHIMA).

"Part of the American Nurses Association's dedication to patient safety and nursing quality comes in the form of advocacy. By creating initiatives that raise awareness both among legislators and the general public, ANA is able to encourage legislation on important issues such as safe patient handling and patients' rights."

Members of a profession have the privilege of having their own standing as a professional represented, advanced, and protected by their professional association. Of course, payment of dues to the association is usually required.

Examples of professional associations in the healthcare field include:

- American Association of Pharmacy Technicians—provides leadership, education, and networking opportunities for this group of professionals.

- American Dental Hygienists' Association—works to support dental hygienists throughout their careers and advance the dental hygiene profession by developing new career paths, expanding opportunities for care, and providing the latest training and information.

- American Occupational Therapy Association—advances the occupational therapy profession through standard-setting, advocacy, education, and research.

- American Public Health Association—addresses public health issues through avenues such as education and advocacy and strengthens the public health profession.

- National Association of Social Workers—aims to advance the careers of social workers, improve their practice, and support the profession.

Chapter 4 Review and Assessment

Chapter Summary

- Healthcare professions include hundreds of specialized jobs that require various levels of training; examples include community health workers, pharmacists, naturopaths, home health and personal care aides, nurse aides, and midwives.

- Becoming licensed or certified in a healthcare field provides benefits such as ensuring employers that you have a certain level of skill and experience and protecting you and your profession from substandard practices; to obtain a license or certification, you must usually undergo training from an approved source, pay a fee, and pass an exam.

- Professional organizations often play a role in advocating for laws related to licensing and may set standards of ethical conduct, in addition to offering continuing education and interpretation of ethical rules.

Vocabulary Matching

1. document that formally recognizes the recipient as having successfully achieved a specific level of training or competence
2. group that consists of individuals who are subject to specific standards regarding training, experience, and ethical rules
3. temporary negation of the rights and privileges granted by a license
4. process for authorizing or approving a facility, program, or person that conforms to formal standards
5. legally authorized permit to work in a given field
6. healthcare workers who deliver services involving the identification, evaluation, and prevention of diseases and disorders; dietary and nutrition services; and rehabilitation and health systems management
7. an official government act that permanently takes away all rights afforded by a license
8. set of rules established to guide the conduct of members of a profession

A. accreditation
B. allied health professionals
C. certification
D. code of ethics
E. license
F. professional organization
G. revocation
H. suspension

Multiple Choice

9. Disciplinary revocation proceedings require the licensee to be provided with _____.
   A. a lawyer
   B. financial compensation
   C. access to files
   D. due process

10. The _____ Data Bank lists all actions that revoke, suspend, or restrict a license for reasons related to the practitioner's professional competence.
   A. Licensed Provider
   B. National Provider
   C. National Provider Status
   D. National Practitioner

Chapter 4 Review and Assessment

Completion

11. Maintaining a license is the responsibility of the healthcare _____.

12. A(n) _____ is not mandatory but can often help you further your career.

13. Continuing _____ may be required to maintain a license or certification.

Discussion and Critical Thinking

14. Review the scenario presented at the beginning of this chapter. What advice would you give Sally? Where should she go to get background information about the providers in her area? What questions should she ask the office personnel prior to making a first appointment?

15. Why are education, skill, and ethical standards established for healthcare professionals?

16. What are three privileges that healthcare professionals have?

17. What is the difference between a certification and a license?

18. Do you think that the licensing requirements for health careers should be the same across all the states? Explain your answer.

19. How do licensing requirements impact the demand for licensed healthcare professionals?

Activities

20. The next time you go to your doctor's office, look for a license posted somewhere in the office. Are there any certificates of specialization on display?

21. Look up your state's requirements to be certified or licensed in a healthcare profession of interest to you. Which professions did you find? What are the requirements for those professions? Give three examples.

22. Find the Bureau of Labor Statistics' *Occupational Outlook Handbook* on the Internet. Explore various healthcare-related jobs, including the requirements for each. Identify two healthcare jobs at the associate's degree level, two at the bachelor's degree level, and two at the graduate level. Prepare a chart that compares the type of school or college, length of instruction, and average cost of each degree.

Case Study

Bruce, a registered nurse, has been licensed with the state's Board of Nursing for over 15 years. He has earned a bachelor's degree in nursing. Bruce works in the cardiac unit of a hospital on the evening shift. He has worked full time in the same unit of the hospital for over 10 years.

Bruce has a good reputation as a nurse, and the doctors in the hospital where he works have faith in him and his abilities. As a result, the doctors have told Bruce and the other high-performing nurses in the unit not to disrupt them with minor orders.

One evening, Bruce spoke to one of the doctors about a patient who was in pain. The doctor instructed Bruce to do what he thought was needed to make the patient more comfortable. The patient's pain increased, so Bruce administered a pain medication. He noted in the patient's chart that a verbal order was received by the doctor. However, Bruce never went back to the physician to obtain the actual medication order. After the medication was given, the patient's condition deteriorated, requiring transfer back to the Intensive Care Unit.

Bruce admitted to the hospital Board that he wrote the order. He also repeatedly stated that this was "common practice" in the unit. Bruce was fired from his position at the hospital. The hospital filed a formal complaint with the Board, stating that Bruce was terminated by the hospital for falsification of medical records and administration of medication without a physician's order. Because Bruce did what he thought was expected, he was fined and lost his job.

Do you think Bruce should have lost his job? What should he have done differently to prevent this problem from occurring? Is the physician responsible for any wrongdoing in this case?

Chapter 5

Civil Liability of Healthcare Practitioners

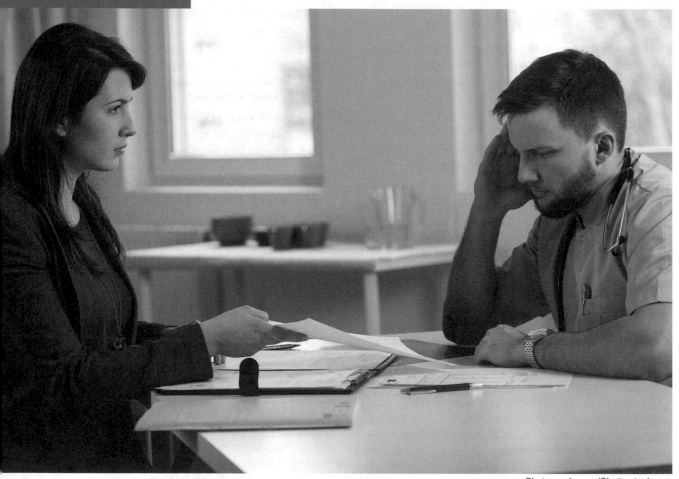

Photographee.eu/Shutterstock.com

Chapter Outline

Civil Law

Torts

Unintentional Torts

Standard of Care

Breach of Duty

Causation

Resulting Loss or Injury (Damages)

Intentional Torts

Compensation for Loss or Injury

Restraining Orders

Contract Law

Product Liability

Defenses to Civil Liability

Ethical Issues Related to Civil Liability

Objectives

- Explain the components of civil law, including unintentional and intentional torts, compensation for loss or injury, restraining orders, contract law, and liability.
- Discuss ethical issues related to civil liability

Key Terms

assault

battery

breach of duty

business disparagement

causation

civil law

civil liability

civil litigation

contract law

defamation

defendant

false imprisonment

fraud

implied contract

intentional infliction of
  emotional distress

intentional torts

invasion of privacy

libel

medical malpractice

money damages

negligence

negligence per se

plaintiff

punitive damages

restraining order

slander

standard of care

statute of limitations

strict liability

tort

Uniform Commercial Code

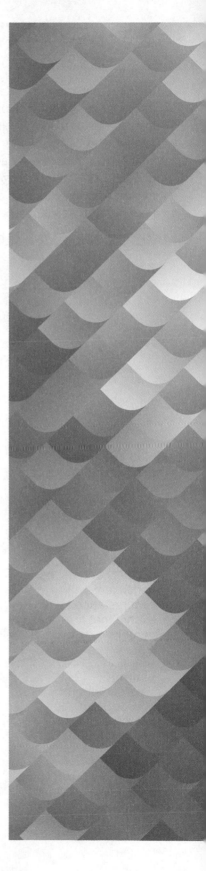

What Would You Do?

Imagine that you are a medical assistant assigned to give an injection to an older female patient who has provided consent but is obviously afraid of needles. The patient allows you to clean the injection site and hold her arm as you prepare to administer the injection. At the last moment, however, the patient tries to pull her arm away. Should you grip her arm and finish the procedure because she had originally agreed to receive the injection? Did she communicate through her behavior that she had revoked her permission and now objects to the procedure? Would you be liable if you let her refuse the injection? Are you violating any ethical standards if you decide what is best for the patient and give the injection despite her apparent objection?

As the old saying goes, to err is human. Even if a healthcare practitioner has good intentions and the necessary skills to conduct a procedure, the outcome may not be as expected. While the employer will assume the responsibility for these errors, healthcare practitioners are responsible for their actions and are held accountable as well.

Medical accidents and injuries can result in a painful process. Not only are these errors difficult for the patients and their families, they are also difficult for the provider due to the emotional response of causing an injury and responding to a lawsuit, if one is filed. This type of litigation is referred to as **civil litigation**.

Civil law is noncriminal law, and it includes both intentional and unintentional situations. Most civil cases involve disputes related to breach of contract, the collection of a debt, monetary compensation for personal injuries, property damage, or family law issues such as divorce. This chapter focuses on civil law as it relates to healthcare.

civil litigation
a formal legal procedure or action in court that determines legal rights and responsibilities

civil law
noncriminal law; typically addresses nonviolent circumstances and events that are perceived as wrongs suffered

plaintiff
a person or group who is accusing another person or group of wrongdoing

defendant
a person against whom an action or claim is brought in a court of law; may also be called a *respondent*

Civil Law

Civil law determines private rights and liabilities. Civil lawsuits usually involve disputes related to rules of conduct between individuals or organizations, which might include injuries or breaches of contracts. In a civil lawsuit, the **plaintiff** (alleged victim who brings an action) typically seeks to recover monetary damages (payments) from the **defendant**, or *respondent* (alleged wrongdoer). The plaintiff might also seek to have the court either compel the defendant do something or prevent the defendant from doing something. Civil law differs from criminal law in that the government prosecutes criminal law, and criminal law may result in incarceration. Criminal law is discussed more fully in Chapter 6.

Historically, United States civil law developed from English common law. This applies to all states except Louisiana, which uses French law or earlier Roman civil law. The US Constitution and most states' civil law derive from English common law (Figure 5.1). Common law was originally based on community rules derived from directives or rights granted by the King of England, such as those derived from the Magna Carta.

This law also came from individual English cases or Parliamentary enactments that have been formalized by legislative action in the form of state statutes throughout the United States. The statutes and rules among the various states are diverse but fundamentally similar. In part, this diversity reflects different community standards and values across the country. This is why, even if you know the laws in one state, you cannot presume to know the laws in another. Due to this diversity of law, attorneys must pass a bar exam and obtain a separate license for each state in which they practice.

Civil liability (legal responsibility) generally involves only money and not *incarceration,* or imprisonment. For example, a defendant in a lawsuit who is found to be liable typically pays money to the plaintiff as restitution (repayment), compensation, or punishment. It is important to note that civil liability can result from actions that the defendant either failed to perform or did not intend to do as well as from wrongful actions. Such actions are called *torts* and are discussed in detail in the next section.

Civil courts may use "injunctive relief" to compel or forbid certain actions. This type of remedy is a form of "equitable relief" that relies on judicial concepts of fairness rather than enforcement of specific laws or legal rules. Failure to obey these rulings may lead courts to find defendants in "contempt of court," which may lead to incarceration.

civil liability
the legal obligation to pay damages or perform another court-enforced action as a result of private wrongs (noncriminal acts) or breach of contract

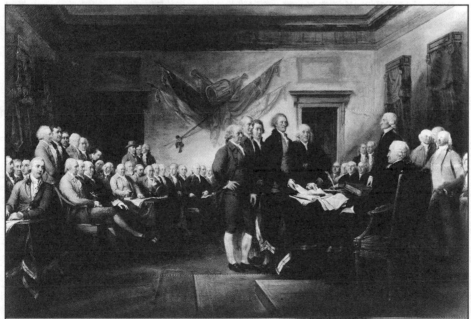

Everett Historical/Shutterstock.com

Figure 5.1   As laws were developed in the United States, the Founding Fathers drew inspiration from English common law.

Civil courts settle disputes between individuals (including corporations). There are several different levels of civil courts. Many jurisdictions have "small claims" courts that are relatively informal and allow individuals to appear without attorneys or juries to settle relatively small financial disputes, often under $10,000. Disputes that are more significant (up to about $25,000) may be addressed in municipal or district courts, which can involve jury trials.

Most states operate county-level courts, or district courts, which can address major financial issues. These courts also may grant equitable relief, which can involve conduct such as restraining orders. These courts are sometimes called *superior courts*. The states also operate courts of appeal and one supreme court to resolve similar issues resolved in different ways at the superior court level. A state's highest court may not be called a "supreme court," however; as the state of New York calls its highest court the *Court of Appeals*. For major interstate or international disputes, or those governed exclusively by federal law such as patent infringement, the federal government operates district courts, federal courts of appeal, and the US Supreme Court (Figure 5.2).

tort
an act of wrongdoing that results in injury to another person or damage to another's property

Torts

A **tort** is a wrongful act that is committed against another person or against property, resulting in harm or economic loss. Tort liability can result from intentional or unintentional conduct, or it can be based on strict liability. *Strict liability* means that a defendant is held responsible for

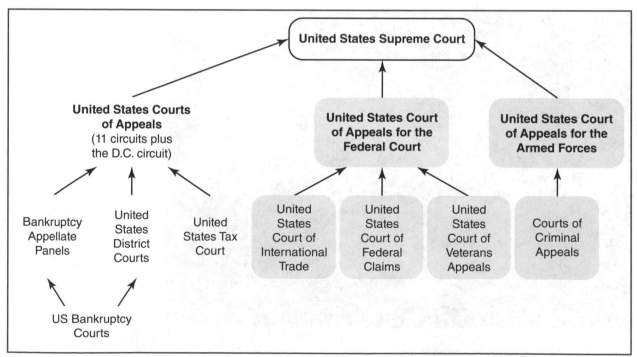

Source: Westlaw Integration Solutions

Figure 5.2 Organization of the US federal court system.

any damage that results from his or her conduct, regardless of how much care was taken or whether the conduct was intended. For the plaintiff to receive a monetary payment for injury suffered, the defendant must be proven to be at fault in some way.

Unintentional Torts

Torts that are committed unintentionally are called *negligence*. **Negligence** occurs when someone who has a duty to protect another person from unreasonable risk of harm breaches that duty, resulting in injury to the other person. Negligence may occur through either action or inaction. A case of negligence through action might include a nurse providing the wrong dosage of a medication. A case through inaction might include a nurse not providing the medication at all.

negligence
the failure to act as a reasonable person of ordinary prudence would act in a certain situation

Although the elements of negligence are the same for healthcare professionals as for other people in the community, negligence directly related to patient care is called **medical malpractice**. Malpractice involves action or inaction related to specialized tasks normally performed by a medical professional in the context of a duty of care for the patient. Intentional inappropriate action is called *malfeasance*, unintentional inappropriate action is called *misfeasance*, and failure to act is called *nonfeasance*. More than one of these may be included in one negligence claim for medical malpractice. For example, a doctor may delay too long to initiate a forceps-assisted birth procedure (nonfeasance), and then use too much force with the forceps (malfeasance).

medical malpractice
the improper, unskilled, or negligent treatment of a patient by a healthcare professional

To establish negligence, a plaintiff must prove that (1) the defendant had a duty to the plaintiff, (2) the defendant breached that duty by not conforming to the standard of conduct that is required, and (3) the defendant's negligent conduct caused (4) damages.

Standard of Care. Standard of care refers to the reasonable degree of caution and actions a person should provide to another person, typically in a professional or medical setting. For example, for a primary care physician or an oncologist (cancer specialist), the standard of care in the case of a cancer patient may include a recommendation of chemotherapy, radiation therapy, or surgery.

standard of care
the degree of caution or actions expected of a person, such as a healthcare practitioner, in the course of professional duties

In the healthcare field, standard of care (expected actions) is often established by the common law standards of reasonable conduct for a person of similar skill and education under similar circumstances. These standards vary by type of work and type of specialty. For example, the standard of care for a nurse practitioner is different from the standard of care for a neurosurgeon. However, standards for both are measured by how a competent nurse practitioner or a competent neurosurgeon would be expected to act under a given circumstance.

Rules of professional ethics generally guide conduct but do not represent standards to measure whether someone has breached a duty. A written ethical rule is not sufficient to determine the standard of care. Expert witnesses in a lawsuit may refer to these ethical rules, but the testimony of experts always determines the standard of care (Figure 5.3).

Expert Witness Testimony in Medical Malpractice Cases

In medical malpractice cases, typical citizens serving on a jury would not know what constitutes proper conduct for a particular healthcare professional. As a result, expert witnesses who are knowledgeable about the specific professional standard alleged to have been breached are often called on to testify. Both plaintiffs and defendants use expert witnesses. The jury (or judge) decides which experts to believe. These experts can describe the provider's duty, the nature of the provider's failure to act in accordance with that duty, and how a competent provider working in the community would have been expected to act under similar circumstances. In most medical malpractice cases, the accused provider would be confronted by experts in his or her specialty area.

For example, suppose a physician prescribed a decongestant to a patient who previously had a stroke. The drug packaging indicated that the decongestant causes adverse effects in patients who have had strokes. If the patient developed complications similar to those experienced by other stroke patients, did the physician commit malpractice? Did the physician breach a duty by not properly balancing the risks of harm versus the potential benefits of the decongestant? Physician experts would be needed to establish the standard of care.

Goodheart-Willcox Publisher

Figure 5.3   People with specialized knowledge in the field serve as expert witnesses in medical malpractice cases.

negligence per se
negligence in which the duty is presumed if the act violated a law intended to protect the public; unlike ordinary negligence, the conduct is automatically considered negligent, and the focus of the suit will be whether the conduct proximately caused damage to the plaintiff

breach of duty
a failure to perform some obligation or promise; the neglect or failure to fulfill the standard of care when one person or company has an obligation toward another person or company

In some instances, specific laws established by the state legislature define the duty or standard of care. Any activities outside the bounds of those laws are either illegal or unauthorized. Not complying with the law is called **negligence per se**. If a healthcare provider is found to have violated the law and damaged someone, a breach of duty is presumed.

Breach of Duty. The term **breach of duty** means that someone has not acted as a reasonable person would be expected to under the same circumstances. A breach is something that must be determined as fact and usually has to be proven in court. First, the appropriate standard of care or duty must be determined. Then the person's conduct must be compared to what was called for by the standard or duty. Finally, it must be proven that the breach, and not something else, caused the injury or loss.

For example, if a pharmacist is expected to warn a patient about side effects of a particular medication and does not, a breach has occurred. Breaches of standard of care happen often. The question is whether the breach matters and causes a negative outcome.

Causation. In some situations, even if you did not conduct yourself according to your duty as a healthcare professional, you may not be liable. Your action or inaction must be the cause of actual, proven damages unless damages can be presumed, as in some defamation cases. In these situations, the idea behind "no harm, no foul" applies. If damage did not occur as a direct result of your breach, you are not liable.

Suppose an operating room nurse provides a surgeon with unsterilized instruments for surgery, and the standard of care is to provide thoroughly sterilized instruments. If the patient died of a sudden heart attack or another condition unrelated to the contaminated instruments, there is no **causation**. In other words, even though the nurse failed to perform up to the standard of care and breached a duty, her actions did not cause the patient's death. Therefore, there would be no damages or liability for negligence. The nurse may be subject to employer discipline, but not civil liability.

While your breach of duty must be a direct and foreseeable cause of damages, it does not have to be the sole cause of damages for you to be liable. This is a complicated part of the law. Your action must be related enough so that the result is foreseeable if you failed to act properly. In many cases, several actions and inactions may contribute to the ultimate injury or harm.

Suppose the unsterilized instruments in the previous example caused a serious infection and the surgeon was aware of it but did not attempt to take appropriate mitigating action, such as administering antibiotics. If the patient died of that infection, both the nurse and the surgeon might be liable because each of them caused at least part of the problem (Figure 5.4).

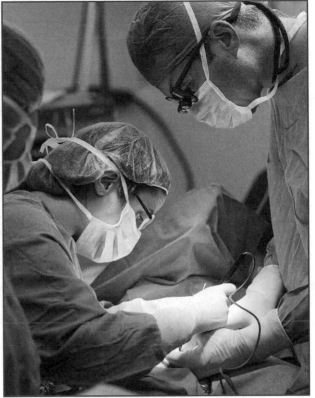

Franck Boston/Shutterstock.com

Figure 5.4 Even if you are not the primary surgeon in an operation, an error that you make could have consequences.

causation
term that describes the relationship between an action or condition and its effect or result

In some instances, causation can be presumed. This is the case when circumstances make the cause of damages obvious. This is often described as "the thing speaks for itself," or in Latin, *res ipsa loquitur.*

Resulting Loss or Injury (Damages). For negligence to have occurred, the plaintiff must show that some form of actual loss or injury was caused by the defendant. This can include physical or emotional injury or loss of value to property. These losses are necessary to calculate compensating monetary awards. Damage awards are discussed more fully following the discussion of intentional torts.

Intentional Torts

Intentional torts occur when a person intends an act and the action causes harm, whether the person intended harm or not. It is important to understand that, in this case, the word *intent* does not mean that you

intentional torts
deliberate civil wrongs

necessarily intended to do harm, but that you intended the action that ultimately caused harm. For example, in the scenario presented at the beginning of the chapter, a medical assistant may be liable for committing assault and battery on the job for giving a person an injection without permission.

Wrongful intentional acts are generally subject to the strongest punishment because they are more easily avoided. For example, you should be able to easily avoid using words calculated to hurt another person's reputation. The practical problem is that liability is associated with your intent to act, not to your intent to cause the resulting harm. You may think that giving an injection is good for the patient and that your actions are well intended. However, if there was no prior patient consent and an injury results from your action, you could be liable because you intended to give the unauthorized shot. Whether or not you were aware of the subsequent injury to the patient does not matter in this case.

In a healthcare setting, the most serious intentional misconduct results from actions that also violate an ethical duty to the patient. Therefore, the example of the unapproved injection also includes a violation of an ethical duty to honor the patient's autonomy. Whenever you are providing services to a patient, the potential for civil claims exists. These claims can include assault and battery, false imprisonment, intentional infliction of emotional distress, invasion of privacy, defamation, and fraud. In many jurisdictions, several of these are also criminal offenses and are discussed in Chapter 6.

battery
the intentional offensive or harmful touching of another person without that person's consent

Battery is the harmful or offensive touching of another person without permission or excuse. This goes beyond accidental touching, such as bumping into someone in an elevator, and generally does not include emergency actions, such as pulling an unconscious person out of a burning house. If you grab and forcefully hold a patient's arm to overcome the patient's fearful objection to the injection, as in the opening scenario of this chapter, you might have committed battery (Figure 5.5).

assault
an intentional attempt to injure or harm another person; no physical contact is necessary for an assault to occur

Assault occurs when a person feels fearful of an imminent battery. This is always viewed from the perspective of the "victim." A healthcare worker might not be afraid of a hypodermic needle, and so will try to show a patient how it might be used. However, this might scare the patient, who has unusual sensitivities or did not want to have the injection and was afraid you were going to give it immediately. If the patient can show that you placed him or her in a position of fear of immediate injury, you may be liable.

false imprisonment
term for the restraint of a person in a bounded area without justification or consent

False imprisonment is the intentional overruling of a person's right to leave. If you intentionally lock a patient in a room while you search for some assistance, you might be liable for false imprisonment, even if it was for only a short time.

intentional infliction of emotional distress
a tort that involves purposeful misconduct that is so extreme that it causes the victim severe emotional trauma

Intentional infliction of emotional distress occurs when someone or something causes severe emotional distress or anguish that goes

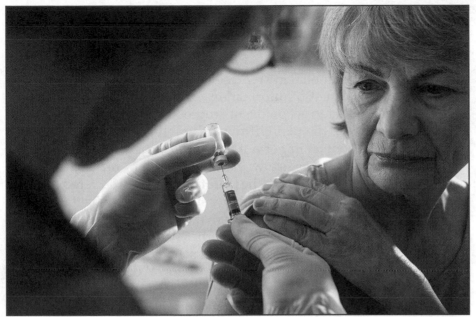

Image Point Fr/Shutterstock.com

Figure 5.5 Forcing someone to undergo a procedure that he or she has objected to, such as a vaccination, is considered battery.

beyond mere embarrassment or angst. This might include something that causes Post-Traumatic Stress Disorder (PTSD) or another clinically diagnosable condition. Outrageous misconduct with a child, in the presence of a parent, might rise to the level of intentional infliction of emotional distress on the parent.

Invasion of privacy occurs when private information is disclosed without consent. In recent years, there has been an increasing amount of legislation at both the state and federal levels that describes the right to privacy. Disclosure of private information can be a violation even if the disclosure was not specifically intended. For example, you might, out of habit, copy an unauthorized individual on an e-mail and thereby disclose a patient's private information.

Defamation causes someone to be shamed, ridiculed, held in contempt, or lowered in the estimation of the community, to lose employment status or earnings, or to otherwise suffer a damaged reputation. Written statements of defamation are called **libel** and spoken statements are called **slander**. Generally, if you assert that the content of your communication is your opinion and not an actual fact, you may be protected by constitutional rights to free speech.

For example, if you say that a doctor is a "quack," your comment may be interpreted as mere opinion. If you make several false statements to support your assertion, your actions may be considered intentional and false shaming of the doctor, causing injury to his or her reputation.

invasion of privacy
intrusion into the personal life of another person without just cause

defamation
any intentionally false communication, either written (libel) or spoken (slander), that harms a person's reputation; decreases the respect toward the person; or induces disparaging, hostile, or disagreeable opinions or feelings against a person

libel
defamation that occurs in a written format

slander
defamation that occurs in a verbal manner

business disparagement
false and injurious statements related to a business; requires proof of a specific economic loss

fraud
the intentionally false representation of a material fact that is calculated to deceive, and does deceive, another person to legal detriment or loss

Other forms of this tort include **business disparagement**, which occurs when communication relates to a business or practice rather than an individual person. This might occur when someone makes a false comment about a hospital committing insurance fraud.

Fraud is the intentional misrepresentation of facts—through words, conduct, or concealment of information—that deceives another person and causes him or her to act on the misrepresentation, resulting in damages. To prove fraud, the plaintiff must show that the defendant knew that a statement about an important fact was untrue.

The plaintiff also must show that the defendant made this untrue statement on purpose to deceive the plaintiff, who then suffered harm by relying on the falsehood. This is a higher standard than what might exist for merely calling someone names or making false statements because fraud involves actual intent to harm another person.

Fraud may occur as part of a planned scheme or result from merely momentary anger on behalf of the perpetrator. Words alone can be as costly as hitting someone on the head. There are numerous examples of patients being purposely misled by "snake oil salesmen." These individuals purposely convinced people to spend sizeable amounts of money on medicinal or other therapeutic remedies for incurable diseases. Victims

 # Career Corner

A medical coding specialist (also known as a medical coder) uses alphanumeric diagnostic and procedure codes to convey information about illnesses and treatment. There are different types of codes for inpatient and outpatient procedures. There are also sets of codes for diagnoses, laboratory procedures, telemedicine consultations, and other services. The codes are tied to the amount of money that providers and facilities are reimbursed for by health insurance carriers. Therefore, proper coding is vital to the revenue and financial stability of a healthcare facility.

Medical coders review medical records to assign the appropriate codes, so they must have an understanding of medical terminology as well as clinical notes and procedures. The coding process also requires knowledge of payer policies and relevant civil and criminal laws.

Inaccurate or incomplete coding can result in missed or reduced payments, costing healthcare providers and facilities revenue. Coding inaccuracies can be considered fraud and may have legal ramifications. Therefore, competent coders are important to a healthcare facility.

Becoming a certified professional coder demonstrates to potential employers that you have a certain level of coding skill and accuracy. Adhering

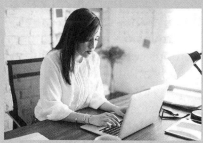

antoniodiaz/Shutterstock.com

to the ethical standards of the profession is also important. The American Health Information Management Association (AHIMA) and other professional organizations have established standards of ethical coding. Conduct some research on how to become a certified coder and the types of courses required.

of these schemes may recover monetary damage awards on their own by bringing civil fraud charges in civil court.

Torts are a complex area of law, and this brief summary provides you with a basic foundation for understanding the topic. Even attorneys who practice regularly in this area may need to occasionally refer to academic treatises such as the "Restatement of Torts (Second)," recent case law, and statutes.

Compensation for Loss or Injury

Compensation for civil liability involves financial payment to the injured party of an amount thought to be equal to the proven damages. This can include out-of-pocket expenses but also "general damages" that can be presumed and calculated, sometimes by a jury. These are termed *compensatory damages* because they are intended to compensate the plaintiff. In the case of minimal damage, nominal damages may be awarded to demonstrate the defendant was at fault but did not cause significant loss.

Damages can be described in a variety of ways but always in terms of **money damages**. For personal injury cases, damages may include medical costs, lost wages, loss of projected future income, and pain and suffering. In situations involving property loss, damages may include the cost of repair, lost profits, and consequential damages that are secondary but foreseeable.

money damages
payments awarded by the court in a liability suit

For example, if a surgeon unintentionally sews a body closed and leaves a clamp inside, some kind of harmful consequence is foreseeable, such as an injury to internal organs. Most damages have to be proven by evidence of loss or cost of care. However, some damages may be presumed, as is often the case with pain and suffering resulting from bodily harm.

In the case of intentional misconduct, a court may award **punitive damages**, which are intended to punish the perpetrator and make an example for others so they will not conduct themselves in the same manner (Figure 5.6). Punitive damages are essentially up to the discretion of the judge. An award of punitive damages is generally established at a level that actually punishes the defendant and involves the judge considering the wealth or financial capacity of the perpetrator. This can have significant consequences, especially if you are operating your own practice or healthcare business.

punitive damages
a type of award that is designed to punish a defendant and deter bad conduct

Civil liability may be caused by individual employees, but damages end up being paid by their employers. This is because most healthcare organizations are held responsible for the civil wrongs of their employees, who are essentially agents of the employer. Usually the responsible supervisor (sometimes called *respondeat superior*) must take responsibility for his or her subordinates and, most of the time,

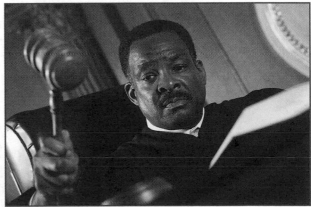

sirtravelalot/Shutterstock.com

Figure 5.6 A judge may decide that punitive damages are appropriate in the case of intentional misconduct.

94   **Unit 2**   The Healthcare Environment

has created the financial capability to pay damages. To hedge against this risk, many employers buy business or malpractice insurance.

Generally, for a court to order a defendant to pay money to a plaintiff, damage or loss must be proven. However, in some cases, damages are presumed. For example, damages have traditionally been presumed in cases that involve defaming another person by declaring they have a horrible disease. In other cases, future damage can be predicted or expected and some civil actions can involve orders from a court to pay future lost income, for example.

Of course, healthcare providers are concerned that malpractice claims can result in the loss of their money to compensate an alleged victim. The possible impact on the healthcare provider's reputation, employability, and continuing maintenance of a license are also concerns. In addition, as described in Chapter 4, the incident might be registered with national databases that track such misconduct. This may affect the healthcare provider's reputation, as well as his or her ability to obtain medical malpractice insurance at a reasonable cost, or to purchase it at all.

Restraining Orders

restraining order
a court order intended to protect an individual from further harm from someone who has hurt him or her

In extreme cases, the plaintiff may restrain the activities of a healthcare provider. This action would be taken in addition to any financial claim by the wronged person. A **restraining order** is a form of equitable relief that is based on a judge's sense of fairness and justice rather than any particular standard set by law. There have been instances of physicians continuing to practice life-sustaining care for a patient against the wishes of family members. In these instances, a restraining order could be brought against the physician.

The famous case of Terri Schiavo, who was considered to be in a permanent vegetative state, involved a husband who went to court to request that the doctor be restrained from providing life-sustaining care so that his wife could be allowed to die a natural death (see Chapter 2).

Situations involving restraining orders also arise in the context of healthcare providers engaged in the manufacturing of products, such as the violation of a patent or trademark. A court could act, as the result of a lawsuit, to order that an individual stop selling products that would lead a reasonable consumer to be confused about which product is authorized to be sold by the holder of a proper patent or copyright privilege. Bayer has brought several such suits to protect its aspirin-related products from sales practices of other companies.

Contract Law

contract law
rules-based statutes and case law related to enforcing promises

Another area of civil law that affects healthcare providers is **contract law**. A contract is essentially an agreement that a court will enforce. Contracts permeate all aspects of general business and healthcare. You can

Copyright Goodheart-Willcox Co., Inc

create a contract through both oral and written promises to do something in exchange for something of value. Sometimes the conduct of the parties establishes an **implied contract**, which is the same as other contracts but requires different proof to show it existed. In healthcare, this is usually a promise to provide services in exchange for money.

There are many sales of products among healthcare organizations as well as commercial businesses. To the extent that a contract involves the sale of goods, the **Uniform Commercial Code** may apply. The code has been adopted, with minor modifications by most states, based on a national model code to facilitate trade (for example, the California Commercial Code). In particular, the code is used to interpret or resolve issues related to implied terms not specifically included in written contracts. The courts are available to enforce the terms of contracts if someone fails to perform what they promised.

As a healthcare provider, you or your employer may establish various conditions, in addition to a fee, in exchange for services. For example, your employer may request to arbitrate any dispute related to care, and patients may agree as a condition of receiving care, thereby relinquishing their right to settle disputes through expensive civil trials.

Before receiving services, patients also may be asked to sign forms, known as *informed consent* forms, that explain the nature of medical care procedures and risks. In addition to recognizing and honoring patients' rights to autonomy and dignity, this form of contract agreement also shifts some risk of liability to the patient. This is equivalent to "assuming the risk" associated with an amusement park ride or buying a car "as is."

Ethical issues can arise in the area of contract law and may necessitate public policy action. For example, hospitals can usually refuse to contract for care with a patient if the prospective patient does not have health insurance. However, federal legislation requires that emergency facilities accepting Medicare stabilize life-threatening situations before transfer or discharge. Nevertheless, uninsured patients are billed for service (Figure 5.7). Ethical issues related to contracts also can arise when a healthcare professional develops contracts with patients, particularly in cases of elective treatment such as cosmetic surgery.

Generally, contracts should be agreed to by people of equal bargaining power. Patients rely heavily on medical providers' opinions and may not be in an equal bargaining position with them. Due to potential patient vulnerability or incapacity, healthcare professionals must be aware that the relationship of parties to a contract can make some transactions invalid, even after the fact.

For example, if the healthcare provider is in a position to be overbearing, not forthcoming, and/or misleading to the extent of committing fraud, then a contract can be found void and

implied contract
an enforceable promise or agreement created by the action of the involved parties without a specific written or spoken agreement

Uniform Commercial Code
set of laws and regulations that govern all commercial transactions in the United States

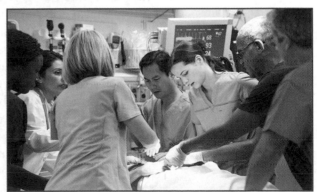

Monkey Business Images/Shutterstock.com

Figure 5.7 Patients experiencing a medical emergency of any kind must be given treatment, regardless of their ability to pay.

unenforceable. Of course, this situation can also mean a breach of ethical standards related to respecting patient autonomy and other ethical doctrines, regardless of the validity of the contract.

Important contract issues are also involved in insurance policies that protect you from loss as a result of financial liability you might encounter. Generally, insurance is a contract between you and an insurance carrier. For a price, an insurance company will pay up to an agreed-upon amount for certain predefined events that impose financial liability on the insurance customer. This issue is addressed more fully in Chapter 8.

As with torts, contract law is a complex issue, and this brief summary provides you with a basic foundation for understanding the topic. Attorneys who practice regularly in this area occasionally consult references such as the "Restatement (Second) of Contracts," which is a secondary academic source summarizing the topic, as well as recent case law and specific state statutes.

Product Liability

Another area involving civil liability for healthcare providers and others is product liability. Manufacturers have a duty to be sure their products do not harm consumers. Liability can arise from negligence (unsafe design or manufacture), breach of warranty, or in some cases, concepts of **strict liability**. When a manufacturer creates a product to be used in commerce, it is fully responsible for the design and manufacturing methods to produce safe products.

strict liability
the imposition of liability that makes a person or company responsible for actions or products that cause damages, regardless of any intent, caution, or preventive acts

Liability as a form of negligence occurs when economic or personal injury results from a poorly designed or poorly manufactured product. Duties also may include warning patients of possible injury and advising patients of specific safety practices related to the product.

For example, if a physician recommends a product (such as a specific wheelchair) for his or her patients and injury occurs, the manufacturer may be liable along with the physician. Even if a prescription headache pill is made correctly, the physician may need to warn the patient that taking more than three pills at a time may result in liver damage.

In the case of a pacemaker (an implanted device to control a patient's heart rate), the manufacturer may have a duty to warn the patient about electrical or radio interference, just as the physician does. As with other negligence cases, the breach of duty must be proved and the specific action being contested must have caused actual loss to the patient.

Liability also may arise for a manufactured product by way of a simple breach of warranty claim. A warranty is basically a form of contract agreement with the consumer that a product will work as promised (usually, as advertised). If the product does not work due to a manufacturing or design problem, a consumer may be able to make a claim for money based on the broken promise.

You are probably familiar with warranty claims or guarantees for any number of products. Generally, warranty claims are limited to actual loss by the actual written terms of the sales or warranty agreement. The customer accepts these terms either explicitly or by implication when he or she purchases the product.

Much of the "fine print" on product labels attempts to limit possible liability from implied warranties that are not specifically written out at the time of sale (Figure 5.8). There are several terms that can be used to limit the expectations of an implied warranty's validity. One such warranty is *merchantable*, which means that a product is of sufficiently reasonable quality and condition to be fit for sale.

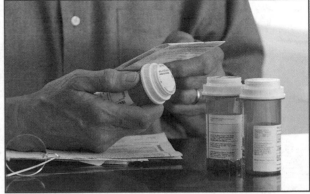

Burlingham/Shutterstock.com

Figure 5.8   Pay close attention to the "fine print" on medication labels, which could alert you to the possible dangers of taking a medication.

One example of a limitation on an implied warranty is the date stamps on medicines indicating the medicine being offered is effective within the sell date for that product. Another warranty is the assertion that a product could be "fit for a particular purpose" intended by the customer when that intent is known to the seller. Limitations can seem contrary to the advertised purpose of a product. In some states, limitations on implied warranties have been eliminated to avoid consumer

Ethical Dilemma

Imagine that you are a sales representative for a very large and profitable pharmaceutical company. You are assigned to a fast-selling medication (Drug A). Sales are excellent, and your commission has been high. However, you find yourself in an ethical dilemma as you read Drug A's marketing information, a journal article, and an internal confidential memo from the company.

The marketing information lists the medication side effects and risks such as dry mouth, headaches, and so on. In the journal article, researchers state that Drug A increases the risk of blindness, which is not listed in the marketing brochure. The internal memo states that employees should not discuss the journal article with anyone. The memo goes on to say that the study was not reputable and that numerous clinical trials have been conducted internally to determine that the drug is safe.

As the sales representative, how do you respond? Should you continue selling the medication? Should you adhere to the request made in the internal memo?

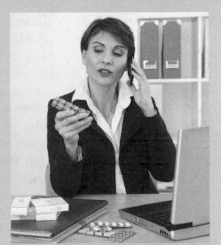

Image Point Fr/Shutterstock.com

confusion. For further reading on this topic, you may refer to the Restatement of Torts (Third), which is an academic summary of the law.

The final area of civil liability for products is the concept of strict liability. Some activities are so inherently dangerous that the law requires those who engage in them to be strictly liable, regardless of how careful they are in their activity. In the medical field, federal Medicaid and Medicare reimbursement rules impose strict liability and deny payment for certain "never events." If providers allow these events to occur when they should never happen, they must take full financial responsibility. For example, if a patient receives too much radiation from seed implants inserted to kill cancer cells, strict liability for the defective product may result.

Defenses to Civil Liability

Proving there is a proper defense to the plaintiff's allegations is important to defending any civil dispute. In negligence cases, this primarily involves proving that you met the level of care for the alleged improper service, that the plaintiff's damages were not caused by you, or that the plaintiff suffered no harm. In tort cases, defenses include that the patient consented or assumed the risk for the damages, that there was an emergency necessitating unusual physical contact or restraint, or possibly unavoidable fear in the mind of the plaintiff. In contract law cases, the plaintiff must have performed or been ready to perform his or her contract obligations before complaining about your failure to perform adequately or in a timely manner.

statute of limitations
a written law that limits the period of time during which a person can assert his or her right to bring a claim, or forever lose the right to bring a claim

The fact that someone has been negligent, commits an intentional wrong, or breaches a contract does not necessarily mean that person will have to pay damages. There is a legally set time limit—called a **statute of limitations**—during which the damaged party can sue. This is the case in all civil matters. When the time limit runs out, a claim can no longer be made. This is based on the concept that if you make a mistake and cause damages, you should not have to worry about that mistake or be confronted with it many years later, when witnesses may not be available or evidence has been destroyed so that you are not able to defend your actions.

While the time period for the statute of limitations varies by state, there is usually a set period during which a person must bring a claim for personal injury resulting from a practitioner's negligence. The statute of limitations also applies, with defined time frames, for written contracts. In some instances, statute limitations do not begin until a person is actually aware of the breach and his or her damages. For example, if a patient finds a sponge embedded in her body five years after surgery, and the sponge is causing substantial problems, she would still be able to sue the medical provider at that point and for a period covered by the statute of limitations.

Ethical Issues Related to Civil Liability

Negligence, breaches of contract, and the committing of intentional torts can raise ethical issues as well as liability issues involving financial damages. Each of these acts represents some form of violation of a personal right. At the minimum, you would have not honored the person's right to autonomy, whether it is related to self-determination or the right to refuse treatment. Ethical issues can arise even if there is not much financial loss or physical injury. For example, all acts of battery on a patient occur without patient consent and therefore are a violation of the patient's autonomy.

Enforcement of professional ethics differs from civil law in that it may subject a person to discipline that may include everything from a private reprimand to loss of a professional license. For example, a professional ethics standard may require cooperation with any investigation into an alleged ethical violation. Failure to do so does not lead to imprisonment, as in the case of violating criminal law. Nor does it usually lead to loss of money unless restitution is involved, but it may contribute to additional discipline being imposed as a result of the investigation into whether ethical standards were violated. This might include a special condition on the right to continue practicing by requiring additional training in professional ethics (Figure 5.9). The violation of a criminal law or incurring civil liability for an injury does not automatically result in a disciplinary response from a licensing agency but certainly may serve as evidence in a disciplinary case raised by the same or related conduct.

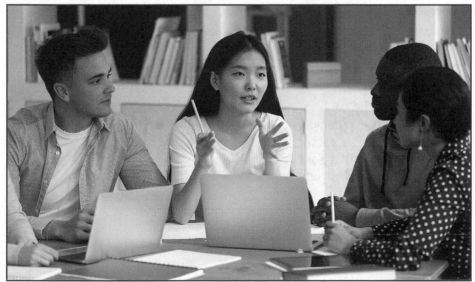

fizkes/Shutterstock.com

Figure 5.9 Ethics training in the workplace may help employees understand certain ethical issues.

Chapter Summary

- Civil law is noncriminal law that includes unintentional and intentional torts, disputes related to breach of contract, debt collection, family law issues, and monetary compensation for property damage or personal injuries.
- Ethical issues related to civil liability for healthcare workers may arise from negligence, breaches of contract, and intentional torts, as well as liability related to financial damages.

Vocabulary Matching

1. written or verbal agreement to a healthcare procedure given after a person understands the benefits and risks
2. person against whom an action or claim is brought in a court of law
3. intrusion into the personal life of another person without just cause
4. intentional attempt to injure or harm another person, possibly without physical contact
5. intentionally false representation of a material fact that is calculated to deceive, and does deceive, another person to legal detriment or loss
6. act of wrongdoing that results in injury to another person or damage to another person's property
7. relationship between an action or condition and its effect or result
8. legal obligation to pay damages or perform another court-enforced act as a result of noncriminal acts or breach of contract
9. failure to act as a reasonable person of ordinary prudence in a certain situation
10. failure to fulfill the standard of care when one person or company has an obligation toward another person or company
11. noncriminal law; law that typically addresses nonviolent circumstances and events that are perceived as wrongs suffered
12. improper, unskilled, or negligent treatment of a patient by a healthcare professional
13. defamation that occurs in a verbal manner
14. set of laws and regulations that govern all commercial transactions in the United States
15. the degree of caution or actions expected of a person, such as a healthcare practitioner, in the course of professional duties

A. assault
B. breach of duty
C. causation
D. civil law
E. civil liability
F. defendant
G. fraud
H. informed consent
I. invasion of privacy
J. medical malpractice
K. negligence
L. slander
M. standard of care
N. tort
O. Uniform Commercial Code

Chapter 5 Review and Assessment

Multiple Choice

16. All of the following statements about civil liability are true *except* _____.
    A. it usually involves money
    B. it may require the wrongdoer to serve prison time
    C. it can result if the person intended or did not intend to do anything wrong
    D. it developed from English common law

17. The legally set time in which a person can sue is called a(n) _____.
    A. legal standard
    B. statute of time
    C. statute of limitations
    D. restraint

18. Defamation that occurs in writing is called _____.
    A. tort
    B. *respondeat superior*
    C. slander
    D. libel

Completion

19. Duty, nonconformity, causation, and _____ are the four essential elements of a negligence case.

20. _____ is the harmful or offensive touching of another without permission or excuse.

21. _____ means shaming someone through an act of communication that will affect his or her reputation.

Discussion and Critical Thinking

22. What is the best way to avoid being found negligent while performing your work?

23. Does the availability of insurance coverage to protect you against malpractice claims increase or decrease your interest in healthcare? Why?

24. Why does the lack of informed consent when treating a patient lead to you being liable for damages? Consider the ethical concept of autonomy in your answer.

Activities

25. Why is violating professional rules of conduct not punishable by incarceration?

26. How can violating a criminal law affect your compliance with professional ethical rules?

27. May a person be found civilly liable and criminally liable for the same conduct? Explain.

28. Read the front page of any newspaper or news website. Find and record a basis for civil liability in one of the articles.

29. Search the Internet to find out if your state limits or caps the amount that may be recovered in a medical malpractice case. Do you think this amount, if any, is too low? Too high? Why?

30. Watch the YouTube video, "Defensive Medicine." Is the fear of malpractice lawsuits killing healthcare in the United States? Write a two-page opinion paper on this issue and support your position through examples.

Case Study

Imagine that you are a private, independent visiting nurse. You have agreed to stop by Mrs. Jones's house each day at 4:00 p.m. to make sure she has taken her medicine, for the fee of $150 per week. On Thursday, you notice that she has not taken her pills from the previous day. You recall that you spent time chatting with her and actually forgot to check that she had taken her dosage that day. You are concerned that she is behind, so you decide to tell her to take two pills today to make up for the missed pills from yesterday. The next day she becomes ill and needs to be hospitalized.

A. Have you been negligent?
B. Have you violated any ethical standards?
C. Are you in breach of contract?
D. Are you liable for Mrs. Jones' hospital bill?

Chapter 6

Criminal Liability of Healthcare Practitioners

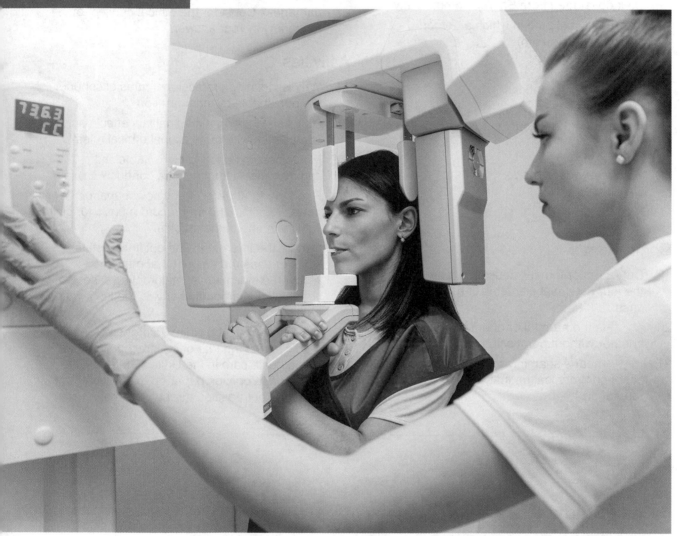

Roman Zaiets/Shutterstock.com

Chapter Outline

Criminal Law: Offenses against the Public

    Criminal Acts

    Criminal Defense

Levels of Intent

Government Healthcare Program Fraud

Failure to Report Crimes or Abuse

Professional Ethics and Criminal Law

Objectives

- Describe the difference between civil liability and criminal punishment.
- Explain the different levels of criminal intent.
- Understand the scope of healthcare program fraud.
- Describe the consequences of failure to report crime and abuse.
- Describe the relationship between professional ethics and criminal law.

Key Terms

conspiracy

crime

criminal law

criminal negligence

due process

felony

general intent

mandatory reporter

misdemeanor

privileged communication

prosecutor

specific intent

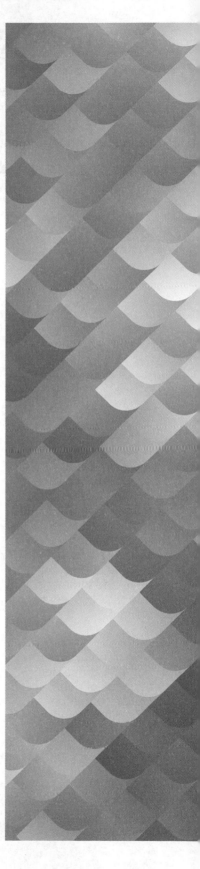

What Would You Do?

Suppose you are a medical assistant working in a small skilled nursing facility. A colleague, who is a mental health counselor, brags to you that he has been treating groups of four patients for one hour, and then submitting Medicare bills for an hour visit with each of the four patients. Is the counselor's action legal and ethical?

Unlike civil law, which involves disputes between private individuals, criminal law involves offenses against the public as a whole. These offenses include specific acts that the government has defined as crimes. Consequently, the government will take action against a defendant who is accused of a crime. City, county/state, or federal governments will be involved, depending on the specific crime.

Criminal Law: Offenses against the Public

criminal law
a system of law consisting of a body of rules and statutes that define conduct prohibited by the government because such conduct is an offense against the state and threatens and harms public safety and welfare

crime
an act, or failure to act, that is deemed injurious of public welfare or morals and for which someone can be punished by the government

Criminal law is a body of rules established by governments to protect individuals and society by regulating the behavior of individuals and groups. The objectives of criminal law include maintaining public safety and order and protecting individuals. A **crime** is an offense against the public, which can be an act forbidden by law or a failure to act as required by law. People who break criminal laws will be held responsible through punishment such as fines and sometimes jail or prison time (Figure 6.1). This system uses punishment as a way to deter criminal behavior.

As described in Chapter 5, healthcare has its own special area of civil law (medical malpractice), but that is not the case in criminal law. Although the vast majority of healthcare workers are honest and capable, opportunities for criminal wrongdoing are abundant because of access to vulnerable patients, personal property, medical supplies, drugs, and funding available through complex medical billing procedures.

When a healthcare worker violates a criminal law, the opponent in court will not be a patient represented by a private lawyer, as would be the case in civil court. Instead, the healthcare worker will be confronted by government lawyers (prosecutors) who represent the public and have extensive government resources at their disposal to prove wrongdoing.

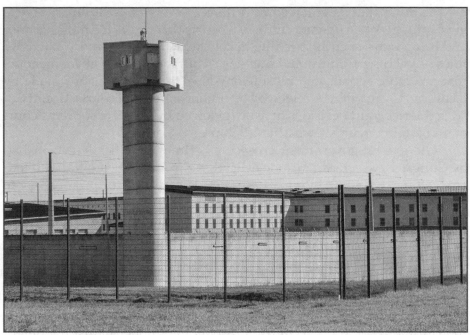

pixinoo/Shutterstock.com

Figure 6.1 One possible consequence of breaking a criminal law is time in jail or prison.

Criminal Acts

A criminal offense is generally classified as either a **misdemeanor** or a **felony**. A misdemeanor can result in fines and imprisonment for up to one year. A felony can result in substantial fines, more than one year in prison, and even death. In many cases, conviction of a felony is also automatic grounds to revoke a professional certification.

Crimes can originate in many forms. Physical abuse, financial exploitation, theft, fraud, gross negligence, and murder are all examples of crimes that occur in healthcare as well as other fields. This chapter addresses some areas of criminal law that are important to understand while conducting healthcare business or delivering healthcare services.

Many acts can be subject to both criminal and civil sanctions and have the same name. For example, criminal assault, battery, and fraud are similar to civil actions discussed in Chapter 5. However, criminal acts are prosecuted in criminal courts, and civil litigation occurs separately in civil courts.

In addition, the level of proof required to find guilt or fix responsibility is higher in criminal courts than in civil claims. Criminal courts can impose fines payable to the government and incarcerate the defendant if the defendant is found guilty. In civil cases, the court may order that money be paid by a defendant to a plaintiff, but it does not impose incarceration.

misdemeanor
a minor crime; maximum punishment includes fines and up to one year in jail.

felony
a serious crime that typically involves violence and is usually punishable by at least one year in state prison or death

Criminal law is enforced at different levels of government. Local governments often operate municipal courts that prosecute minor crimes and infractions, such as speeding tickets, which do not require extensive fines or jail time. County- and state-level courts prosecute misdemeanors that are more serious and most felony-level crimes. Decisions made by local courts can often be reviewed by higher state-level courts. County or state district court decisions may be reviewed by the state supreme court or, in certain circumstances, the US Supreme Court.

The federal government prosecutes crimes specifically established by Congress, which can include everything from Medicare fraud to federal felony drug smuggling. These crimes can lead to fines, orders to re-pay money (called *restitution*), and incarceration in federal prisons. Federal courts are organized by districts that do not align directly with state boundaries. Federal court rulings can be appealed, in certain circumstances, to the US Supreme Court.

Criminal Defense

prosecutor
a representative of the government who brings charges and leads government efforts to prove the guilt of a defendant in court

due process
the legal requirement that the government provide fair treatment through the normal judicial system

In criminal cases, a **prosecutor** represents the public against the defendant, who is the person or entity accused of a crime (Figure 6.2). As with all defendants, a healthcare provider accused of a crime has certain rights under the US Constitution and the constitution of the state in which the prosecution occurs. These include the rights to both procedural and substantive **due process** granted by state law and the Amendments to the Constitution.

Due process is the legal requirement that the government must provide fair treatment through the normal judicial system. *Procedural due process* means the defendant is treated fairly and has the right to be notified of the charges, have a speedy trial, and present a defense against those charges. *Substantive due process* affords a person the rights established by the Bill of Rights, including fundamental attributes of liberty.

As noted previously, a significant difference between civil and criminal law is the level of proof required. In most civil matters, proof must be convincing enough for the jury to believe merely that the facts "more likely than not" justify liability. In criminal matters, however, proof must convince all jurors "beyond a reasonable doubt." This standard means that jurors have no rational basis for doubting guilt or that any doubt that exists is unreasonable. Proof must be presented in a criminal trial without relying on the defendant, who has a right to not prove anything or present any information that would make him look guilty (incriminate himself).

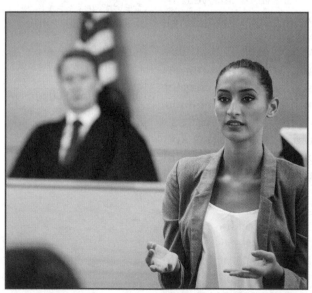

wavebreakmedia/Shutterstock.com

Figure 6.2   A prosecutor is a lawyer who represents the public against a defendant.

The defendant also has the right to prevent certain individuals from testifying, depending on their relationship with the defendant. For example, the law encourages open communication in husband-wife, physician-patient, attorney-client, and clergy-penitent relationships. In many cases, the defendant's statements made in confidence to the other party in one of these relationships can be kept private.

These statements, called **privileged communications**, cannot be used without the defendant's permission. The law allows this to encourage wrongdoers to open up and perhaps receive advice to obey the law from trusted sources. It also derives from constitutional rights to privacy and ethical considerations of patient autonomy. In the landmark case of *Roe v. Wade*, 410 US 113 (1973), which defined guidelines for legal and illegal abortions, the US Supreme Court acknowledged that the physician-patient relationship is one which evokes constitutional rights of privacy.

While healthcare providers have legal and ethical duties to protect patient privacy, the right to invoke (initiate) the privilege for a doctor or other medical professional *not* to testify against a patient/defendant does not belong to the provider. That privilege belongs to the patient/defendant, who must invoke it to prevent disclosure of information by current or former providers.

The traditional physician-patient relationship has been extended in many states to include other licensed healthcare providers, such as psychotherapists, nurse practitioners, and physician assistants. Often, medical personnel supporting the physician, such as a nurse or medical assistant, may be included as extensions of the doctor's privilege if they are required to be present so the doctor can work with the patient.

Although a defendant's right to privileged communication is an important one, it is not absolute and so may be limited in certain

privileged communication
information exchanged between people who are in certain recognized relationships, such as a physician-patient relationship, that cannot be disclosed without the consent of the protected party

Career Corner

Forensic science technicians examine potential physical evidence to support prosecution of a crime. Both physical and chemical analysis may be involved in this process. Fingerprints, bodily fluids, bullets, and hair are a few of the items that may be studied. The technician may take photographs of the crime scene. Results of any tests the technician performs are documented in written reports. Regular activities for forensic technicians also include preserving evidence, testifying in court, and discussing evidence collection and their findings with attorneys and law enforcement personnel.

A degree in science from a four-year college or university is required for these positions in the field. Examples of possible required courses include physics, biology, microbiology,

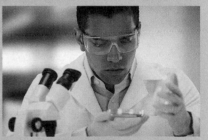
Rocketclips, Inc./Shutterstock.com

chemistry, medical technology, and genetics. On-the-job training is generally required.

circumstances. For example, if the defendant tells the healthcare provider that he intends to take actions that would cause self-injury or injury to others, the healthcare provider has a duty to report that information. Other exceptions also may apply and vary from state to state.

Levels of Intent

criminal negligence
the failure to use reasonable care to avoid consequences that threaten or harm the safety of the public and that have a foreseeable outcome

general intent
a mental plan to do something that is against the law whether the specific results that eventually occur were meant to happen or not

specific intent
a conscious intention and premeditation to do something that is prohibited by law and will cause a specific harm or result

A healthcare provider does not always have to be purposefully trying to break a law to violate a law. That's because general intent and strict liability (described in Chapter 5 in relation to civil liability) are also found in criminal law. As previously explained, strict liability means a person will be held responsible for the outcome of an act regardless of personal intent. Strict liability is rare in criminal law, but it does exist for crimes such as statutory rape, in which even a reasonable belief that the minor is an adult is not a defense. Strict liability can also arise with laws related to accuracy of medical billing.

Crimes can be classified into three levels of offenses: (1) **criminal negligence**, (2) **general intent**, and (3) **specific intent**. The first level, criminal negligence, is a heightened level of negligence beyond that of a simple breach of duty. It is an act that is characterized as careless, inattentive, willfully blind, or reckless. Criminal negligence is a statutory offense that mainly occurs in situations involving the death of an innocent party, such as a motor vehicle accident, but it has been applied to healthcare workers in certain situations. For example, if a healthcare worker gives a patient an unauthorized prescription drug, causing a lethal outcome, the worker could be found criminally negligent (Figure 6.3).

The second level of crimes includes those that involve general intent. This means the acts were intended, but the results were not. For example, assault is usually a general intent crime. A nurse administering a vaccination does not usually intend to create fear in a patient, although the act might do just that. Likewise, a surgeon may intend to operate on a patient, but choose the wrong leg, causing an unintended result. That surgeon could be prosecuted for battery.

The third level is specific intent crimes, in which both the act and the result are intended. For example, if a hospital orderly takes a patient's wallet and intends to keep it, the act could be considered theft or larceny. State and federal legislation defines which crimes require specific intent. These include most serious crimes, such as burglary and murder. It is usually up to a jury to determine if the standard for the required level of intent has been met to find the defendant guilty of the charges in a particular case.

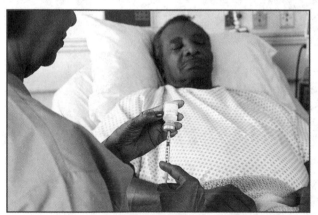

Monkey Business Images/Shutterstock.com

Figure 6.3   Healthcare workers must be careful when administering medication, as an error could harm a patient and cause a worker legal trouble.

Government Healthcare Program Fraud

In the United States, government healthcare benefits are available to a number of special groups. These include people over 65 years of age, disabled persons, veterans, the poor, Native Americans, members of the military, and members of Congress. While not universally available, large-scale programs such as Medicare (for older adults and the disabled) and Medicaid (for the poor) have become important sources of revenue for healthcare professionals. Several of these specific laws are explained in more detail in Chapter 7.

The complexity of these programs and the availability of predictable revenue from them have led to widespread and well-publicized criminal activity by providers who try to exploit the system for personal gain. In 2018, the federal budget for Medicare alone totaled over $593 billion, providing a tempting target for criminal activity. In response to these crimes, the government has established extensive rules and procedures to help reduce fraud and abuse. The Centers for Medicare and Medicaid Services (CMS) budgeted over $2.1 billion for attempts to reduce fraud during 2018.

While it may seem that fraud relates to money or other property, it also can apply when fraudulent conduct induces patient consent or reliance for unnecessary care. Criminal fraud is a violation of law and ethical standards because it involves both violation of patient autonomy and malfeasance.

Because fraud has become so widespread, issues such as "errors" in billing are being addressed by requiring a strict liability standard. This means that "intent" is assumed in certain circumstances. For example, when submitting claims to Medicare, Medicaid, or other government healthcare programs, a designated person must sign and certify that the billing is accurate (Figure 6.4).

If you are the healthcare professional who is responsible for certifying invoices at your workplace, the government is relying on you to be sure that the billing is correct. If the billing is incorrect, you will be held personally responsible. The burden is on you to know the healthcare program's rules, or you may be presumed to have acted improperly on purpose.

Clearly, this is a heavy burden and can catch someone unaware. The government must prove guilt, of course, but presumption of intent can make a defense difficult. Failure to accurately certify billing claims can lead to loss of income, loss of reputation, possible loss of credentials, and incarceration in federal prison. This is why most healthcare employers designate certain

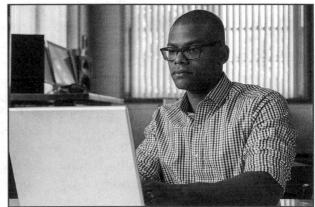

Burlingham/Shutterstock.com

Figure 6.4 Someone, such as a hospital administrator or business manager, may be assigned to certify billings.

staff members—such as the chief financial officer, business manager, or facility administrator—to certify billings.

Clearly defined roles for administrative specialists allow them to take particular care of critical administrative tasks and help clinicians focus on patient care. A healthcare professional's ethical duty is to be ready and able to provide proper care. This can mean knowing the rules of government healthcare programs and following them carefully.

In fiscal year 2018, the federal government brought 572 criminal prosecutions for healthcare fraud against 872 defendants. In addition, the Health and Human Services Inspector General brought 679 criminal actions for Medicare and Medicaid crimes and recovered 20.2 million dollars.

The problem is so bad that, in addition to criminal penalties, the federal government has established an exclusion list that prohibits future participation in Medicare and Medicaid for individuals who have actually committed financial fraud or lied while engaged with the programs. Not only are these individuals personally excluded, but the federal government prohibits employers from engaging the services of these individuals.

conspiracy
an agreement made by two or more people to perform an illegal or harmful act

The crime of **conspiracy** is sometimes associated with fraud. Conspiracy occurs when two or more people agree to commit an unlawful act. If you are involved in conversations with anyone who is considering committing fraud, or any other crime, you can be charged with conspiracy even if you change your mind and withdraw before fraudulent behavior occurs.

In 2018, the owner of 20 home health agencies in Florida, Rafael Arias, was convicted of Medicare fraud conspiracy. The defendant had recruited others to falsely claim they operated separate facilities that were in fact owned and operated by Arias. He was sentenced to 20 years and required to pay more than $66 million in restitution.

Failure to Report Crimes or Abuse

In contrast to civil law, employers are not necessarily responsible for the crimes of their employees. Generally, criminal acts are considered unforeseeable, and the responsibility lies with the individual who commits the crime. However, individuals can be prosecuted for aiding or abetting a criminal act, even though their actual conduct was otherwise not criminal.

For example, providing a coworker with a ride to the bus station may be innocent enough, unless you know your coworker is fleeing after stealing drugs from the hospital where he or she is employed. While the law does not require you to report a crime, you may have some difficulty explaining the difference between "not reporting" and "aiding" the alleged criminal, depending on the situation.

mandatory reporter
a person who has a legal requirement to report an event or issue to someone else; might include reporting child or elder abuse

Furthermore, as a healthcare professional, you may have a special legal obligation to report certain crimes. For example, many state laws require healthcare workers, teachers, and others—so-called **mandatory reporters**—to report suspected child and elder abuse and neglect (Figure 6.5). Most states penalize mandatory reporters who knowingly fail to report when there is suspicion of abuse or neglect. Failure to report child abuse is a misdemeanor in most states. On the other hand, 19 states and the Virgin Islands provide for prosecution if someone falsely reports abuse. Many states have similar laws related to reporting elder abuse.

The duty to report also may override physician-patient privilege in certain criminal situations. For example, imagine that a doctor provides medical care to a gunshot victim who has fled the scene of a crime. The doctor may be accused of aiding or abetting a felony, or being involved in a criminal conspiracy, if this treatment is not reported to authorities as required and the suspected felon escapes. A famous example is Dr. Samuel Mudd, who treated John Wilkes Booth after the assassination of President Lincoln. Mudd waited until he was being questioned by authorities to report his contact with Booth and the treatment he

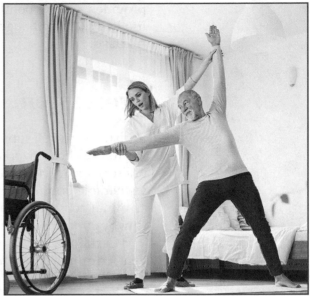

Halfpoint/Shutterstock.com

Figure 6.5 Healthcare workers have a responsibility to keep vulnerable populations such as the elderly safe. This includes reporting suspected abuse.

Ethical Dilemma

Suppose that a healthcare provider has been assigned to care for an elderly male patient who has just been admitted to the rehabilitation center. As the healthcare provider helps the patient get comfortable in his room, she notices that the patient has significant bruising. The patient's adult son, who is his caregiver, brought the patient in and is sitting in the waiting room.

When asked about the bruising, the patient first insists that the healthcare provider promise to keep everything confidential. He seems reluctant to reveal any information, but the healthcare provider continues to ask. The patient eventually reveals that his son is rough with him when he needs assistance and sometimes hurts him by accident. The patient lives in his son's home and relies on him for financial support.

What should the healthcare provider do? What is the healthcare provider's duty in this situation, given the threat to the patient? How might you determine if this healthcare provider is a mandatory reporter?

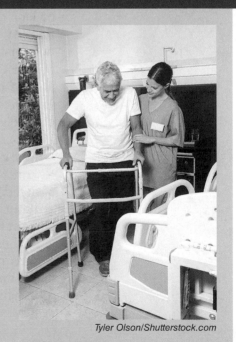

Tyler Olson/Shutterstock.com

provided during Booth's escape. Mudd was convicted and sentenced to life in prison, although he later received a presidential pardon and was released.

Professional Ethics and Criminal Law

So, isn't everyone subject to criminal laws? Why is criminal law important to healthcare workers? One consideration is that healthcare workers often work in close proximity to vulnerable patients. Working with a vulnerable population provides greater opportunities or temptations for criminal activity, but also subjects healthcare providers to greater scrutiny by supervisors, patients' families, and colleagues.

Certain routine business practices may be designed, in part, to prevent criminal acts. These include requiring patient consent, property recordkeeping, drug inventories, and other aspects of a healthcare worker's daily routine. In addition, the healthcare field itself is increasingly involved in new types of activities that require new determinations of the boundaries of law and ethical conduct.

For example, the killing of another human being is called *homicide*, which is not always a crime. Homicide may be excused, for instance, in a non-negligent accident or as a result of justified self-defense. Not being guilty of a crime, however, does not necessarily mean being free of criticism. Many patients have a deteriorating condition from which they could die. Medical providers are not necessarily at fault for the death, but they are held to professional rules and laws to provide care expected of competent providers under the same circumstances. Misdiagnosis or lack of proper care may be negligent (malpractice) and result in civil liability or professional discipline. However, unless there was recklessness or criminal intent involved, a death itself does not result in criminal liability.

Of course, in your normal workday as a healthcare provider, you will probably not struggle with legal or ethical issues related to homicide (Figure 6.6). As you may recall from Chapter 2's discussion of the Hippocratic Oath, the earliest version forbids a physician from taking a life in any way. However, certain healthcare providers may now need to confront the ethical issues and changing legal standards related to assisted death (euthanasia), mercy killings, assisted suicides, and living wills in which the patient requests that no unnatural means be used to sustain life.

These types of issues have brought healthcare and decisions regarding death together more frequently. Just as ethical standards have developed over the years, so has the law. However, while advances in science and ethics may affect their view of whether certain medical practices should no longer be considered crimes, healthcare providers must wait for the laws to actually change to avoid being subject to prosecution. Similarly, you might consider whether your own ideas of morality still align with changing standards of professional ethics.

If you are found guilty of a criminal act, there is some likelihood you also will be subject to ethical review by an oversight authority. If you have an independent credential, you may be charged directly with ethical violations. If you are employed by a person or organization that holds its own license, it may act as an employer to protect its own license or even its contract with other licensed persons or organizations. In fact, losing your license or job may have more impact on your life than paying a fine, serving short-term incarceration, or being on criminal justice system probation for a period of time.

There are several ethical decision-making models that can be useful when you are faced with difficult professional decisions. Figure 6.7 provides a partial list of codes of ethics from various healthcare fields that can assist in ethical decision-making. All of these sources are available on the Internet.

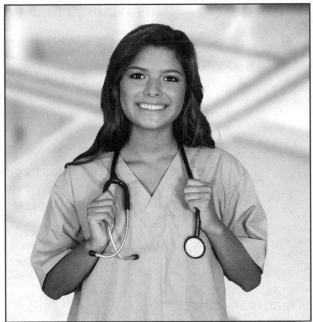

Rob Marmion/Shutterstock.com

Figure 6.6 Although a healthcare worker won't encounter life-and-death situations every single day, related questions of ethics are becoming more common.

Examples of Codes of Ethics for Healthcare Practitioners

- American Association of Medical Assistants Code of Ethics
- American Chiropractic Association Code of Ethics
- American Medical Association Code of Medical Ethics
- American Nurses Association Code of Ethics for Nurses
- American Physical Therapy Association Code of Ethics for the Physical Therapist
- American Registry of Radiologic Technologists Standards of Ethics
- American Society for Clinical Laboratory Science Code of Ethics
- Certified Nursing Assistant Code of Ethics
- National Association for Health Professionals Code of Ethics & Standards of Practice

Goodheart-Willcox Publisher

Figure 6.7 Most healthcare professions have developed their own codes of ethics, specific to their profession.

Chapter Summary

- Civil law involves disputes between private individuals, whereas criminal law involves offenses against the public as a whole.

- Criminal intent is classified into three levels: criminal negligence, general intent, and specific intent.

- Because of the immense governmental budget for healthcare programs and the predictable revenue that results, government healthcare program fraud is widespread.

- Individuals can be prosecuted for aiding or abetting a criminal act, even if their actual conduct was not criminal, if they do not report a crime or instance of abuse.

- Adhering to professional ethics is important to all healthcare practitioners because they work with a vulnerable population, providing both greater opportunities for criminal activity and greater scrutiny by society.

Vocabulary Matching

1. person who has a legal requirement to report an event or issue to someone else; might include reporting child or elder abuse
2. an act, or failure to act, that is deemed injurious of public welfare or morals and for which someone can be punished by the government
3. information exchanged between people who are in certain recognized relationships, such as a physician-patient relationship, that cannot be disclosed without the consent of the protected party
4. legal requirement that the government provide fair treatment through the normal judicial system
5. serious crime that typically involves violence and is usually punishable by at least 1 year in state prison or death
6. minor crime; maximum punishment includes fines and up to 1 year in jail
7. agreement made by two or more people to perform an illegal or harmful act
8. conscious intention and premeditation to do something that is prohibited by law and which will cause a specific harm or result
9. failure to use reasonable care to avoid consequences that threaten or harm the safety of the public and that have a foreseeable outcome
10. mental plan to do something that is against the law, whether or not the specific results that eventually occur were meant to happen
11. system of law consisting of a body of rules and statutes that define conduct prohibited by the government because such conduct is an offense against the state and threatens and harms public safety and welfare
12. representative of the government who brings charges and leads government efforts to prove the guilt of a defendant in court

A. conspiracy
B. crime
C. criminal law
D. criminal negligence
E. due process
F. felony
G. general intent
H. mandatory reporter
I. misdemeanor
J. privileged communication
K. prosecutor
L. specific intent

Multiple Choice

13. Three employees working in a medical office billed health plans for services that were not provided, and then shared the money between them. This is considered _____.
    A. due process
    B. consensual fraud
    C. conspiracy
    D. civil fraud

14. Mandatory reporters are required to report _____.
    A. illegal drug use
    B. billing fraud
    C. employee theft
    D. child abuse

15. Crimes can be classified into three levels of offenses, which include all of the following *except* _____.
    A. general intent
    B. unexplained intent
    C. specific intent
    D. criminal negligence

Completion

16. A criminal offense is generally classified as either a(n) _____ or a felony.

17. The _____ enforces criminal laws.

18. The right to a speedy trial is referred to as _____.

19. Conviction for the most serious crimes requires proof of _____ intent.

Discussion and Critical Thinking

20. When a person is medically determined to be in a permanent vegetative state, is it unethical or a crime to intentionally let the person die by withholding life-sustaining care? Why or why not?

21. If a healthcare employee releases a patient's personal health records to the press without authorization, is the employer subject to criminal culpability?

22. What are three reasons for the existence of Medicare fraud?

23. If you are called to testify about what you told one of your patients, may you disclose the information, even if it might be privileged?

24. Why is it more difficult to obtain a criminal conviction than a monetary judgment?

Activities

25. Search the Internet for the "60 Minutes" report on Medicare fraud. Watch the report, and then write a one-page reaction paper that includes suggestions for reducing Medicare fraud.

26. Write a five-paragraph essay about why you think death with dignity laws do not exist in many states.

27. Use the Internet to find and read section RCW 70.245.190 of the State of Washington's Death with Dignity Law as it applies to healthcare workers. Explain your reaction to the law in one paragraph.

Case Study

Imagine you are a visiting nurse providing daily care to a woman who is recovering from a car accident. You notice that the patient has a new injury to her hand. When you ask the patient about this, she asks you to keep the conversation confidential. Then she confides that she injured her hand yesterday after slapping her 8-year-old daughter in the face.

The patient is concerned about being charged with abusing her daughter, so she asks if you can get her prescription pain medicine for her hand without letting her doctor know. Do you think that, if you got the prescription, you could continue to develop communication with the woman and help her stop being violent? What crimes and ethical issues might this involve? Should you share your concerns about this patient's request with your supervisor?

Chapter 7

Federal Statutes and Regulations That Impact Healthcare

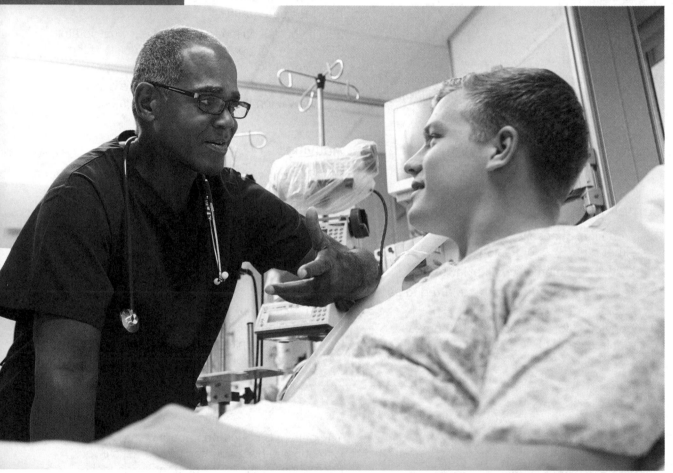

Monkey Business Images/Shutterstock.com

Chapter Outline

The Patient Protection and Affordable Care Act

Medicaid and Medicare

Medicaid

Medicare

Fraud and Abuse

The Health Insurance Portability and Accountability Act

The Americans with Disabilities Act

The Rehabilitation Act

The Emergency Medical Treatment and Active Labor Act

The Health Information Technology for Economic and Clinical Health Act

21st Century Cures Act

Objectives

- Describe the Patient Protection and Affordable Care Act and explain the controversy over the act.
- Explain Medicare, Medicaid, and related laws.
- Describe the Americans with Disabilities Act (ADA) and explain who is covered by the act.
- Explain the purpose of the Rehabilitation Act and the Emergency Medical Treatment and Active Labor Act.
- Explain how HIPAA and HITECH work to ensure privacy protection.
- Summarize the provisions of the 21st Century Cures Act.

Key Terms

21st Century Cures Act

Americans with Disabilities Act (ADA)

Anti-Kickback Statute

Emergency Medical Treatment and Active Labor Act (EMTALA)

False Claims Act

Health Insurance Portability and Accountability Act (HIPAA)

Patient Protection and Affordable Care Act (ACA)

Public Health Service Act

Rehabilitation Act

Stark Anti-Referral Law

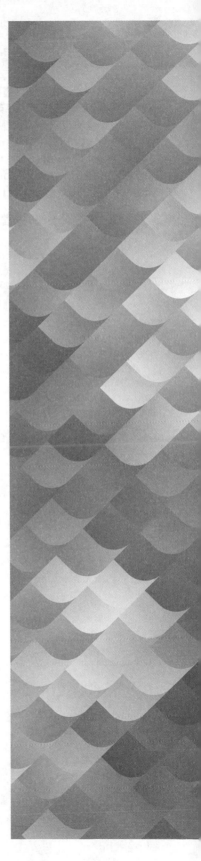

What Would You Do?

Suppose you recently completed a medical assisting program and started your first job in a wonderful community clinic. You live in a small rural town, and the physician you work for is the one who delivered you. Now you are expecting your first child and want her to deliver your baby. But you have noticed that she is billing patients for services she has not provided. She has also billed for patients she has not seen at all. The first few times you saw this, you thought it was an error, but now you see it often. You are concerned that this physician is behaving illegally and unethically. What should you do?

Public Health Service Act
law that structured the United States Public Health Service as the primary division of the US Department of Health, Education, and Welfare, which later became the United States Department of Health and Human Services

State statutes comprise a large portion of laws applicable to healthcare, yet laws and regulations at the federal level also have a major impact on healthcare. The **Public Health Service Act** of 1944 contains a significant portion of federal healthcare law. The act primarily focuses on the Department of Health and Human Services (HHS). The HHS administers hundreds of programs and contains 11 operating divisions with various objectives, such as providing financial assistance to low-income individuals, conducting medical research, providing healthcare and advocacy services, and enforcing laws and regulations related to human services.

These divisions include the Administration for Children and Families, the Food and Drug Administration, and others. There are also several agencies within HHS that are focused specifically on healthcare, including the National Institutes of Health (NIH), which is involved with medical research, and the Centers for Disease Control and Prevention (CDC), which helps to protect the nation's health.

In addition to the Public Health Service Act, many other federal laws affect the delivery of healthcare. The Patient Protection and Affordable Care Act (ACA), passed in 2010, was designed to provide comprehensive health insurance reforms. A number of other laws have established direct medical care programs for special populations, including the military, veterans, and even Congress itself. This chapter describes a few of the many programs that affect a great number of patients and that may affect you personally and professionally.

Patient Protection and Affordable Care Act (ACA)
law that was passed to help decrease the number of Americans who do not have health insurance and help reduce the overall cost of healthcare

The Patient Protection and Affordable Care Act

The **Patient Protection and Affordable Care Act (ACA)** was signed into law on March 23, 2010 by President Barack Obama. The law was challenged (and is still being challenged at the time of this publication) all the way to the Supreme Court by many states that claimed it was unconstitutional. One of the major reasons the law has been so controversial is its requirement that everyone purchase health insurance (Figure 7.1). This was a requirement for all individuals who did not have health insurance coverage. If people did not purchase health insurance, they were charged a health insurance tax. This requirement of the ACA has been eliminated.

On June 28, 2012, the US Supreme Court determined that this requirement was equivalent to a tax because the Internal Revenue Service (IRS) was designated as the agency to collect it. Therefore, the Supreme Court found

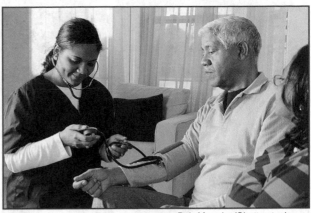

Rob Marmion/Shutterstock.com

Figure 7.1   The Affordable Care Act was passed to ensure that more Americans have health insurance and access to medical care.

this provision of the law constitutional. However, as part of this same ruling, the Supreme Court found that a provision requiring states to participate in an expanded Medicaid program exceeded federal authority. This provision, but not the entire law, was determined to be unconstitutional. The ACA continues to be implemented and challenged throughout the country.

The ACA expanded coverage for low-income Americans by creating an opportunity for states to extend Medicaid eligibility, effective January 1, 2014. The expansion applied to individuals who have incomes up to 138 percent of the federal poverty level. This change allows states to provide Medicaid coverage for low-income adults who do not have children without requiring a waiver. States have the option to receive additional federal funding for this expansion, but participation is not required. Some states have opted out of the expansion.

The following additional changes have occurred as a result of the ACA:

- **Extended Coverage for Young Adults.** Group health plans and health insurance companies offering group or individual health insurance coverage that provides dependent coverage of children must make coverage available for adult children up to 26 years of age.

- **Eliminating Pre-Existing Condition Exclusions.** Group health plans and health insurance companies may not create exclusions for pre-existing conditions in coverage for children and adults. This means that health plans and insurance companies cannot deny coverage to anyone based on an existing medical problem.

- **Prohibiting Cancellations (Rescissions).** The ACA prohibits insurance companies from cancelling insurance coverage when an individual gets sick. These are known as *abusive*

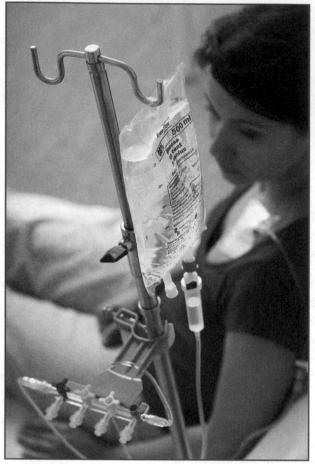

Image Point Fr/Shutterstock.com

Figure 7.2 The ban on lifetime or annual caps on healthcare was designed to help people who require extensive care, such as cancer patients who need expensive chemotherapy treatments.

rescissions. Insurance companies do this to avoid covering the cost of an individual's healthcare needs. Group health plans and health insurance companies offering group or individual insurance coverage are now prohibited from cancelling coverage once the enrollee is covered, except in cases of fraud or intentional misrepresentation. Enrollees must be notified before their coverage is cancelled.

- **Health Insurance Exchange.** Each state has developed a health insurance exchange or defaulted to the federal exchange. A health insurance exchange is a marketplace in which individuals and small businesses can purchase health insurance.

- **Medicaid Expansion.** States that elected to participate in the Medicaid expansion changed their eligibility requirements to receive Medicaid coverage. In states that have expanded Medicaid coverage, people can qualify based on income alone.

- **Banning Lifetime/Annual Caps.** Health insurance companies cannot establish financial limits on the payout amount for their members on a lifetime or an annual basis (Figure 7.2).

- **Business Health Insurance Tax.** Companies with 50 employees or more, and with at least one full-time employee, must provide health insurance or pay a tax to the government.

- **Preventive Services.** Certain preventive services are considered essential benefits; co-payments, co-insurance, or deductibles cannot be required.

Medicaid and Medicare

The Centers for Medicare and Medicaid Services (CMS) is a division of HHS that directs the Medicaid and Medicare programs. Medicaid provides healthcare benefits to the poor, and Medicare provides healthcare insurance to those who are eligible. People eligible for Medicare are 65 years of age or older who have paid taxes for a minimum required period, and those younger than 65 years of age who have a particular disability or end-stage renal disease.

Medicaid

Medicaid is a federal program funded by both federal and state funds, yet the program is administered only by the states. The states establish eligibility criteria to determine who can qualify for Medicaid benefits. As a result, not all people with low incomes qualify. Some states provide healthcare for low-income individuals who do not meet the federal Medicaid eligibility criteria. If available, these programs can be accessed through state health insurance exchanges and may be supported by tax subsidies. The criteria for Medicaid eligibility often include factors such as pregnancy, blindness, or disability and may depend upon the individual's age, income, assets, resources, or lawful immigration status.

Although state law determines eligibility and distribution of Medicaid services, federal law limits state discretion. For example, federal law forbids states from reducing state welfare benefits based on the receipt of federally funded Medicaid services. Undocumented immigrants and immigrants who are in the United States on a temporary basis (those who have temporary work visas or student visas, for example) are not eligible for Medicaid in most states, regardless of how long they have been in the United States. However, emergency treatment is available to all immigrants, regardless of their legal status. Legal and undocumented immigrants who meet all eligibility requirements can receive Emergency Medicaid. This service covers the costs of emergency medical treatment.

Medicare

Unlike Medicaid, which provides medical benefits, Medicare is an actual insurance program that provides coverage for hospital and medical services. Funding for the Medicare system comes from taxes and fees paid by eligible individuals. All workers pay taxes to support this program during their careers and, when eligible to participate, most people must pay a monthly premium for the medical services portion of Medicare. An optional prescription drug plan (Medicare Part D) covers prescription medication (Figure 7.3).

Fraud and Abuse

There are several federal laws related to healthcare business practices that are considered to be fraud and abuse. Fraud consists of intentional acts of deception. Abuse refers to improper acts that are not consistent with standard practice

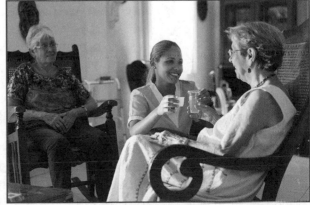

Diego Cervo/Shutterstock.com

Figure 7.3 Some Medicare plans pay for medication that older adults need.

and may result in over-utilization of overpayment. The following laws seek to reduce the amount of fraud and abuse that occurs in the healthcare field.

False Claims Act
law that prohibits any individual or business from submitting, or causing someone else to submit, a false or fraudulent claim for payment to the government; allows individuals to sue on behalf of the government on knowledge of past or present fraud against the federal government

The **False Claims Act** imposes liability on people and companies (typically federal contractors who sell goods to or perform services for the government) who defraud governmental programs. Because the federal government pays such large amounts of money to healthcare institutions, this act has been increasingly applied to the wider healthcare field. Examples of actions that fall under this act include filing false expense reports to a government agency, giving or receiving kickbacks, overstating charity cases, and knowingly selling defective products to the government.

Under the False Claims Act, healthcare providers who knowingly make fraudulent or false claims to the government are fined $5,500 to $11,000 per claim. They also must pay three times the amount of the damages caused to the federal program. To violate the False Claims Act, actual intent to defraud the government is not required.

The False Claims Act includes a provision that allows people who are not affiliated with the government to file a lawsuit on behalf of the government (also known as *whistleblowing*). In legal terms, whistleblowing is referred to as a *qui tam*. The whistleblower does not need to be personally harmed by the alleged false claim, but people filing under this provision stand to receive a portion of any recovered damages.

Once the *qui tam* is filed, the government has the option to join the action as a plaintiff. If the government joins, the whistleblower is entitled to 15 to 25 percent of any award or settlement. If the government decides not to join, the whistleblower can receive between 25 and 30 percent of the award or settlement. This payment acts as an incentive for individuals to assist the government with identifying fraud. Whistleblowers are protected from retaliation when they file their lawsuits.

Anti-Kickback Statute
a criminal statute that prohibits the exchange (or offer to exchange) of anything of value in an effort to receive the reward of federal healthcare program business

The **Anti-Kickback Statute** and **Stark Anti-Referral Law** are two laws that are particularly important to the creation of business partnerships between healthcare facilities. Violations of these laws may result in monetary penalties, Medicare claims not being paid, liability under the Federal Claims Act, and exclusion from the Medicare program.

Stark Anti-Referral Law
law that prohibits physician referrals of designated health services for Medicare and Medicaid patients if the physician or an immediate family member has a financial relationship with that entity

The Anti-Kickback Statute prohibits the offering, paying, soliciting, or receiving of anything of value in return for rewards or referrals, or to generate federal healthcare program business. For example, pharmaceutical companies are not permitted to offer products, services, or money to physicians in return for promoting their products or drugs (Figure 7.4). Other examples include offering discounted medical goods or services for providing referrals. The penalties for violating this law are both civil and criminal.

The Stark Anti-Referral Law governs physician self-referral for healthcare services. The law prohibits physicians from referring Medicare and Medicaid patients to any organization with which the doctor or his or her immediate family has a financial relationship, unless an exception applies. The belief is that a physician may not make the best medical decision if he or she has an economic interest.

If a physician violates this law, he or she may have to pay up to $15,000 in penalties for each claim and three times the amount of the improper collection. Violations of the False Claim Act may also come into play in these situations. Mandatory exceptions to this law were created to promote patient convenience, efficiency, and care continuity. So, for example, if a physician is part of a group practice, there is an exception that allows the physician to refer patients to providers and services within the group.

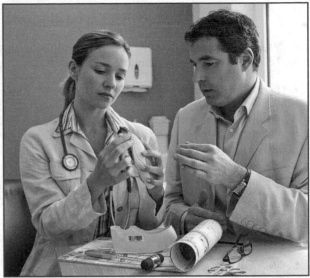

Image Point Fr/Shutterstock.com

Figure 7.4   It is illegal for physicians to make promises of sales to pharmaceutical representatives in exchange for money.

The Health Insurance Portability and Accountability Act

The **Health Insurance Portability and Accountability Act (HIPAA)** includes the Privacy Rule and the Security Rule. HIPAA provides federal protections for protected health information (PHI) held by covered entities and provides patients with rights related to their health information (Figure 7.5). These rights include patients determining who can view and receive their health information. At the same time, the Privacy Rule permits the disclosure of PHI that is needed for patient care and other important purposes. The original intentions of this legislation were the standardization and simplification of information transmission and cost savings. HIPAA applies to all forms of individuals' PHI, including oral, written, and electronic.

If an entity is not covered, it does not have to comply with HIPAA's Privacy Rule or the Security Rule. Examples of non-covered entities include employers, many schools, law enforcement agencies, state agencies (such as child protective services), and life insurance carriers.

Health insurers and providers who are covered entities must comply with patients' rights to:

- ask to see and/or receive a copy of their health records
- have corrections incorporated into their health records

Health Insurance Portability and Accountability Act (HIPAA)
law that aims to protect the confidentiality and security of healthcare information and help control administrative costs

HIPAA Regulations and Covered Entities		
Entities that must follow the HIPAA regulations are referred to as *covered entities*. The Privacy Rule and Security Rule apply only to covered entities, which include the following.		
A Healthcare Provider	**A Health Plan**	**A Healthcare Clearinghouse**
a provider of services who conducts certain business electronically, such as electronically billing health insurance companies *Examples:* • chiropractors • clinics • dentists • doctors • hospitals • nursing homes • pharmacies • psychologists	with certain exceptions, an individual or group plan that provides or pays the cost of medical care; includes many types of organizations and government programs *Examples:* • health insurance companies • health maintenance organizations (HMOs) • government programs that pay for healthcare (military and veteran health plans, Medicare, Medicaid)	entities that process nonstandard health information they receive from another entity into a standard format (standard electronic format or data content), or vice versa *Example:* • billing service that processes or facilitates the processing of data from one format into a standardized billing format

Source: US Department of Health & Human Services

Figure 7.5   Covered entities must follow HIPAA's Privacy Rule and Security Rule.

• receive a notice that informs them of how their health information may be used and shared

• decide if they want to give permission before their health information can be used or shared for certain purposes (such as marketing)

• obtain a report that explains when and why their health information was shared for certain purposes

The Privacy Rule sets limits on who can look at and receive health information. Patient information can be shared to ensure treatment and care coordination, to pay doctors and hospitals for healthcare services, to protect the public's health (if a patient has a contagious disease, for example), and to make required reports to the police (such as reporting gunshot wounds).

Health information cannot be used or shared without obtaining the patient's written permission unless this law allows it. For example, without patient authorization, providers generally cannot give patient information to employers, use or share information for marketing or advertising purposes, or share private notes about a patient's healthcare.

The Security Rule is related to electronic protected health information (e-PHI). This rule ensures confidentiality of all e-PHI that the covered entity receives, maintains, and transmits. The standards in this rule require covered entities to adhere to administrative, physical, and technical safeguards to protect e-PHI.

As a healthcare professional, if you are working for a covered entity, you will be responsible for understanding and following all of these HIPAA Privacy and Security Rules. Failure to conform to the HIPAA Privacy Rule could result in civil or criminal penalties. HIPAA violations can range from a single patient's record being viewed by a healthcare worker without good reason to massive breaches of thousands of patients' health records. Healthcare providers need to be aware of HIPAA at all times. Even something as seemingly harmless as leaving a fax on a desk or speaking about a patient in an elevator can be a violation of HIPAA.

As patient information becomes easier to share across the continuum of healthcare, there is a greater responsibility to protect that information. Patients must be informed about practices for use and disclosure of their information. They must also give written consent to the use and disclosure of their information for treatment, payment, and healthcare operations. HIPPA also gives patients the right to access and edit their health information.

Career Corner

Speech-language pathologists (also referred to as *speech pathologists*) focus on disorders related to human communication and work with patients of all ages. These professionals help prevent, evaluate, diagnose, and treat communication and swallowing disorders. These disorders can be caused by stroke, emotional problems, brain injury, hearing loss, physical abnormality, developmental delay, and cerebral palsy.

Speech pathologists diagnose and evaluate speech problems, such as fluency (stuttering), articulation, language comprehension, and voice disorders. These professionals design and carry out comprehensive treatment plans. Speech pathologists work closely with teachers, physicians, psychologists, social workers, rehabilitation counselors, and other members of interdisciplinary teams. They do not work directly under medical supervision, meaning they have a great deal of autonomy.

A master's degree, along with a supervised clinical program for graduate students, is typically required to become a speech pathologist. In these clinical programs, supervised work provides the opportunity for students to gain hands-on experience with patients and clients who have speech or communication problems.

Speech pathologists are typically required by employers to obtain the American Speech-Language-Hearing

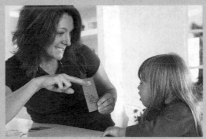
Monkey Business Images/Shutterstock.com

Association Certificate of Clinical Competence. To earn this certificate, one must complete a master's degree and a supervised clinical fellowship as well as pass a national examination. If college teaching is the goal, then a doctorate degree is usually needed. A doctorate degree is also typically required to conduct research in this field or have a private practice.

Americans with Disabilities Act (ADA) law that prohibits discrimination against people with disabilities in employment, transportation, public accommodation, communications, and governmental activities; also establishes requirements for telecommunications relay services

The Americans with Disabilities Act

The **Americans with Disabilities Act (ADA)**, enacted in 1990, prohibits discrimination based on a person's disability. To be considered disabled and protected under the ADA, an individual must have a physical or mental impairment that substantially limits his or her life activities. These activities include walking, talking, seeing, and learning. The ADA does not specifically name all of the covered impairments, but common examples of disabilities include using a wheelchair, needing to utilize assistive devices such as canes and walkers, blindness, deafness, a learning disability, and some mental illnesses. Four key sections of the ADA that relate to healthcare are described in Figure 7.6.

Healthcare-Related Sections of the Americans with Disabilities Act (ADA)		
Title I	Equal Employment Opportunities	This title is designed to eliminate barriers that would deny qualified individuals with disabilities access to the same employment opportunities and benefits available to those without disabilities. Employers must reasonably accommodate the disabilities of qualified applicants or employees, unless an undue hardship would result. This title prohibits discrimination in recruitment, hiring, promotions, training, pay, social activities, and other privileges of employment. It restricts questions that can be asked about an applicant's disability before a job offer is made.
Title II	Public Services	This title prohibits discrimination based on disability by public entities. It requires that state and local governments give people with disabilities an equal opportunity to benefit from all of their programs, services, and activities by providing equal access. This includes access to services and activities such as public education, recreation, healthcare, voting places, social services, courts, and town meetings.
Title III	Nondiscrimination by Public Accommodations and in Commercial Facilities	This title mandates accessibility in all types of businesses that serve or are open to the public, including medical offices and facilities. It also includes places such as hotels, zoos, restaurants, funeral homes, recreation facilities, movie theaters, daycare centers, convention centers, and health clubs.
Title IV	Telecommunications	This title addresses telephone and television access for people with hearing and speech disabilities. It requires common carriers (telephone companies) to establish interstate and intrastate telecommunications relay services (TRS) 24 hours a day, 7 days a week. TRS enables callers with hearing and speech disabilities who use text telephones (TTYs or TDDs), and callers who use voice telephones, to communicate with each other through a third party communications assistant. Title IV also requires closed captioning of federally funded public service announcements.

Source: US Department of Justice

Figure 7.6   Titles I-IV of the ADA secure specific healthcare-related rights for people who have disabilities.

ADA mandates, in part, that all healthcare facilities be accessible to people with disabilities (Figure 7.7). This requirement includes offices that specialize in mental health, vision, dental, or alternative care. Accessibility applies to both physical and communication access.

Healthcare facilities should address physical access issues such as the following:

- having accessible paths into and through the facility
- wide and easy-to-open doors
- accessible examination and/or treatment rooms and equipment
- appropriate reach ranges
- accessible restrooms and dressing areas

A facility's physical structure should not prevent access to areas such as waiting rooms, lobbies, doorways, and restrooms. Ramps or elevators should be offered as alternatives to stairs, and doorways, waiting rooms, and lobbies should be spacious enough to accommodate wheelchairs. Providers should ensure safe access to scales, exam tables, and chairs. Patients cannot be charged for the inclusion of any required services or devices.

Communication access includes auxiliary aids, services, and other types of program access. Healthcare providers must ensure that they can effectively communicate with people who have a range of disabilities. Examples of

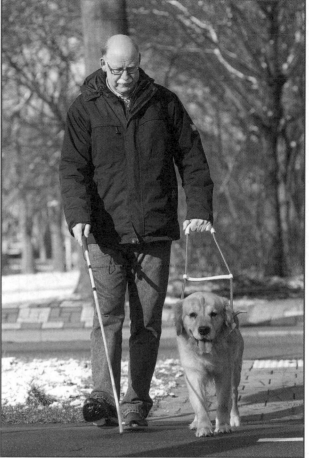

Jeroen van den Broek/Shutterstock.com

Figure 7.7 To make their facilities accessible to everyone, hospitals are required to allow service animals into the facilities.

such disabilities include people who have hearing or seeing difficulties, speech difficulties, or learning disabilities. Healthcare professionals may use a variety of auxiliary aids and services to help facilitate communication, such as a service that provides sign language interpreters or telephone interpretation service centers.

People with disabilities should have access to the same goods and services as people without disabilities. If this is not possible, healthcare providers should modify their policies or procedures. For example, healthcare providers must make an exception to a "no pets allowed" policy for patients with service animals. Additionally, staff should provide assistance whenever needed, such as helping to open doors. If accommodations cannot be made, the provider should refer patients to providers who do offer accessibility.

Healthcare facilities should include signs to help people with disabilities. Figure 7.8 identifies the symbols required for use by the ADA regulations.

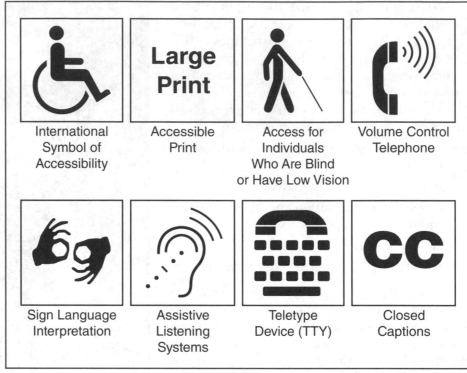

Goodheart-Willcox Publisher

Figure 7.8 Disability access symbols.

Ethical Dilemma

A 10-year-old girl is admitted to the hospital. She has a brain injury and was transferred to the rehabilitation unit after ankle surgery. As a result of her brain injury, she is unable to speak or see. The girl's mother has insisted that the girl be handfed pureed food instead of being tube fed, as the mother believes that it is one of her daughter's few pleasures in life. It takes the mother an hour to feed her each time.

The hospital staff is busy and concerned about the three-hour hand-feeding requirement. The clinical staff believes that the tube feeding will provide the nutrients the child needs, so the hand feeding is not clinically necessary. There is no medical reason to prevent the child from eating pureed food.

1. Does the hospital have an ethical obligation to feed the child by hand? Do they have a legal obligation? Why or why not?

2. Is this a reasonable accommodation? Why or why not?

3. Is it ethical for hospital staff to spend three hours a day

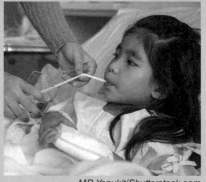

MR. Yanukit/Shutterstock.com

feeding the child if it is not clinically necessary, as that is time taken away from other patients?

The Rehabilitation Act

The **Rehabilitation Act** of 1973 prohibits discrimination based on disability in programs run by federal agencies, programs that receive federal financial assistance, federal employment, and the employment practices of federal contractors. In 1998, Congress amended the Rehabilitation Act of 1973 so that it required federal agencies to make their electronic and information technology accessible to people with disabilities. The law applies to all federal agencies. For example, pictures on web pages now need to have text embedded in metadata (hidden background information) in a format that allows screen readers to describe the picture to visually impaired persons.

Rehabilitation Act
law that prohibits discrimination based on disability in programs run by federal agencies, programs that receive federal financial assistance, federal employment, and the employment practices of federal contractors

The Emergency Medical Treatment and Active Labor Act

In 1986, Congress enacted the **Emergency Medical Treatment and Active Labor Act (EMTALA)** to ensure public access to emergency services regardless of ability to pay. The law was intended to prevent the practice of patient dumping. The term *patient dumping* describes the transfer of patients, for financial reasons only, from private to public hospitals without consideration for their medical condition or stability for the transfer. The laws states that:

Emergency Medical Treatment and Active Labor Act (EMTALA)
a law created to ensure public access to emergency services regardless of ability to pay

> "In the case of a hospital that has a hospital emergency department, if any individual comes to the emergency department and a request is made on the individual's behalf for examination or treatment for a medical condition, the hospital must provide for an appropriate medical screening examination within the capability of the hospital's emergency department, including ancillary services routinely available to the emergency department, to determine whether or not an emergency medical condition exists."

Hospitals that are participating in Medicare and that offer emergency services are required to provide a medical screening examination (MSE) when a request is made for examination of or treatment for an emergency medical condition (EMC) regardless of an individual's ability to pay. This obligation applies only to Medicare-participating hospitals, which include most of the hospitals in the United States, but it does not apply only to Medicare patients. This obligation applies to any individual, even if he or she is not a United States citizen.

EMTALA imposes the following three legal duties on hospitals:

1. Hospitals must perform an MSE on any person who comes to the hospital and requests care to determine whether an EMC exists (Figure 7.9).

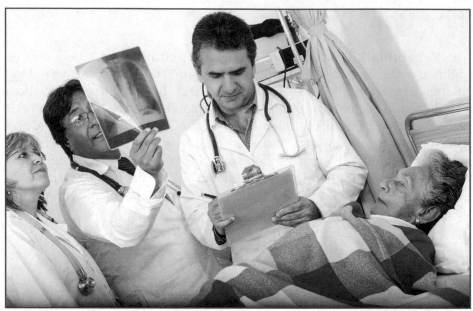

ESB Professional/Shutterstock.com

Figure 7.9   A medical screening exam is necessary for every person who enters a hospital seeking care.

2. If an EMC exists, hospital staff must either stabilize that condition to the extent of their ability or transfer the patient to another hospital with the appropriate capabilities.

3. Hospitals with specialized capabilities or facilities (burn units, for example) are required to accept transfers of patients in need of such specialized services if they have the capacity to treat them.

The Health Information Technology for Economic and Clinical Health Act

The American Recovery and Reinvestment Act (ARRA) of 2009 invested in the nation's infrastructure to stimulate the economy. The ARRA included the Health Information Technology for Economic and Clinical Health (HITECH) Act, which seeks to create a paperless national health information network. To achieve this, the HITECH Act provided more than $40 billion to assist and provide incentives for physicians and hospitals to adopt electronic health records (EHRs).

Because an expansion in the exchange of electronic protected health information (e-PHI) is expected, the HITECH Act also widens the scope of privacy and security protections available under HIPAA and increases the potential legal liability for non-compliance with its rules.

The HITECH Act increases civil penalties for willful neglect and expands the reach of HIPAA's data privacy and security requirements. These requirements now apply to the business associates of those entities that are subject to HIPAA. Business associates include accounting firms, billing agencies, law firms, or other companies that provide services to HIPAA-covered entities.

21st Century Cures Act

The **21st Century Cures Act**, signed into law in 2016, promotes and funds the acceleration of research into preventing and curing serious illnesses. It also accelerates drug and medical device development, attempts to address the opioid abuse crises, and tries to improve mental health service delivery. The act includes a number of provisions that push for greater interoperability, adoption of electronic health records, and support for human services programs.

21st Century Cures Act act that promotes and funds research into preventing and curing serious illnesses, including mental illnesses

Highlights of the bill include changes in the protection of health data. The HHS will be charged with revising health information privacy rules to allow:

- researchers to use protected information for research purposes
- researchers to remotely access health information
- individuals to authorize future use of their information for research

The bill encourages the use of electronic health record systems to collect data with the goal of enhancing research and treatment. It creates the Serious Mental Illness Coordinating Committee, targeting tracking of advancements in the treatment of serious mental illnesses and emotional disturbances.

The Cures Act also addresses the Medicaid same-day billing issue. It allows Medicaid patients to see multiple professionals on the same day for different services, such as primary care and mental health services.

Chapter Summary

Federal laws and statutes address the following aspects of healthcare:

- Help ensure quality and accessible care to the elderly, poor, and disabled and provide the same quality of care for disabled people as for non-disabled people.
- Protect individuals' health information and minimize opportunities for healthcare fraud.
- Prevent patient dumping.
- Provide electronic resources for research endeavors.

Vocabulary Matching

1. protects the confidentiality and security of healthcare information and helps control administrative costs

2. prohibits discrimination based on disability in programs run by federal agencies, employers, and contractors, and programs that receive federal financial assistance

3. ensures public access to emergency services regardless of ability to pay

4. decreases the number of Americans who do not have health insurance and helps reduce the overall cost of healthcare

5. prohibits discrimination against people with disabilities in employment, transportation, public accommodation, communications, and government activities

6. prohibits individuals and businesses from submitting fraudulent claims for payment to the government

7. prohibits physician referrals of Medicare and Medicaid patients to health services in which the physician or an immediate family member has a financial interest

8. prohibits the exchange of anything of value in exchange for the award of federal healthcare program business

9. made the United States Public Health Service the primary division of the US Department of Health, Education, and Welfare, which later became the Department of Health and Human Services

10. accelerates research into preventing and curing serious illnesses

A. 21st Century Cures Act
B. Americans with Disabilities Act
C. Anti-Kickback Statute
D. Emergency Medical Treatment and Active Labor Act
E. False Claims Act
F. Health Insurance Portability and Accountability Act
G. Patient Protection and Affordable Care Act
H. Public Health Service Act
I. Rehabilitation Act
J. Stark Anti-Referral Law

Multiple Choice

11. Which act creates the Serious Mental Illness Coordinating Committee?
    A. 21st Century Cures Act
    B. HITECH Act
    C. Mental Health Act
    D. Public Health Service Act

12. A physician specializing in sports medicine owns a physical therapy clinic. He refers patients only to his physical therapy business because he believes that it is the best one. He may have violated the _____.
    A. Commerce Clause
    B. False Claims Act
    C. Health Insurance Portability and Accountability Act
    D. Stark Anti-Referral Law

13. A patient arrives at the emergency room and does not have health insurance. The hospital then transfers the patient to another facility because she does not have the ability to pay. This is a violation of the _____.
    A. Americans with Disability Act
    B. Emergency Medical Treatment and Active Labor Act
    C. Affordable Care Act
    D. Health Insurance Portability and Accountability Act

Completion

14. A(n) _____ is a person who is protected from retaliation for reporting perceived wrongdoing.

15. The name of the law that allows people access to their health records is _____.

16. The _____ Act provides incentives for utilizing electronic health records.

Discussion and Critical Thinking

17. Review the scenario presented at the beginning of this chapter. What would you suggest that the medical assistant do? Incorporate information on ethics from Chapter 2 in your response.

18. What steps should healthcare personnel and healthcare facilities take to assist people with disabilities?

19. Explain the Emergency Medical Treatment and Active Labor Act (EMTALA), Health Insurance Portability and Accountability Act (HIPAA), and Health Information Technology for Economic and Clinical Health (HITECH) Act. What is the main purpose of each?

20. Why was the HITECH Act needed to expand the use of electronic health records?

21. Do you think that Medicare should be available to everyone? Why or why not?

22. Why was the ACA so controversial?

Activities

23. Visit a hospital. Notice what features are there to make access easier for people with disabilities. What could make access difficult? Do you observe any HIPAA violations? If you cannot visit a hospital, search the Internet for regulations requiring hospitals and other facilities to make their facilities accessible. Write a one-page description of your findings.

24. Search the Internet for information about the Patient Protection and Affordable Care Act. Write a two-page paper describing the debate surrounding the act. After examining the pros and cons, explain whether you support the act and why. Support your decision with evidence from your research.

Case Study

Marcy worked at a hospital as an admitting clerk for the emergency department. She heard on the news that a famous person had been in the emergency department and was later admitted. She was curious about why the person was admitted, so she looked up his medical record.

Two days later, Marcy was asked to meet with the Director of Human Resources.

The Director stated that she knew Marcy had looked into the patient's file and that her access of the medical records was not related to her job because the patient had been admitted when she was off duty. Marcy was fired and escorted out of the hospital.

Did the hospital act legally? If so, what was the basis for their decision? Would it have mattered if Marcy was working when the person was admitted?

Chapter 8

Managing Risk in Healthcare

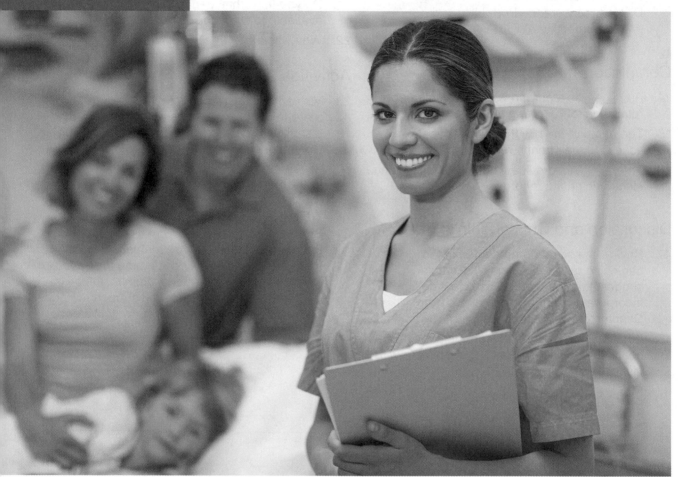

wavebreakmedia/Shutterstock.com

Chapter Outline

Competence
> Complying with Evolving Laws
> Avoiding Errors

Obtaining Informed Consent

Forms of Medical Practice

Insurance and Risk Management
> Understanding How Insurance Works
> Managing Defense and Settlements
> Reporting Claims
> Understanding Covered Conduct
> Deciding to Self-Insure

Risk Management Programs

Legislation to Limit Malpractice Claims

What do Do When Problems Arise

Objectives

- Describe elements of competence that reduce a healthcare practitioner's risk of malpractice or medical error.
- List and describe forms of healthcare practices.
- Describe the role of insurance in healthcare.
- Explain the role of risk management programs in healthcare.
- Identify legislation passed to limit malpractice claims.
- List actions that should be taken when risks arise.

Key Terms

defensive medicine
general liability insurance
insurance
professional malpractice insurance
risk
risk management
scope of practice
vicarious liability

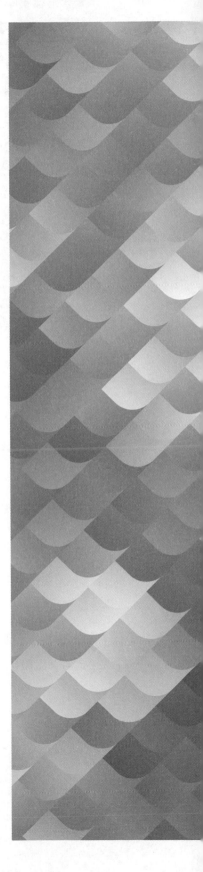

What Would You Do?

risk
the possibility of loss or injury

Risk, the possibility of loss or injury, is an inherent part of life. No matter where you work, there will be risks to yourself and to others. Of course, the first step in reducing risk is to use common sense. That is, you should rely on experience and exercise caution to avoid harming yourself or others.

Because workplace problems develop on a daily basis, businesses have safety programs, policies, and procedures to reduce risk and encourage employees to take care of themselves and others. The insurance industry provides ways for businesses to protect themselves from common risks. In many ways, the healthcare field is no different from any other business. Healthcare professionals work with healthy people to maintain and improve health and well-being, as well as with people who already have illnesses or injuries. In all cases, ill or healthy, healthcare workers confront the same issues and everyday possibilities of injury, harm, or offense that any typical retail or commercial business would.

However, there also are particular risks that arise in the healthcare field that you need to understand. Those unique risks might include a clinician's failure to read a scan from a routine screening or a medical office's inadvertent data breach. Understanding these risks can help you protect yourself and your patients, whether you are an employer or an employee.

Competence

From the healthcare perspective, in addition to using common sense, the first line of defense against risk is being competent. Put simply, competence reduces risk. Working within your scope of practice, following the standard of care, ensuring that your skills are up to date, keeping yourself informed about laws that regulate your work, and making sure you comply with those laws will dramatically reduce your chances for practicing unethically.

Competence will help you avoid many common situations that cause patients to sue, such as making a misdiagnosis, performing a procedure incorrectly, carrying out a questionable order, not listening to and responding appropriately to patient requests, and not complying with employer policies and procedures (Figure 8.1).

When seeking healthcare, patients often arrive when they are already in a state of distress, injury, or illness. This can create a stressful environment, but competence is a good tool for managing that stress. As long as the healthcare provider acts in a way that a reasonably competent and similarly trained professional would under the same circumstances, there should be no liability for a dire patient outcome.

Complying with Evolving Laws

One aspect of competence is staying informed about legal developments that affect your healthcare practice. For example, because of new developments in the electronic health records field, you should keep abreast of regulations from the Health Insurance Portability & Accountability Act (HIPAA) and Occupational Safety and Health Administration (OSHA) that govern workplace rules.

Failing to comply with evolving laws can increase your chances of being found liable for losses. Being out of compliance with a law is considered not upholding your duty. As discussed in Chapter 5, this can increase the

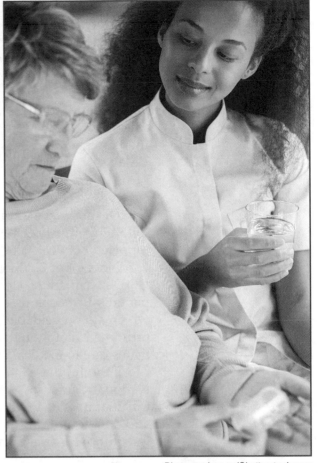

Photographee.eu/Shutterstock.com

Figure 8.1 Competence is important to avoid errors in the healthcare field.

chances for a claim of negligence under a concept called *negligence per se,* which occurs when you violate a law and an injury results. The law establishes a duty on your part, and being in violation means that you have breached a duty of care. If you happen to be involved in medical research, certain laws may require independent reviews by Institutional Review Boards (see Chapter 2) before you begin your study. Failure to follow procedure when conducting research can lead to violations of privacy rules and other laws.

Avoiding Errors

Previous chapters have addressed the notion of being mindful of ethics, training, and education, as well as the practice of due care under given circumstances. These concepts lead to proper care and minimization of risk. However, even when ethics and standards of care are followed, errors still occur.

For example, mishaps occur regularly in healthcare settings, and many of these are preventable. A landmark study by the Institute of Medicine (IOM) in 1999, called *To Err is Human*, found that between 44,000 and 98,000 patients are killed in hospitals each year due to preventable adverse events caused by treatment itself and not an underlying condition. Since that time, more than 100 new reports have been written and administrative attention has been focused on the issues raised in the IOM report. The Patient Safety and Quality Improvement Act of 2005 was enacted to encourage the development of voluntary, provider-driven initiatives to improve the quality and safety of healthcare. A standardized national reporting system for medical errors is needed, because many errors still go undetected.

Despite some improvement in practice and certain geographic areas following the 1999 IOM report, the rate of harm from hospital stays reported between 2000 and 2007 was 25.1 per 100 admissions. According to a November 2010 study by the Office of the Inspector General of the US Department of Health and Human Services, about 1 in 7 Medicare patients in hospitals experience a serious medical error, 44 percent of which are preventable. In 2016, a Johns Hopkins University safety expert estimated that more than 250,000 deaths occur each year in the United States due to medical error.

Despite these statistics, few injured patients file lawsuits. The National Center for State Courts (NCSC) conducted an analysis of medical malpractice litigation in state courts. A 2010 study by LaFountain and Lee found "rarely does a medical malpractice caseload exceed a few hundred cases in any one state in one year." This is, in part, due to prompt efforts by defendants and their insurers to settle claims arising from obvious errors to reduce cost and publicity.

Even with the best care and education, factors such as sudden distraction, failure of previously reliable products, and inaccurate information from patients can all lead to errors in practice (Figure 8.2). Therefore, when you sense that something may potentially go wrong, you should immediately notify your supervisor.

In addition, seek out employer-designated risk management staff, if available. You also can consult with professional practice management advice groups or professional ethics hotlines. It is also common practice for professionals to consult with peers who have had similar or greater experience in a given situation.

Obtaining Informed Consent

Part of conducting competent practice is obtaining informed consent from the patient. Obtaining patient consent is the responsibility of the

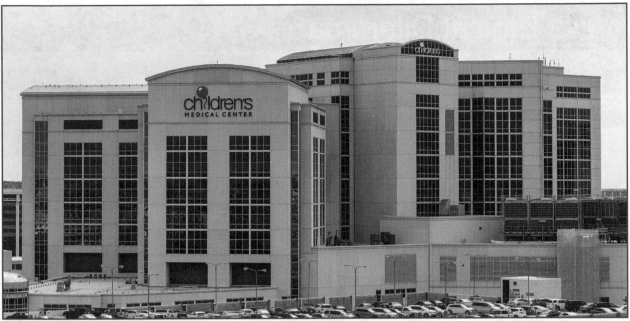

CasoyMartin/Shutterstock.com

Figure 8.2 Errors still occur even in the most careful and prepared hospitals.

physician. Even though forms may be signed and clinical notes may assert that the patient was in fact competent, information received or the validity of the consent may be incorrect.

There may be a shared responsibility to ensure that the patient's consent is valid and continues over time. Even if you are assisting the professional who originally obtained the consent, you may have an ongoing responsibility to report any concern you have regarding the validity of a patient's consent. This responsibility usually stems from employer policy and procedures or your own certification. If there is an error with a patient's consent, or if treatment continues or exceeds what the patient agreed to, there may be liability. It is for this type of situation that **insurance**, malpractice insurance in particular, has been developed to minimize risk to the provider.

Informed consent is actually a form of risk reduction in which the patient takes some responsibility for the service provided. This does not mean that the provider will have no liability or that there will be no argument about the quality of service. However, there is at least some basis for arguing that the patient was willing to take the risk and that both the patient and provider shared important information, while the physician upheld the ethical duty for recognizing patient autonomy. Chapter 9 discusses informed consent in more detail.

insurance
a contract that states that one party (the insurance company) will pay for certain types of monetary loss in the event of loss or damages occurring from some predefined categories of risk in return for the payment of money in advance, called a *premium*

Ethical Dilemma

Imagine that you are a nurse and a patient asks you to help him remove his oxygen mask. He says that he knows he will not live much longer, and he does not want to continue to have his life sustained via the oxygen life support. You are concerned that the patient does not understand the consequences of removing the oxygen, so you explain to him that doing so could lead to oxygen deprivation, brain damage, paralysis, discomfort, and death.

The patient indicates that he understands the risks but wants to live free of the machine for a while if he is going to die anyway. You are concerned that if you agree to help him, it may be against the law, your professional ethical standards, your employer's policies, your supervising physician's orders, and your own moral ethics. You also are concerned that this decision could subject you to a maltreatment claim for implementing the patient's request rather than continuing normal care practices.

If you refuse to obey the patient's request, are you violating his right of autonomy and placing your own self-interest first? After all, the patient is permitted to refuse medical care. Does patient informed consent relieve you of potential liability? Should you refuse because he will die soon and is unlikely to sue you for refusing to honor his request? Should you talk to your supervising physician before acting?

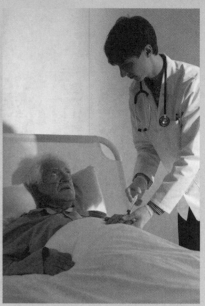

Photographee.eu/Shutterstock.com

Forms of Medical Practice

One way in which healthcare professionals can limit the risk to their personal assets is by choosing which business structure or employment status to use while providing services to the community. There are several different practice models, including employee, sole practitioner, partnership, or corporation.

If you are providing healthcare services as an employee, as long as you work within the bounds of your professional competence and in the line of duty as an employee, your employer will be responsible for any liability that arises from your conduct. You may still be liable for ethical violations, but injury to a patient will generally come under the legal concept of *respondeat superior*. This concept means that the employer must answer for any civil fault under a "master-servant" relationship with employees and thus is responsible for your conduct.

scope of practice
the range of procedures and actions an individual is permitted to perform; based on education, experience, competence, and formal training

It is important that you understand the limits of your permitted **scope of practice** so that you are not found to be outside your employer's responsibility. Scope of practice is generally framed by your required level of education and experience, the extent to which regulating organizations authorize your type of work, and any additional limits your employer may place on what tasks you may perform. For example, if you were trained in the military to perform certain medical procedures in an emergency, but you are not licensed to do so by the state you practice in, performing those procedures would be outside your scope of practice.

Most employers will require you to practice only within the scope of your training and licensing and may even be more restrictive to reduce their own risk. This is why employers carry insurance that involves both **general liability insurance** for business activities and also malpractice coverage for staff members who are working for the organization. The employee-employer relationship does not mean that, as an employee, you will never be sued individually. However, you always have the defense that you were serving as a mere employee and therefore did not have independent responsibility for any mishap.

Nevertheless, an employee may still be subject to license revocation or other disciplinary action for unprofessional or unethical conduct. If you are a licensed healthcare professional, you are always personally responsible for acting with your own independent judgment and training within your scope of practice. You cannot allow an unlicensed person, even the president of the company employing you, to make professional judgments for you.

If you are a sole practitioner, you will be fully liable for your work, but you also will have the most autonomy in choosing how, when, and where to work. Sole practitioners often carry general liability insurance and malpractice insurance to reduce financial loss to themselves if they are found responsible for civilly damaging a patient in a way that requires them to pay money damages.

Similarly, partnerships, which are agreements between two or more people to work together as a team, establish joint liability (Figure 8.3). This means that each partner is liable for the acts of all the others. Generally, licensed professionals may only create partnerships in which they intend to practice with other people holding a similar license. This prevents people from acting on behalf of a licensed professional in a specialty that they do not have the right to practice.

In partnerships, liability flows to each individual, so the error of three or four individuals may flow entirely onto one partner who may have sufficient personal assets to pay for the damages. This form of organization may actually increase your exposure to risk from participating partners under a concept called **vicarious liability**. Under this theory, you can be held responsible for the acts of partners or other people associated with you based on your relationship, and not specifically on your own conduct.

general liability insurance
insurance that protects against injuries and property damage resulting from general risk associated with business or property ownership, such as "slip-and-fall" accidents

vicarious liability
liability for loss or damages of one person or entity attributable to another person based on their relationship, even if the second person or entity was not directly involved in causing the loss

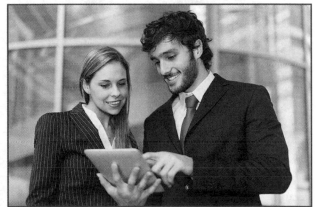
Minerva Studio/Shutterstock.com

Figure 8.3 Partnerships allow several people to share liability for errors that may occur in a business.

During the past few decades, laws have been passed to authorize limited liability partnerships, in which individual partners are not liable for the individual acts of other members of the partnership. This legislation reduces your exposure to risk, but you would still want to carry insurance to cover your own individual liability.

Finally, you can protect yourself by forming a professional corporation, a limited liability corporation, or a general corporation that has its own existence and takes on its own legal responsibility. These organizations are formed by following formal procedures established by states and generally involve paying an annual fee or tax and filing a separate return for the corporation. You will still be responsible for your own mistakes, but not for the errors of your associates beyond the assets of the corporation. Liability will attach to the corporation itself and the assets owned by the company, rather than to the individual practitioners' own individual assets.

defensive medicine
patient care that involves conducting more tests or treatment than would be called for if litigation or malpractice was not of particular concern

Insurance and Risk Management

Insurance is a complicated concept that is defined by the terms of the written insurance policy itself. There are a number of important aspects of insurance policies that you should understand before you make presumptions about what insurance will or will not cover.

Studies have found that the practice of **defensive medicine** occurs when healthcare providers are not confident in their insurance coverage or are concerned about increasing insurance premiums. In these cases, providers have been found more likely to report frequently ordering otherwise unneeded diagnostic procedures, referrals, or prescriptions. Of course, your primary concern should be the minimization of risk of loss not only to protect yourself, but also to minimize any injury or loss to your own patients.

Insurance is a way for you to shift the risk of financial loss from yourself to a company that is willing to share your risk, for a price. Most businesses carry general liability insurance that covers business problems such as fire and loss of property. Malpractice insurance is a specialized form of insurance that covers errors due to a failure to provide competent service (Figure 8.4). The basic idea is that most people and businesses will be careful, and most professionals will not incur losses, so insurance companies can spread their losses among their insured customers.

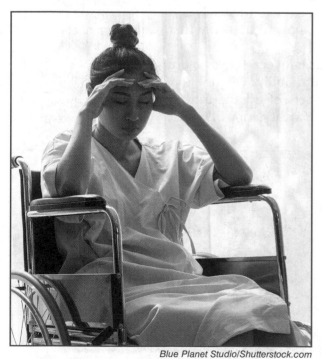

Blue Planet Studio/Shutterstock.com

Figure 8.4 Malpractice insurance is important because it protects healthcare professionals and facilities when errors occur.

Insurance is typically supervised by state oversight agencies, but healthcare-related insurance policies are essentially individual contracts between healthcare providers and insurance companies. The actual written terms of the contract agreement govern the rules of how insurance protects you. You will want to carefully consider and understand the terms of **professional malpractice insurance**. That is your first step in minimizing your risk by way of insurance.

professional malpractice insurance
a contract between an insurance company and a healthcare professional under which the company will pay for certain types of monetary liability created if the professional makes errors when treating a patient

Understanding How Insurance Works

Generally, you have a duty to cooperate with your insurance carrier and to conduct yourself according to the terms of your insurance contract. You also should understand that fees for the lawyers carrying out your defense might be deducted from the amount your policy covers. For example, if you have a $500,000 insurance policy and the lawyers' fees are $100,000, the amount of money available to pay actual damages to a patient could be reduced to $400,000. In other words, the more expensive the litigation costs, the less money there is to pay the actual claim against you.

It is also important to know that, except in certain states, the patient can sue for any amount of money consistent with the damages suffered. The patient is not restricted by the amount of insurance you have. If you have a $500,000 insurance policy and a $2 million successful claim against you, your insurance might cover $400,000 ($500,000 less $100,000 in litigation expenses), and you might be liable for the remaining $1.5 million.

Managing Defense and Settlements

Many insurance policies contain a clause that requires the insured person to let the insurance company manage any defense or settlements. Most policies also require the insured person to cooperate with the insurance company in whatever action it takes. Even if you think you are not liable for the alleged failure, you may be required to participate in potentially burdensome and time-consuming preparation and sharing of records.

Additionally, your insurance company may agree to settle the case for a certain sum of money simply to avoid the likely higher costs of going to trial. You may be surprised to find that you are being asked to accept a malpractice settlement negotiated by your insurance company to avoid litigation expense, especially if you personally felt you were not at fault.

Reporting Claims

Time can be an important factor when it comes to insurance coverage. For example, there is usually a set time period during which a claim must have occurred and been reported to the insurance carrier. This means that you must report your knowledge of a problem before the insurance policy term lapses, or you will not be covered. Upon renewal, many policies include the date when the policy first became active and the date through which it will remain active as long as the coverage has been continually in place.

Understanding Covered Conduct

Understanding insurance also involves knowing the types of conduct that are covered by your policy. General professional negligence, for example, is often covered. However, certain types of conduct cannot be covered by insurance as a matter of public policy. Actions involving fraud and sexual discrimination are often not covered, because state and federal legislatures do not want insurance companies to compensate wrongdoers involved in serious misconduct.

Deciding to Self-Insure

Requirements for carrying insurance vary by state and by medical specialty. In some circumstances, you may not be required to have insurance. However, some states require minimum insurance coverage for certain types of practitioners to enable them to participate in the state program to cap liability (Figure 8.5). In addition, some employers require certain practitioners to carry their own minimum insurance.

Nevertheless, in most situations, you may self-insure. That means you are prepared to pay for any potential claims made against you out of your own resources. Generally, people do this because traditional insurance is for the benefit of the person purchasing insurance, not for the party that was injured or suffered loss. Therefore, you may continue to carry your own risk without insurance, but you may not be able to mount an effective defense quickly or be in a position to settle claims effectively.

In some cases, you may obtain insurance policies that have very high deductibles, such as $35,000, that are "stop-loss" policies. These types of policies prevent you from having to pay for very large claims, even if you are prepared to pay for smaller claims out of your personal assets. Plaintiffs' attorneys are usually eager to identify the amount of insurance you might actually carry to determine whether the litigation they are pursuing will result in actual monetary payments to the plaintiff and themselves. If you have an insurance policy that has a high deductible, the plaintiff may assume you will be pressured to settle quickly and cut your losses.

Alternatively, if you have no insurance, the plaintiff also may believe you will be pressured to settle early to preserve your personal assets. However, if you are very lucky, the plaintiff may not consider it worth the cost to take you to court if there is little money available.

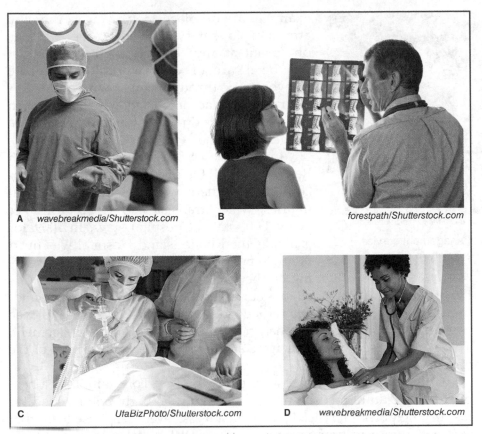

A   wavebreakmedia/Shutterstock.com   B   forestpath/Shutterstock.com

C   UtaBizPhoto/Shutterstock.com   D   wavebreakmedia/Shutterstock.com

Figure 8.5   Practitioners in various healthcare fields must obtain a minimum of insurance coverage in some states. Examples: A—surgeon; B—chiropractor; C—nurse anesthetist; D—physician assistant.

Risk Management Programs

Some major healthcare businesses and many insurance companies operate preventive **risk management** services for their employees and policyholders. The programs are designed to provide expert assistance in reviewing procedures and business practices. The goal is to identify areas that could be improved to reduce the risk of causing harm to others and incurring liability to yourself, your employer, and the company. Therefore, these programs focus on prevention, which can certainly be cost-effective.

Typically, these services include an on-site visit from a specialist who will review forms and procedures and discuss any areas of possible improvement (Figure 8.6). Other approaches include Internet-based instruction and telephone-based call centers that provide additional information on maintaining good practice standards and effective business practices designed to minimize errors.

A risk management program may include assessment of a workplace's culture, with suggestions for how to possibly change it. For

risk management
a program or practice to examine causes of loss and to design or implement preventive actions or methods to reduce loss once a cause is identified

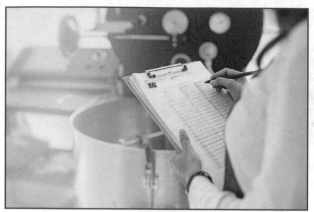

Mila Supinskaya Glashchenko/Shutterstock.com

Figure 8.6   One type of risk management service involves a specialist writing the facility to make recommendations.

example, a workplace may want to increase attention to safety and decrease a focus on "profit at any cost." It is important that you be aware of your workplace's culture to avoid risk through your own conduct. A culture of blame or one in which people in higher positions do not listen to others can be problematic.

In 2017, the US Administration for Health Resources and Quality estimated that from 2010 to 2015 there were 3.8 million hospital injuries, which translates to 115 injuries per every 1,000 patient hospital stays. In 2009, for example, the Rhode Island Hospital was fined $150,000 by the state health agency for operating on the wrong finger of a patient. This was the fifth incident of its kind to occur at that hospital in two years, including three operations on the wrong sides of patients' brains. Employee warnings about procedures had not been addressed by management. These "wrong site" incidents were attributed to the work culture of the hospital.

Culture also can have positive effects on risk. For example, if a hospital has a culture focused on safety, incentives might be provided for identifying potential risks. Having an adverse event response team that is focused on developing systems for prevention rather than on blame also can be helpful (Figure 8.7).

Protocols and standards of practice can be useful in risk reduction for an individual practitioner. However, a broader, continuous quality improvement program has been recognized as playing an important part

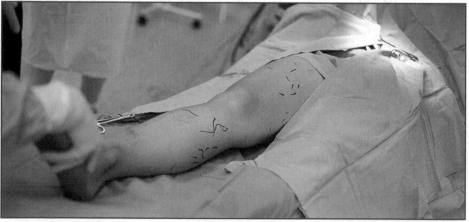

UVgreen/Shutterstock.com

Figure 8.7   The marks shown on this patient's leg signal to the surgeon which leg requires the operation.

in safe healthcare delivery. The US Department of Health and Human Services' Health Resources and Services Administration (HRSA) has developed a Quality Toolkit to assist healthcare organizations with their quality improvement (QI) efforts. The tools and resources in this kit are used for implementing data collection and performance measurement techniques that can be integrated into existing organization practices to improve delivery of care.

HRSA indicates that a successful QI program begins with an honest and objective assessment of an organization's current culture, its commitment to improving the quality of its care and services, and its readiness for change. Understanding an organization's strengths and weaknesses regarding QI is a good starting point to assess its readiness for change. Of course, change itself always has its own risks, so undertaking or participating in a QI program is not a guarantee that malpractice or errors will be eliminated.

In addition to quality improvement, employer-sponsored educational programs that help staff remain competent in their fields can be useful for reducing risk. For example, a nursing home may develop staff training courses in fall prevention. Tools such as a fall predictive risk assessment also would be helpful.

 ## Career Corner

Occupational health and safety technicians inspect and collect data on workplace safety and health conditions. These professionals examine workplaces for potential hazards and help to ensure that safety regulations both exist and are followed. They conduct tests and measure hazards to help prevent harm to employees, property, the environment, and the general public. These professionals work in various settings, such as offices, factories, mines, hotels, food service sites, and hospitals. They often travel as they visit and examine different worksites.

Employers typically require an associate's degree for entry-level positions in this field. Some government agencies require a bachelor's degree in healthcare administration or healthcare management. Many employers also prefer to hire employees who have obtained certification in the field. This might include the Occupational Health and Safety Technologist certificate, which is offered by the Council on Certification of Health, Environmental, and Safety Technologists.

To advance in this field, occupational health and safety technicians can obtain certification as Safety Trained Supervisors, which will prepare

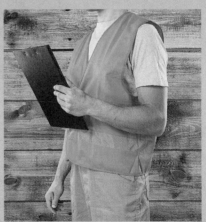

Billion Photos/Shutterstock.com

them for a management position. Another way to advance in the field is to earn a graduate degree in healthcare administration or healthcare management.

Legislation to Limit Malpractice Claims

The impact of insurance and healthcare litigation on the overall cost of healthcare is a controversial issue. Several states have tried to address this issue by enacting so-called "tort reform" laws that limit the amounts of malpractice claims. For example, legislation in California has limited general damages claims against physicians to $250,000. However, because many other states have not accepted this approach to reducing healthcare provider risk, insurance costs have generally continued to rise, as has litigation in many jurisdictions.

What to Do When Problems Arise

If you are caring for a patient and determine that an error has been made, the first action you should take is to ensure the health of the patient. Document the error immediately in the patient's file and create an incident report. In addition, if the error could potentially be attributed to you, consider making notes for your own potential malpractice defense and keep them in a pre-litigation file for personal use with your attorney. These notes may be used later to help refresh your memory of the incident. The notes also may be protected as attorney work product in certain circumstances.

Of course, you need to follow the policies of your employer and, as necessary, communicate with your employer's risk management staff, attorney, or insurance carrier. If you are an employer, confer with your professional advisors and insurance company when an incident occurs.

Never destroy any notes or records, either paper or electronic, that you feel will be damaging, as this will only make the situation worse (Figure 8.8). You always need to cooperate with your employer and insurance company. You also should be prepared to deal with the problem for up to several years while it is resolved in settlements or litigation.

In the absence of serious injury, formal legal action may be avoided by engaging in honest communication with the patient

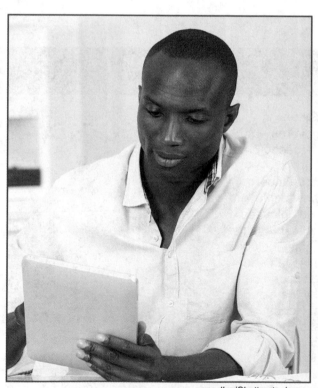

goodluz/Shutterstock.com

Figure 8.8 Notes and records can serve as important documents in lawsuits.

accompanied by an explanation and/or apology. It is important to remember that if you are an employee, your employer has a vital role in resolving these types of problems, and any steps you take should be in accordance with your supervisor's policies and approval. After formally resolving the situation with the patient, your employer may ask you to take remedial training or other steps to avoid future errors.

Hiding medical errors not only injures the patient, but doing so is unethical, violating client autonomy and your duty to do no harm (Figure 8.9). This type of behavior can be criminal and may involve additional civil liability for fraud or other claims. "To err is human," so you need to be competent at handling situations in which you were not as competent as possible.

It is important that you also be aware of procedures that may be affecting patient health. Medical errors and mistakes may not always be the fault of a single individual. Sometimes they may be due to delivery system procedures or policies that have adverse consequences. One example is the development and spread of drug-resistant bacteria caused by overuse of drugs resulting from the practice of defensive medicine. Between 20 and 50 percent of all antibiotics prescribed in hospitals are either not needed or inappropriate.

Another example is patient visiting practices, where bacteria may be inadvertently carried to patients from outside the facility. An individual practitioner may not have actually caused the infection but must be aware of the possibility and observe and report possible issues.

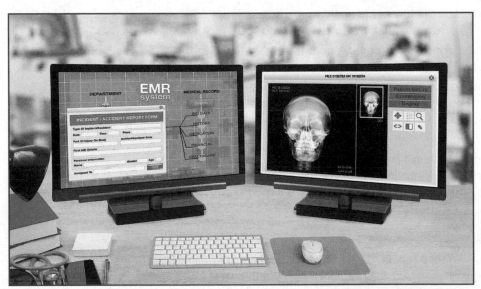

Figure 8.9 If a medical error occurs, it must be recorded in the patient's medical record. Hiding or failing to record a medical error can be considered a criminal act.

Chapter 8 Review and Assessment

Chapter Summary

- Risk can be reduced by providing competent care and using common sense.
- Your status as an employee or independent provider may have some effect on your liability for errors.
- Insurance does not reduce the risk that you will be found liable for error, but it can help you meet the financial liability that may result.
- Major medical providers and some insurance companies have developed programs to help reduce risk.
- Risk of providing care has been limited in some states, where malpractice claims have certain defined limits.
- In case of a problem, first ensure that the client is properly cared for; then maintain good documentation and communicate effectively with your employer, other providers, and the patient.

Vocabulary Matching

1. range of procedures and actions an individual is permitted to perform based on education, experience, competence, and formal training
2. contract between an insurance company and a healthcare practitioner under which the company will pay for certain types of monetary liability if the practitioner makes errors when treating a patient
3. insurance that protects against injuries and property damage resulting from risk associated with business or property ownership, such as "slip-and-fall" accidents
4. program or practice that specifically examines causes of loss and then designs and implements preventive actions to reduce loss
5. patient care that involves conducting more tests or treatment than would be called for if litigation or malpractice was not of concern
6. liability for loss or damages of one entity attributable to another entity based on their relationship, even if the second entity was not directly involved in causing the loss
7. the possibility of loss or injury
8. contract that states that an insurance company will pay for certain types of monetary loss in the event of loss or damages occurring from predefined categories of risk in return for a premium payment

A. defensive medicine
B. general liability insurance
C. insurance
D. professional malpractice insurance
E. risk
F. risk management
G. scope of practice
H. vicarious liability

Multiple Choice

9. The first line of defense against risk is _____.
   A. perfection
   B. competence
   C. insurance
   D. error

10. According to a study from the Department of Health and Human Services, what percentage of medical errors is preventable?
   A. 83
   B. 100
   C. 44
   D. 29

11. Which of the following statements about malpractice insurance is true?
    A. It will pay for all claims against you.
    B. It is required in all states.
    C. It may be required by your employer.
    D. It is available to everyone.

12. Which form of business can help protect you from losses caused by your business associates?
    A. partnership
    B. a sole proprietorship
    C. a private business
    D. a corporation

Completion

13. _____ insurance protects against injuries and property damage resulting from general risk associated with business or property ownership.

14. Insurance defense costs can _____ the amount of insurance available in your policy to pay claims.

15. _____ liability occurs when a person's loss is attributable to someone else based on a relationship.

16. _____ is the ethical principle that is related to informed consent.

Discussion and Critical Thinking

17. If you are asked to form a business with a friend, does it matter if you and your friend hold different types of licenses? Why or why not?

18. Will insurance fully protect you from malpractice claims? Why or why not?

19. If you wrongfully injure a patient, could your business partner be forced to sell his house to pay money damages?

20. Watch the YouTube video, "Hospital Errors: The High Risk of Medical Mistakes." Then discuss what the hospital could have done to reduce the risk of the infant receiving medication intended for her mother.

21. What is the difference between general liability insurance and malpractice insurance?

22. Under what circumstances may you be legally liable for another practitioner's errors?

23. Does malpractice insurance protect a provider from discipline for violating professional rules of conduct? Explain.

24. How does fear of litigation increase healthcare costs?

Activities

25. Search the Internet to determine if professional liability insurance is available for a field in which you might hope to work. Does this influence which field you might select for a career?

26. Does your state limit the amount a patient can claim for damages against a physician? Search the Internet for information about this and write an essay that describes whether you think your state has established a good policy.

Case Study

Dr. Smith was examining the MRI image of his patient who complained of neck and back pain. He also reviewed the written report of the radiologist who conducted the MRI exam. Dr. Smith immediately noticed, as had the radiologist, that there was a buildup of extensive calcium deposits on his patient's spine around the seventh vertebrae. Dr. Smith concluded that this was the source of the patient's pain, and he acted on this conclusion. The radiologist who prepared the initial MRI report had not indicated any other abnormality. It turned out that the patient was actually suffering from a rare bone infection at the second vertebrae that was not noticed by Dr. Smith or the radiologist. The infection spread and the patient went to another doctor to seek treatment. After recovering, the patient sued Dr. Smith and the radiologist. Assuming that Dr. Smith made an error, how should he respond?

Chapter 9

The Patient-Professional Relationship

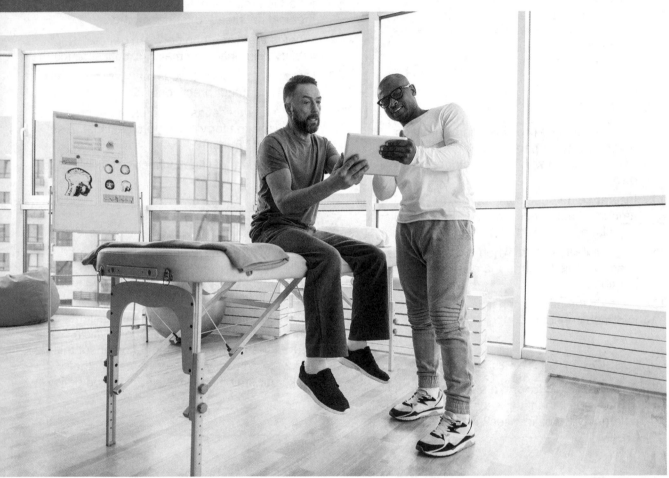

Dmytro Zinkevych/Shutterstock.com

Chapter Outline

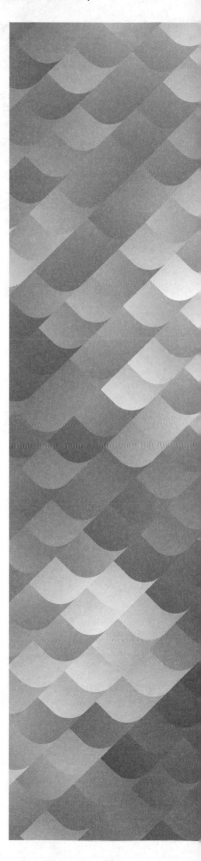

Objectives

- Describe what informed consent means, when it is needed, and how it can be given.
- Explain why confidentiality between a provider and a patient is important and when it can be broken.
- Articulate the role of medical professionals in terms of patient advocacy.
- Explain legal and ethical challenges that arise when a patient refuses medical treatment.
- Provide the legal definition of abandonment and the legal reasons a patient-provider relationship can end.

Key Terms

abandonment
decision-making capacity
express consent
extension doctrine
implied consent
informed consent
notifiable diseases
surrogate decision maker

What Would You Do?

Imagine that you are a clinical social worker hanging out at the beach on a Sunday afternoon. A middle-aged man is in the water threatening to drown himself. He is standing in water that comes up to his chest. You try to console him and talk him out of it. You explain that you are a professional who can help him. He tells you to stop talking to him. What should you do? Should you consider his statement as non-consent to treatment? What if you continue your efforts and he does drown himself? What legal and ethical issues come into play?

The patient-professional relationship is unique, complex, and fundamental to providing and receiving quality care, which leads to improved health outcomes. The Internet and cultural shift have changed this relationship. Patients are no longer passive recipients of care. Many patients are informed about and involved in their care, want to know more about their conditions, and seek to exert greater control. These patients often come to their medical appointments armed with information and website printouts.

To enhance patients' health outcomes, all parties involved must understand the essence of the patient-professional relationship, and the relationship itself must be strong. Achieving better outcomes requires mutual respect and clear articulation of expectations by both parties. This can help prevent misunderstandings related to trust, privacy, confidentiality, communication, expectations, professional duties, and boundaries.

This chapter provides general information about traditional legal issues inherent in the patient-professional relationship. Many of these legal issues stem from healthcare professionals' ethical obligations to patients and are closely related to ethics in general. As you read this chapter, think about the ethical issues discussed in Chapter 2.

Informed Consent

implied consent
a patient action that leads to the presumption that medical care has been authorized

express consent
the verbal or written authorization of care

Before a physician or healthcare professional may provide care to a patient, permission must first be granted. This permission, called *consent*, is defined as a voluntary agreement made with decision-making capacity. In the healthcare setting, when a patient allows a professional to change a bandage or take a blood pressure reading, he or she is giving consent.

Consent can be given in two forms: implied or expressed. **Implied consent** is determined by a patient's action that leads to the presumption that medical care has been authorized. For example, a patient scheduling an appointment for a mammogram implies consent to have that procedure performed. **Express consent** is the verbal or written authorization of care. For example, when a patient responds "yes" to receive an immunization at a medical clinic, he or she is giving verbal express consent (Figure 9.1). When a patient signs a consent form, he or she is giving written express consent (Figure 9.2).

Consent must be given before a healthcare professional may touch a patient. If consent is not given first, then non-consensual touching is considered to have occurred. Offensive non-consensual touching is considered battery even when not related to medical care. Medical battery, as discussed in Chapter 5, is defined as the intentional violation of a patient's rights to direct his or her medical treatment. Therefore, when a patient is treated without informed consent, medical battery has occurred. Laws governing medical battery vary from state to state.

Usually, battery charges are brought when there is a disagreement about whether the patient agreed to or refused treatment. Even when treatment involves a life-saving procedure, or when seemingly minor contact occurs, it can be deemed offensive or harmful. If consent is not given, then the treatment can be considered against the patient's will, even if a healthcare professional does not mean to cause harm.

In 1914, US Supreme Court Justice Benjamin Cardozo stated, "every human being of adult years and sound mind has a right to determine what shall be done with his own body." Cardozo's statement represents the current doctrine of professional ethics, in which a person's right to consent to medical treatment is an important aspect of medical care.

Presenting crucial pieces of information, such as risks and confidentiality, is very important because it provides the patient with comprehensive health information and also protects the provider from liability issues. The **informed consent** process is legally enacted in all 50 states. It is considered

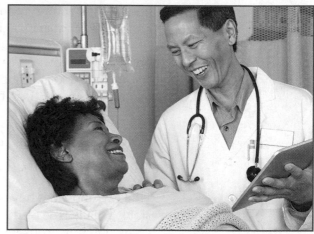

Monkey Business Images/Shutterstock.com

Figure 9.1 When a patient verbally agrees to a procedure, he or she has given express consent.

informed consent
consent obtained from a patient after explaining the benefits and risks of a procedure or course of action

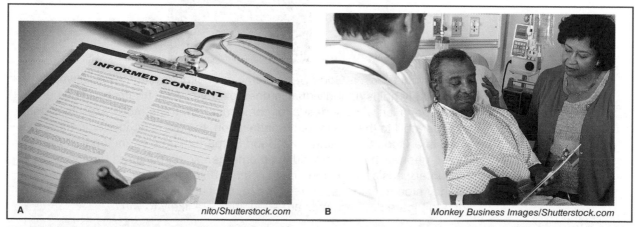

A   *nito/Shutterstock.com*   B   *Monkey Business Images/Shutterstock.com*

Figure 9.2 Expressed consent can also be given in writing, usually via a consent form (A). Signing a consent form (B) means you have agreed to a medical procedure.

both a legal requirement and an ethical obligation to present information and allow a patient to give consent.

What if the patient lacks the capacity to make intelligent decisions on his or her own? For example, what happens if the patient is unconscious or intoxicated but requires emergency treatment, such as surgery, to save his or her life? These kinds of issues are discussed below.

Exceptions to the Requirement of Informed Consent

All laws and rules have exceptions, and these exceptions vary from state to state. This is true of the requirement to obtain informed consent. In some cases, obtaining consent from the patient is not realistic. One well-recognized exception that allows non-consent to medical treatment is medical emergencies. In a medical emergency, for example, a patient may be unconscious, disoriented, sedated, or otherwise incapable of giving consent. Under these circumstances, the law generally allows professionals to presume that the patient would want his or her life and/or functions to be preserved. In the case of an unconscious patient in an emergency, the concept of implied consent is also extended to so-called "Good Samaritans" (Figure 9.3).

decision-making capacity
the patient's ability to make a specific decision at a point in time

Assessing a Patient's Decision-Making Capacity

Decision-making capacity (DMC) refers to the patient's ability to make a specific decision at a point in time. Medical DMC exists when the patient is able to comprehend information about the medical condition

---

Good Samaritan Law

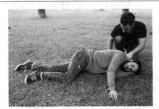

In medical terms, a *Good Samaritan* is a healthcare professional who voluntarily helps an individual in need of emergency treatment. The help must be given without desire for compensation. If the medical professional sends a bill to the victim for compensation, the act is no longer considered one of a Good Samaritan. The Good Samaritan Law offers legal protection to someone who renders aid in an emergency to an injured person on a voluntary basis. A common myth is that healthcare providers will be sued if they stop to help a stranger in need, but such lawsuits are uncommon. If healthcare professionals are sued, they are likely to win.

alex cambero rodriguez/Shutterstock.com

Figure 9.3   An explanation of the Good Samaritan Law.

and its consequences, to reason and consider various options, to make a choice consistent with his or her values and beliefs, and to communicate this choice consistently over time. These decisions are based on the patient's cognitive and physical functioning and the situation in terms of risks and outcomes. The ethical issues of autonomy, beneficence, and informed consent need to be considered.

The principle of autonomy requires a healthcare professional to respect a patient's decision. However, a patient's ability to make sound decisions about his or her health may be impaired by illness or medications. The patient may make choices that are not in his or her best interests and inadvertently cause harm.

As you may recall from Chapter 2, the ethical principle of beneficence requires a professional to act in the patient's best interests. A professional may make decisions that go against the patient's will to protect the patient from harm. Sometimes, tension arises as professionals attempt to maintain patient autonomy and beneficence while determining the best course of action.

Ultimately, the one who decides a patient's decision-making capacity is the attending provider. According to the University of California San Francisco School of Medicine, there are three questions that professionals should consider when determining whether a patient has decision-making capacity. These include whether the patient understands the information given, whether the patient comprehends the consequences of his or her decisions, and whether the patient is using logic to make a decision.

There are tools to help healthcare professionals determine whether the patient is able to direct his or her healthcare. These tools, which may include flowcharts and patient interviews, can be helpful in a non-emergency situation. In an emergency situation, however, there may not be time to consult with others, such as mental health specialists or lawyers. In an emergency, the professional must quickly make the best decision he or she can.

Religious beliefs are accepted by healthcare professionals as valid reasons for an adult to refuse medical treatment. Nevertheless, it must be established that the patient held the same religious beliefs before the proposed treatment and that he or she is not experiencing delusions.

Surrogate Decision Makers

A **surrogate decision maker** is a person who has been entrusted by the once competent patient to make decisions on the patient's behalf when the patient is not able to make those decisions (Figure 9.4). The moral principle behind a surrogate is respect for autonomy and beneficence. The decision maker must reasonably decide

surrogate decision maker
a person who has been entrusted by a once competent patient to make decisions on the patient's behalf when he or she is unable to make those decisions

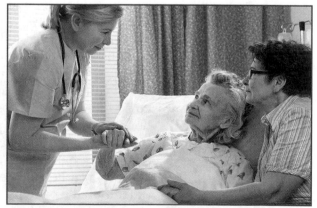

Alexander Raths/Shutterstock.com

Figure 9.4 An elderly patient might choose a son or daughter to be a surrogate decision maker.

which medical procedures the patient would have wanted and what a reasonable person would do in the given circumstances.

The Extension Doctrine

Sometimes, when a patient is undergoing a procedure for which he or she provided consent, additional issues that were not previously known arise and must be dealt with immediately. If it is not feasible at that time to obtain consent for further treatment from the patient, will the provider be held liable for performing this additional procedure? The **extension doctrine** states that if a professional deems an additional procedure to be medically necessary, then the original consent can be extended to cover the unexpected issue.

Consider this example. Dr. Young discovered a hernia on patient Tonya Kennedy while performing an appendectomy. When Dr. Young made this discovery, Kennedy was already under anesthetic and there was no authorized person present to speak on her behalf. Young decided that the hernia must be fixed as part of the appendectomy operation. Had Young not done so, the hernia would have continued to get worse and Ms. Kennedy's health would have been jeopardized.

After the operation, Ms. Kennedy stated that she had to undergo considerable pain and suffering on account of the hernia operation. She filed a civil suit to recover damages for personal injuries resulting from an alleged unauthorized operation performed by the defendant, Dr. Young. The courts could rule in Dr. Young's favor and drop the charges because the extension doctrine applies.

extension doctrine
statute that allows a healthcare professional to extend a patient's original consent to a procedure in an extenuating circumstance when further issues occur during the original procedure

Confidentiality

Confidentiality is central to creating and sustaining trust between healthcare professionals and patients. As discussed in Chapter 2, the original source of a doctor's duty to maintain confidentiality is the Hippocratic Oath. Patients have a right to expect that information about them be held in confidence by their healthcare providers. Confidentiality allows patients to fully disclose information about their conditions without fear of others learning that information.

If full disclosure does not occur, then the professional may not be able to correctly diagnose and treat the patient. In return for the patient's honesty, the healthcare professional must not share confidential information without the patient's express consent unless it falls within one of the exceptions to the rule. These include court orders and threats of self-harm.

When a healthcare professional discloses information to a person other than the patient without the patient's consent or a court order, he or she has committed a breach of confidentiality, even if done accidentally. This disclosure can occur in many ways, including electronically, orally, by fax, or by phone (Figure 9.5). The method of the breach does not matter.

Exceptions to the Confidentiality Rule

In certain circumstances, it is legal to share confidential patient health information. Whenever possible, patients should be informed about such disclosures, but their consent is not required.

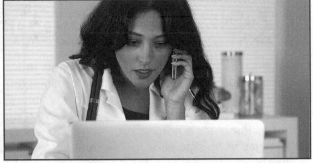

Rocketclips, Inc./Shutterstock.com

Figure 9.5 Healthcare professionals must be careful that the information they share over the phone is not confidential.

Court Order

Patient records are sometimes opened to third parties because of a court order, but information may be shared only as outlined in the order. For example, the court may permit prosecutors who are investigating a provider for criminal activity to examine that provider's records. A court also may allow prosecutors to examine the medical record of a patient who is being investigated for a crime. In these situations, the courts have concluded that an important public good is served by the breach of confidentiality.

Statutory Requirement

Every state requires that certain conditions be reported to legal authorities. This type of breach is generally viewed as being in the best interest of the public, and that interest overrides the patient's confidentiality. For example, gunshot injuries, child sexual abuse, and elder abuse are reportable conditions in most states.

The duty to report these conditions does not always apply to physicians only. In cases of child abuse, for example, various types of healthcare professionals are considered mandatory reporters and therefore are required to notify authorities about these situations (see Chapter 6 for a detailed discussion of mandatory reporting). Healthcare professionals also may be required to share medical records and/or appear in court.

Another example of statutory requirement is the notification of certain serious communicable diseases. Public health agencies, such as county health departments and the Centers for Disease Control and Prevention, monitor the incidence (new cases) and prevalence (the total number of cases) of certain diseases. This monitoring process requires access to medical information.

There are numerous **notifiable diseases**, such as the measles and human immunodeficiency virus (HIV), that healthcare professionals and laboratories must report to certain agencies to protect the health of the public. Healthcare professionals are open to both criminal and civil penalties if they do not report injuries or diseases specified by statute. Those who fail to report also may have their license revoked or suspended.

notifiable diseases conditions that are required by law to be reported to government authorities

Ethical Dilemma

Legislation has been established that allows parents to assertively intervene with nature and take advantage of science to create a child or terminate a pregnancy. While this can be a positive experience for all involved, there are some ethical challenges.

Does the decision to artificially create a child give a woman a greater right to terminate the pregnancy if it is determined early that the embryo is, for instance, female instead of male? What are your duties as a practitioner? Does the mother's autonomy and decision to abort require you to provide treatment? When do assisted conception and right to abortion procedures become genetic selection, and does it matter?

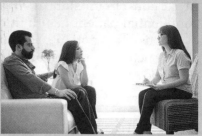

antoniodiaz/Shutterstock.com

Threats of Self-Harm

If a patient threatens harm against himself or herself, there can be ethical and legal reasons for disclosing that information to a third party to help prevent that harm from occurring. For example, if a patient threatens suicide, the healthcare professional must breach confidentiality and disclose the name of the person and the information about the potential harm to a third party. Justification for the breach of confidentiality exists if the professional had reason to believe that this disclosure would help prevent the harm.

Endangered Third Parties

Endangered third parties are involved in dangers such as infectious disease and violence that will harm people other than the patient. Healthcare professionals have a duty to warn third parties when they have reason to believe that a patient may harm them.

For example, if a patient informs a healthcare professional of the intent to cause bodily injury to an ex-spouse, the professional has a duty to warn the person at risk. This is why some practitioners inform patients at the beginning of professional relationships that they will be obliged to disclose threats of harm.

There are still questions related to the duty to warn people about diseases such as tuberculosis and HIV. In some states, certain diseases may be reported to a public health agency that will warn people of possible exposure to a communicable disease. In these situations, a physician's duty to warn is, in practice, limited to reporting his or her affected patients to the relevant state agency.

Confidentiality for Minors

Confidentiality for minors is different from confidentiality for adults in terms of both ethics and the law. In most cases, healthcare professionals should involve the parents or legal guardian(s) in the treatment of and decision-making process for minors.

However, there are certain decisions that minors can make without the consent of their parents or legal guardian(s). For these decisions, minors are entitled to the same confidentiality as adults. These decisions and the age at which they can be made vary by state. For example, in Illinois, children who are 12 years of age and older may receive treatment for sexually transmitted infections, drug use, and alcohol use without parental notification or consent.

Patient Advocates

A patient advocate serves as a liaison between the patient and anyone who is involved in the patient's healthcare. The advocate may be the patient's point of contact with healthcare professionals. The advocate also may communicate with social service agencies, legal counsel, and insurance companies on the patient's behalf (Figure 9.6). In general, the patient advocate ensures that the patient receives the medical attention he or she needs. The advocate also seeks to protect the patient from any discrimination in the workplace due to a medical condition.

Because patients are not always able to advocate for themselves due to illness or other reasons, all caregivers have the responsibility to be patient advocates. This means that healthcare professionals also must act as patient advocates. The duty of patient advocacy is a fundamental element of the patient-professional relationship and derives from the ethical principle of beneficence. Healthcare professionals must place the interests of their patients first. If healthcare professionals are not advocates, then there can be very serious consequences, including a patient's death.

Patient advocacy can be accomplished by caregivers within their areas of expertise and responsibility. For example, a nurse can alert the physician about an order for a medication that the patient is allergic to, a nurse's aide can report patient neglect or unsanitary conditions, a surgical technician can insist that surgical

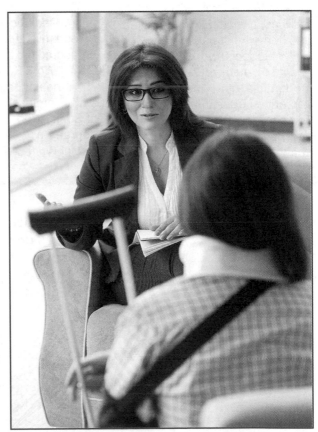

Elnur/Shutterstock.com

Figure 9.6 Healthcare professionals have a responsibility to advocate for their patients.

Career Corner

Social workers work with individuals, families, and communities. They can have roles as educators, therapists, researchers, managers, supervisors, teachers, advocates, and administrators. Social workers can be found in many different settings, such as public agencies, private businesses, hospitals, schools, private practices, police departments, nursing homes, and prisons. Clinical or public health social workers can offer their services in any facility that provides care to patients. This includes hospitals, emergency rooms, hospices, nursing homes, rehabilitation facilities, assisted-living facilities, and home health agencies.

The social work profession has its own ethical standards, credentials, state licensing, and accredited education programs. To become a social worker, a degree in social work from an academic institution with an

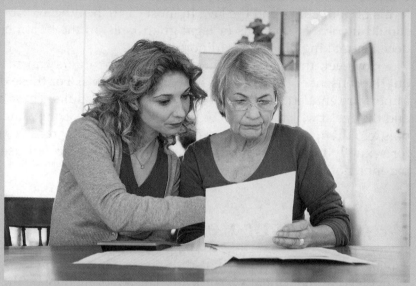

Image Point Fr/Shutterstock.com

accredited social work program is required. The program must be accredited by the Council on Social Work Education.

The undergraduate degree for this profession is the Bachelor of Social Work (BSW). Graduate degrees include the Master of Social Work (MSW), the Doctor

of Social Work (DSW), and the PhD. An MSW is required to provide therapy. Academic programs involve coursework and practical field experience. Most states require practicing social workers to be licensed, certified, or registered, although state requirements vary.

equipment be sterilized properly before use, and a physical therapist can submit additional documentation if an insurance company denies medically necessary treatments.. In addition to individual advocacy efforts, several organizations provide patient advocacy services, such as the National Patient Advocacy Foundation and Compassion & Choices.

Refusal of Medical Treatment

Healthcare providers are trained to save lives. So what if patients do not want treatment or do not want their life saved? What if a patient prefers to end his or her life rather than endure the pain and suffering of a medical condition?

When patients refuse life-sustaining or emergency treatment, the healthcare professional must choose between two unappealing options:

(1) to not provide beneficial treatment, or (2) to force treatment on a competent but unwilling patient. Both of these actions have potential ethical and legal consequences. Providing lifesaving treatment when a competent patient has declined treatment can result in lawsuits for battery, medical negligence, and lack of informed consent.

When treatment is refused, providers need to decide whether the patient has a sound decision-making capacity. This includes determining if the patient understands the consequences of refusing treatment. In some cases, allowing for death with dignity may be just as important as saving a patient's life.

Abandonment

In healthcare, the term **abandonment** refers to termination of the patient-professional relationship in a manner that denies the patient necessary medical care. This occurs when a professional withdraws treatment without giving the patient reasonable notice or providing a competent replacement (Figure 9.7). To be considered abandonment, the relationship's termination must have been brought about by the professional only. Abandonment does not occur if the relationship is terminated by mutual consent, by the dismissal of the professional by the patient, or if the healthcare professional gives appropriate notice to the patient.

abandonment
termination of the patient-professional relationship in a manner that denies the patient necessary medical care

Abandonment also can occur with nurses and other allied healthcare professionals. For example, if a nurse fails to give reasonable notice that he or she intends to terminate the employer/employee relationship or contract, which will lead to serious impairment in the delivery of professional care to patients, then patient abandonment can occur.

Abandonment can be intentional or inadvertent. *Intentional abandonment* is legally riskier because a jury may choose to award punitive damages as punishment for intentionally putting a patient's health at risk. For example, intentional abandonment can occur if the provider terminates the relationship because he or she has not been paid for services. This is viewed by juries as a weak reason to abandon a patient.

Inadvertent abandonment can occur because of misunderstandings, such as a physician who does not have backup coverage while attending to another medical emergency. If a provider works with a medical group, for example, and the colleague who is supposed to be on call does not show up, then the provider may need to abandon his or her patients to handle emergency calls.

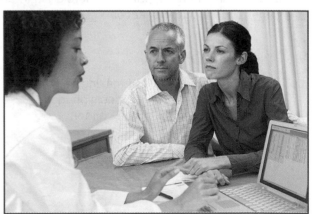

Monkey Business Images/Shutterstock.com

Figure 9.7   If a healthcare professional terminates care without giving his or her patient sufficient notice, this is called *abandonment* and can lead to legal proceedings.

Chapter Summary

- Informed consent is a patient's consent to a procedure or course of action after being informed of its risks and benefits.
- Confidentiality between a patient and a healthcare provider is intended to allow the patient to feel comfortable providing sensitive information that the provider may need in order to diagnose and treat a problem.
- All healthcare professionals are, to some extent, patient advocates.
- When a patient refuses medical treatment, the healthcare provider is faced with both legal and ethical issues.
- If a healthcare provider ends a patient-provider relationship in a way that denies the patient necessary medical care, the provider can face accusations of abandonment.

Vocabulary Matching

1. statute that allows a healthcare professional to extend a patient's original consent to a procedure in an extenuating circumstance when further issues occur during the original procedure
2. person who has been entrusted by a once competent patient to make decisions on the patient's behalf when he or she is unable to make those decisions
3. patient's ability to make a specific decision at a point in time
4. patient action that leads to the presumption that medical care has been authorized
5. termination of the patient-professional relationship in a manner that denies the patient necessary medical care
6. conditions that are required by law to be reported to government authorities
7. verbal or written authorization for care
8. consent given after a patient understands the risks and benefits of a treatment or course of action

A. abandonment
B. decision-making capacity
C. express consent
D. extension doctrine
E. implied consent
F. informed consent
G. notifiable diseases
H. surrogate decision maker

Multiple Choice

9. If a patient is incapable of making healthcare decisions, then a(n) _____ decision maker may make decisions for the patient.
   A. temporary
   B. provisional
   C. surrogate
   D. conditional

10. A doctor who is performing surgery on a patient determines that another procedure needs to be done in addition to the procedure for which patient consent was obtained. The _____ could apply to this situation.
    A. consent doctrine
    B. extension doctrine
    C. expansion doctrine
    D. augmentation doctrine

11. Infectious diseases that must be reported to public health agencies are called _____ diseases.
    A. notifiable
    B. reportable
    C. mandatory
    D. cautionary

Completion

12. Implied consent and _____ are the two types of consent.

13. The _____ law protects healthcare professionals who attempt to assist a person who is not their patient in an emergency situation.

14. A physician is frustrated with a patient who has not paid her bill. The physician decides to stop treating the patient and informs staff not to schedule any further appointments for her. This physician may be liable for _____.

Discussion and Critical Thinking

15. Review the scenario presented at the beginning of the chapter. If you were the clinical social worker, what should you do in this situation? Should you continue trying to talk to the man? Should you be concerned about any legal or ethical violations? If yes, describe the violations that might be involved.

16. Why is consent required before a patient receives medical care? What forms of consent are acceptable?

17. Define the term *abandonment* and explain appropriate reasons and the process for a provider to discontinue care.

18. In what situations, if any, can a healthcare professional breach a patient's confidentiality?

19. Religious beliefs are accepted as valid reasons for an adult to refuse medical treatment. Do agree with this? Explain your reasoning.

20. Explain the ways in which informed consent can be given, and provide examples.

21. What is the purpose of the extension doctrine?

22. Describe ways in which healthcare professionals can be patient advocates.

Activities

23. When Donald "Dax" Cowart was 25 years old, he was severely burned in a propane gas explosion. Dax had third-degree burns over 68 percent of his body. Two psychologists found Dax competent and able to refuse care. Dax's physicians argued that he lacked decision-making capacity (DMC) and so could not reject treatment. Mr. Cowart is now a lawyer who advocates for patients' right to refuse care. He asserts that his right to refuse treatment and die was violated. Read the case study about Dax on the University of Washington School of Medicine website. Watch the YouTube video called "Dax Cowart 2002 1." Then consider the following questions.

    Should people like Dax be allowed to die? If so, when should they be allowed to die? If not, why should people have to go through painful treatments and experience a lesser quality of life? What role do patient advocates play in this scenario? Write a paper that includes your responses to these questions, incorporating laws and ethics to support your views.

Case Study

An 80-year-old man is diagnosed with diabetes while in the hospital. He also has Alzheimer's and his decision-making capacity is determined by lucid intervals, during which he is considered capable. Oral medications are not effective at controlling his blood sugar levels, so you also prescribe him insulin injections. You tell him this and instruct the medical staff that he should be given insulin three times a day. In the morning, the patient agrees to receive the shots. In the evening, when the patient is disoriented, he does not want the insulin injection. When the patient is again lucid and cannot recall the events of the evening, he agrees to receive the insulin. Is the patient competent to make his own medical decisions? What should be done to ensure that the patient receives his insulin injections on time?

Chapter 10

Health Information Technology

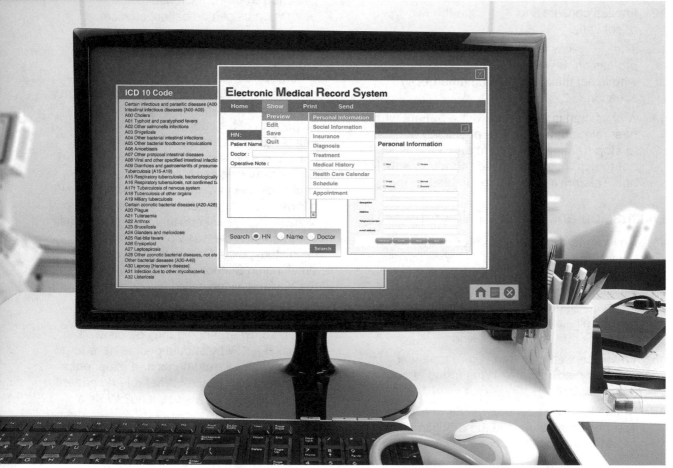

pandpstock001/Shutterstock.com

Chapter Outline

The Use of Health Records

Electronic Medical and Health Records

Legal Implications of Electronic Health Records

Telehealth and Telemedicine

Legal Implications of Telemedicine

Legal Implications of Telehealth

Regulating Mobile Technology

Sharing Data for Research

Reporting a Security Breach

The Privacy Act

The Health Insurance Portability and Accountability Act (HIPAA)

The Health Information Technology for Economic and Clinical Health (HITECH) Act

Data Disposal Laws

Objectives

- Describe the use of electronic medical records and electronic health records, and the legal implications of their use.
- Explain the legal implications of telemedicine, telehealth, and the use of mobile technology in healthcare.
- Identify the pros and cons of sharing data for research and the related legal issues.
- Explain how security breaches can be prevented and how to respond to them when they do occur.
- Describe laws pertaining to the disposal of personal identifying information and other sensitive data.

Key Terms

breach
discovery
e-discovery
electronic health record
electronic medical record
encryption
health information technology
interoperability
personal health record
protected health information
sanctions
telehealth
telemedicine

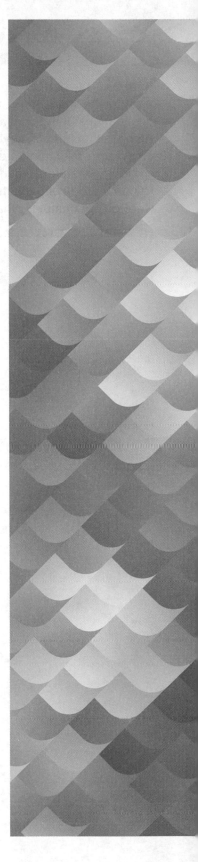

What Would You Do?

Suppose a thief throws a rock through the window of an occupational therapy clinic. Along with monitors, keyboards, and other equipment, a desktop computer is stolen. Records from hundreds of patients were on the computer that was stolen. The data included personal information such as names, addresses, dates of birth, phone numbers, and email addresses. Information related to medical diagnoses and procedures also was included. The data was not encrypted. Because the data was housed on a computer in the building, did the clinic violate any laws? Imagine that you are the clinic's manager. What steps should you and the organization take in response to the theft?

This is an exciting time of change in the field of healthcare. The way that healthcare is being delivered and managed is rapidly changing due to technological advances. New systems and devices are making it much more convenient for healthcare providers and organizations to locate, share, and store patient information. The concept of healthcare providers carrying around folders is obsolete. Instead, they are carrying smartphones and tablets and logging into electronic medical records systems. Technology is revolutionizing healthcare, and this change is happening quickly. However, new challenges come with this opportunity.

health information technology
term for the technical aspects of processing health information

Health information technology (HIT) is the overarching term used to describe the secure management of health information exchanged across computerized systems and between consumers, healthcare providers, insurance companies, healthcare and government organizations, and other entities. This includes many types of health information ranging in complexity from a simple electronic mail (email) exchange between a provider and patient to a situation in which a physician several thousands of miles away provides care to a patient using videoconferencing software (Figure 10.1).

HIT capabilities and utilization have experienced tremendous growth in the recent decade for a variety of reasons. Growth has occurred due to advances in technology, the need to reduce healthcare costs, the lack of healthcare providers in certain specialties and geographic regions, the desire to improve quality of care, patient expectations, and federal funds being allocated to healthcare technology.

HIT has the potential to improve health at the community level. If the data collected by HIT is aggregated, the information can be used to track infectious diseases to prevent and treat outbreaks; assist with developing and improving public health programs and services; gain knowledge about the causes and treatment of illness; and help prevent illness through education, improved services, research, and targeted intervention efforts.

The evolution of HIT creates new challenges as well because the privacy of patients needs to be protected. Laws related to the transfer of information and methods of providing services are changing. New laws have been created and existing ones have been altered and expanded.

This chapter describes two major areas of HIT and the related legal and ethical issues: electronic medical and health records and telehealth. These technologies have altered the way services are delivered and information is shared and utilized. The chapter also addresses data sharing for research and the process of reporting security breaches.

Overall, while HIT promises to improve quality, reduce cost, and increase access to care, it presents the practitioner with the ability to violate established ethical and legal standards instantly and on a massive scale unimagined by earlier generations. Specific rules are evolving to address the new technology, but the general laws and ethics remain essentially the same.

The Use of Health Records

In past generations, patients were not allowed access to their personal health records. This stemmed from a paternalistic belief that the doctor knows best, the records belonged to the doctor, and people would not understand the information anyway. However, it is now established that the medical information about a patient belongs to that patient. The provider owns the information regarding the business aspects of delivering care and has responsibility for the storage and care of the patient information in its custody.

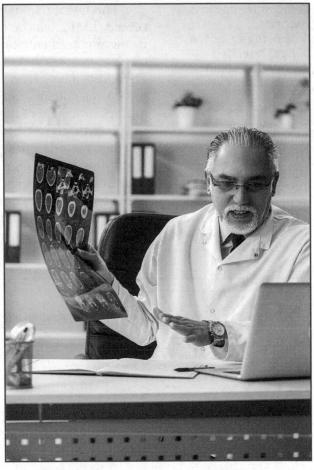

Elnur/Shutterstock.com

Figure 10.1 Health information technology includes many formats, such as videoconferencing, through which healthcare workers interact with patients and technology.

Electronic Medical and Health Records

The Health Information Technology for Economic and Clinical Health (HITECH) Act was created by Congress to stimulate the adoption and utilization of **electronic health records** (EHR) in the United States. The HITECH Act states that, between 2011 and 2015, healthcare providers were offered financial incentives for demonstrating meaningful use of EHR. The act also provides grant money for workforce training in HIT to support health-related IT infrastructure.

electronic health record
an electronic record of health-related information about an individual that conforms to nationally recognized interoperability standards and that is created, managed, and consulted by authorized clinicians and staff in more than one agency

electronic medical record
an electronic record of health-related information about an individual that is created, managed, and consulted by authorized clinicians and staff within one healthcare organization

interoperability
the ability of systems to work and communicate with each other, usually achieved by conforming to standards

The term *EHR* is often confused with the term **electronic medical record** (EMR), but the terms have different meanings. An EMR is the electronic replacement for paper medical charts. It is essentially the physician's own notes that record an encounter with a patient in his or her office. Therefore, it is a record of that one medical visit. An EHR is an aggregated record of a patient's health information over a period of time. It documents multiple encounters that occur in various healthcare delivery settings.

Essentially, an EMR records care that occurs in one setting, while an EHR records multiple providers administering multiple services in multiple settings (Figure 10.2). For example, the EHR may include information from radiology reports, laboratory results, office visits, and visits to the emergency department. For this to occur, the computer systems of different organizations need to be able to communicate with one another. This capability is referred to as **interoperability**.

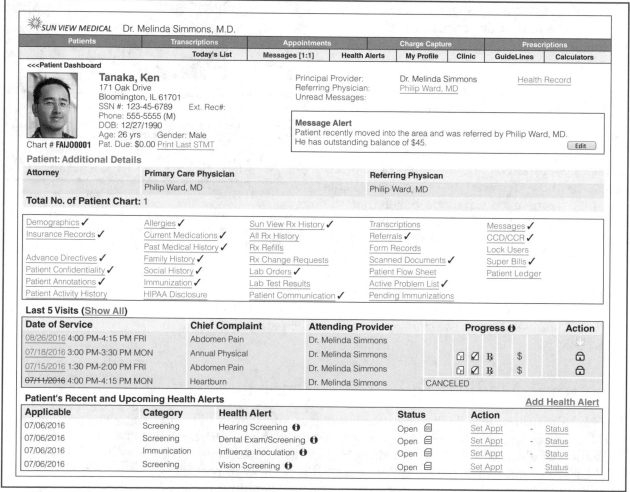

Goodheart-Willcox Publisher

Figure 10.2   An electronic health record usually includes a face page, shown here, which shows a patient's contact information, insurance information, and medical history.

Another term associated with EMR and EHR is the **personal health record** (PHR). A PHR is a collection of information about your health. An electronic PHR simply replaces the box or folder of medical papers that you may already keep for yourself. Because a PHR is kept in an electronic format, it can be accessed at any time on a computer, protected website, or external device that you can carry with you.

The difference between PHR, EMR, and EHR is that you own and control the information contained in the PHR. Some of the information in your PHR may be provided by your health plan or your doctor, but you also may enter information on your own. Doctors and healthcare facilities have control over EHR and EMR maintained in the office, while individuals have control over PHR.

One argument for implementing EHR is that electronic records potentially enhance patient care and therefore minimize malpractice lawsuits. Yet EHR can create new practice standards that have implications for malpractice claims. Standards for timeliness of care, accuracy, security, and privacy may affect the practitioner who uses or does not use EHR and HIT in general. These new standards mean that a provider who implements EHR may experience benefits related to malpractice. Likewise, a provider who chooses not to implement EHR may experience disadvantages as a result of that choice.

The Medical Records Institute conducted a survey in which almost 20 percent of respondents reported receiving malpractice insurance discounts because they implemented EHR. Almost half of respondents reported that using an EHR system reduced their perceived likelihood of encountering a malpractice claim. Twenty percent of respondents with EHR were involved in a malpractice case, and more than 50 percent of them reported EHR as helpful in their defense. The reasons include, but certainly are not limited to, improved automated notifications of laboratory or other test results, improved information transfer between providers, and the ability to read the providers' notes (handwriting can be illegible).

While EHR systems can be helpful to providers, they also can pose challenges if steps are not taken to protect data and thus ensure patient privacy and confidentiality (Figure 10.3). There also is a continued dispute over the ownership of health data, which is discussed further in the section about sharing data for research.

personal health record
an electronic record of health-related information about an individual that conforms to nationally recognized interoperability standards and is controlled by the individual

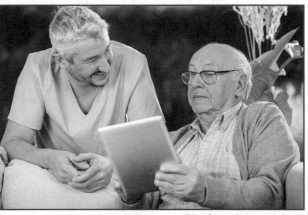

Tyler Olson/Shutterstock.com

Figure 10.3 Healthcare workers such as this home health aide need to ensure that information they access and store through electronic media is secure.

Legal Implications of Electronic Health Records

In an article for the *New England Journal of Medicine*, authors Mangal-murti, Murtagh, and Mello noted that the legal risks and benefits of EHR vary between the stages of implementation and mature use. A facility experiences different medical and legal concerns when the EHR system is first being implemented than when the system is more mature and has been utilized for some time.

Some of the legal issues that they identified in the implementation stage include:

- incomplete transfer of documents
- errors made by new users that may lead to incorrect or missing entries
- problems, or bugs, with the overall system that can lead to errors
- inconsistent use by clinicians that can lead to miscommunication and missing documentation
- missed information due to information overload or not knowing where to find it
- misuse or misinterpretation of clinical decision support tools (such as practice guidelines or medication alerts)

Once the implementation stage has passed, the benefits of EHR become clear. In the mature stage, during which staff members have been using EHR for some time, these benefits include:

- a reduction of errors in care
- adherence to clinical support recommendations, which may improve patient care and protect clinicians from liability
- improved documentation that may prevent errors and help provide a defense against malpractice claims

While this is not an exhaustive list, it does show that there tend to be more risks during the implementation phase and more protection during the mature phase.

If a malpractice claim is filed, the **discovery** process in litigation that involves EHR is different from the process with paper files. During the discovery process, each party is permitted to request information about the case from the other. In medical cases, this usually involves sharing clinical information. Now that many types of business records exist in electronic formats, the term **e-discovery** has become more prevalent.

In April 2006, the US Supreme Court approved amendments to the Federal Rules of Civil Procedure that were aimed at the unique aspects of e-discovery. These amendments took effect on December 1, 2006, and they apply to all litigation in the federal court system. These

discovery
term that describes the pretrial stage of litigation in which both parties of the lawsuit identify information about the case

e-discovery
a process in which electronic data is searched for, located, and secured for the purpose of using it as evidence in a civil or criminal legal case

Ethical Dilemma

One of Dr. Ross's patients was admitted to the emergency room after experiencing a reaction to his medication. The Chief Medical Officer (CMO) of the hospital reviewed the case and saw that the patient was allergic to the medication that Dr. Ross prescribed. The CMO asked a health informatics professional to review the technological breakdown of this prescription.

The CMO wants to know if Dr. Ross was alerted about his patient's allergy. The hospital uses a decision support system that can issue alerts in case of a medication allergy, if a patient is due for a test, or another specified condition. A health informatics professional, who works with health-related IT systems, can check this system to better understand errors. After reviewing the patient's history, the health informatics professional tells the CMO that Dr. Ross overrode the alert

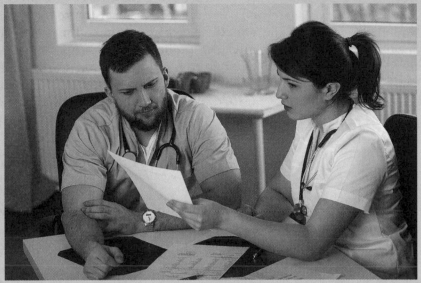

Photographee.eu/Shutterstock.com

about the patient's medication allergy.

With this information, the CMO meets with Dr. Ross to discuss the error. Dr. Ross becomes defensive, saying that he went to medical school and the computer did not. He explains that this patient was a rare accident. Dr. Ross says

he does not like the alerts, stating that there are too many of them and that they just waste time.

Is Dr. Ross behaving unethically by ignoring the alerts? Should the CMO insist that Dr. Ross review the alerts and note why he elects to override them?

amendments change trial preparation and data management practices. For example, the amendments affect how data is stored and how long it is retained.

For the first time, as a result of these amendments, electronic records explicitly included emails and instant message interactions as likely records to be archived and produced when relevant. State courts handle healthcare litigation such as malpractice claims. The states are using the federal e-discovery rule as a foundation for their laws.

It is best to learn about e-discovery laws prior to a claim being filed so that you and your organization can establish ways to adhere to the requirements if a claim is filed. This will likely involve the development of policy and procedures related to data management and storage. Examples include the timing of when emails are deleted and how data is organized so that electronic information can be easily retrieved and produced during the e-discovery process.

Failure to disclose or produce relevant information can result in **sanctions**, which are punishments. If the information was unintentionally lost, perhaps through normal destruction processes that occurred prior to knowledge of impending litigation, then an exception may be made. However, if relevant information was destroyed after learning of impending litigation, sanctions could be applied.

sanctions
a term that, in criminal law, describes the punishment for a criminal offense

Telehealth and Telemedicine

telehealth
the use of a telecommunications system to deliver health-related services and information

telemedicine
the use of technology to facilitate clinical care at a distance

The terms **telehealth** and **telemedicine** are sometimes used interchangeably, but they have different meanings. Telehealth (also known as *eHealth*) is the delivery of health-related services and information using telecommunications technologies. Telehealth includes long-distance encounters that use technology such as remote patient monitoring, virtual support groups, health websites, and social media technologies to provide health information (Figure 10.4).

Telemedicine is limited to the use of technology for facilitating clinical care at a distance, while telehealth encompasses all applications of technology in the healthcare field, such as health behavior support groups (Figure 10.5). Types of telemedicine include the following:

- **Telepsychiatry**—gives patients access to psychiatric services through technology such as videoconferencing

- **Teleradiology**—the transmission of X-rays, computed tomography (CT) scans, or magnetic resonance images (MRIs) using email, websites, or other technology

- **Telepathology**—allows images of pathology slides to be sent from one location to another for diagnostic consultation

- **Tele-ICU**—creates a link between a remote critical care team and an intensive care unit (ICU) in a different location to provide consultation to assist the ICU bedside team in providing care to the patient

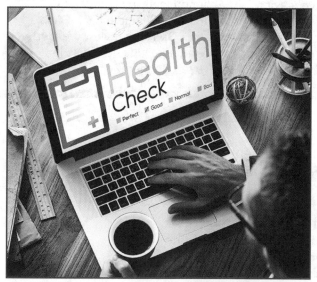

Rawpixel/Shutterstock.com

Figure 10.4 Telehealth includes various technological ways of spreading health information, including websites.

The same standards of care for treating patients by the bedside apply to treating patients from a distance using telemedicine.

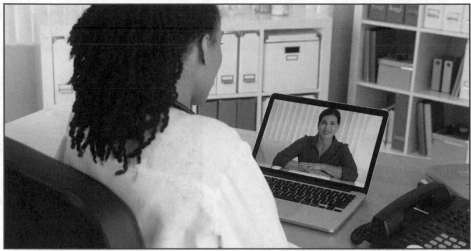

Rocketclips, Inc./Shutterstock.com

Figure 10.5   Through telemedicine, healthcare providers can reach patients who may be housebound or live in remote areas.

Legal Implications of Telemedicine

The legal challenges involved in using telemedicine include the issue of practicing medicine across state lines. For example, say a physician physically practices medicine in his home state but would like to provide tele-ICU services to patients in five other states. If licensure were required in all six states, the doctor would be required to complete one in-state and five out-of-state licensure applications. This process entails completing six sets of accompanying documentation and paying six registration fees.

To assist with addressing this barrier, the Interstate Medical Licensure Compact (IMLC) has been established. The IMLC agreement allows providers in the compact states to practice telehealth in multiple states. As of 2019, 25 states are part of the IMLC, which gives physicians an expedited means of applying for a license to practice telehealth in member states.

Another agreement, the Physical Therapy Compact, developed by the Federation of State Boards of Physical Therapy for physical therapists and physical therapist assistants, became effective on July 9, 2018. Nine states are active as of 2019. Another 12 states have enacted legislation but are not yet processing licenses.

The interstate compact process has allowed for interstate practice among member jurisdictions but has not solved all related legal complexities. For instance, practitioners may need to consider the complexity involved in working in states that do not have the same time period during which patients may bring malpractice claims (defined as *statutes of limitations*). In addition, insurance companies may not cover all

Career Corner

Health informatics professionals have various roles and responsibilities, and the field includes opportunities for people with a broad range of interests and skills. For example, people with technical interests can be designers, developers, programmers, or focus on security. Those with clinical interests can be researchers or workflow designers. People who like game design can create health-related games. Researchers can conduct evaluations of technologies, assess quality improvement, or assess cost effectiveness. There also are many sub-specialties in this field, including public health, consumer, clinical, pharmaceutical, biomedical, and nursing informatics.

The educational background required for these positions ranges from a certification to a doctorate degree. Professional organizations, community colleges, and universities offer certifications. Colleges and universities also offer bachelor's and graduate degrees in health informatics.

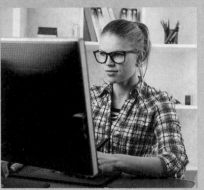

Stasique/Shutterstock.com

jurisdictions, nor do all insurance policies cover telemedicine. Further, there may be practical considerations of how to engage with lawyers licensed in different states and attending court hearings in distant geographic locations.

States also regulate nursing licenses and place similar restrictions on interstate care performed by nurses. The Nurse Licensure Compact helps solve the problems associated with interstate licensing. The Nurse Licensure Compact is a process through which states authorize a nurse licensed and residing in a Compact (home) State to practice in other Compact (remote) States without obtaining additional licensure. Therefore, nurses only need to be licensed once, and their licensure is then recognized in the Compact States. As of 2019, there were 34 Compact States that use this process.

The privilege given through the Nurse Licensure Compact requires nurses to comply with the laws and regulations of the state in which they practice nursing or provide care (where the patient is located). Nursing practice includes patient care as well as all nursing practice as defined by each Compact State's practice laws. The Nurse Licensure Compact affects only licensure and practice among those states that have joined the Compact. The nurse must maintain a nursing license in any non-Compact State to practice in that state, even if the nurse resides in a Compact State.

Legal Implications of Telehealth

Telehealth includes a wide range of technologies for various purposes (Figure 10.6). Healthcare professionals may use applications on their smartphone or tablet to look up drug dosing information, review lab and radiology data, or access other medical information. Telehealth examples also include pedometers, asthma monitors, electronic educational resources, and telecoaching. These technologies enhance collection and access to health information by both patient and practitioner.

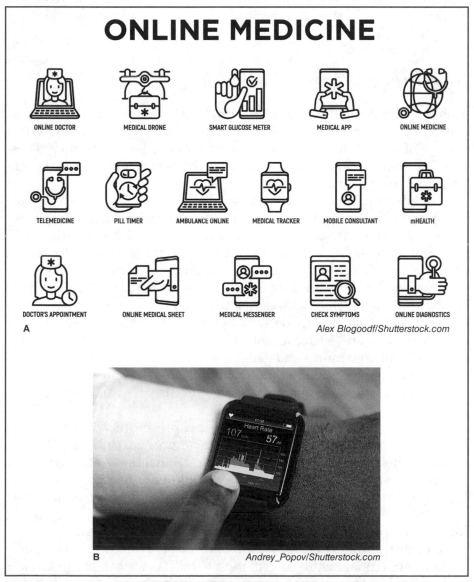

Alex Blogoodf/Shutterstock.com

A

B   Andrey_Popov/Shutterstock.com

Figure 10.6 A—Icons have been developed to show at a glance the various types of telehealth and telemedicine applications available at healthcare facilities. B—Individuals can keep track of their own heart rate, activities, and other health information using a smartwatch.

What are the liability issues related to telehealth? Are non-physicians and physicians liable for posting inaccurate health information on the Internet or dispensing it through electronic communication? Is the developer of a medical application liable if it fails to include vital information?

Many websites, mobile applications, and other electronic modes of communication that provide or transmit medical information include a disclaimer or terms of use. However, these disclaimers may not be enough to protect the validity and enforceability of online agreements and other electronic transactions. Although websites and other telehealth modalities contain terms and conditions that are intended to reduce or eliminate their liability, the laws related to electronic transactions are changing.

Regulating Mobile Technology

mHealth
healthcare-related applications that can be used on smartphones, tablets, and other wireless devices

Mobile technology—also known as **mHealth**, *mobile health*, and *mobile applications*—is another form of telehealth. The term *mHealth* describes the use of mobile devices for medical and public health practice. These mobile devices include smartphones, patient monitoring devices, tablets, and other technology.

Mobile applications are designed for both practitioners and consumers. Practitioners might use drug reference resources, medical image databases, remote access to a patient's medical record, and medical decision support tools (Figure 10.7). Consumers use mHealth apps for a wide range of health activities such as medication reminders, monitoring (such as blood glucose levels or calorie consumption), and the delivery of health information (such as weight loss or healthy pregnancy tips).

mHealth strategies are designed to broaden access to care, improve quality of care, and increase self care, prevention, and early detection abilities. Time constraints and geographic barriers are removed, as these applications can be used anytime and anywhere. They are typically used for diagnosis or disease monitoring. Tests for diseases can be done in the privacy of a patient's home.

These applications also can give people more autonomy over their care. Patients can now check their own heart rate at home or monitor their exercise levels. mHealth applications also have the ability to improve access to care for people who are homebound or live in remote regions. mHealth can be used to improve patient care and safety. For example, some applications are designed to track the location of people with dementia. Medical applications are becoming a central component of medical care, but they are also potentially exposing personal health information to both physical loss of devices and technology-based exploitation from third parties.

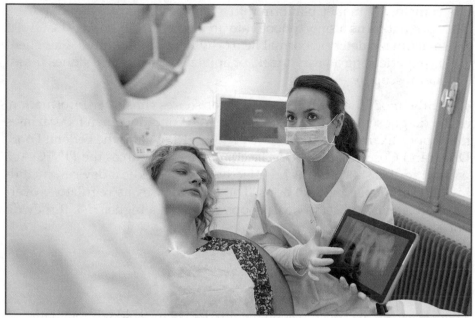

ALPA PROD/Shutterstook.oom

Figure 10.7   Medical apps can be convenient and informative for patients and providers.

Who regulates these applications? What if they fail to detect a disease or send important alerts? The laws surrounding medical applications are still being developed. Who is liable if harm is done— the application developer? Does the case fall under product liability laws?

Certainly not all mobile applications cause alarm if they malfunction. If an application that tracks physical activity or provides access to a medical textbook malfunctions, it is not a life-threatening situation. However, some applications can contribute to serious injury or death. If an application fails to measure blood sugar levels properly or does not include complete side effects of a medication for physicians, serious harm could occur. Some people argue that it is illogical to treat an application malfunction as the cause of a harm because other symptoms would alert the person that something is wrong, even if the application indicates otherwise.

In November 2011, the Food and Drug Administration (FDA) announced that it would regulate certain mHealth applications. This included apps that

- are used as an accessory to an FDA-regulated medical device (an app could enable a healthcare professional to view medical images on a tablet and make a diagnosis)

- transform a mobile platform into a regulated medical device (an app that turns a smartphone into an electrocardiography (ECG) machine to detect abnormal heart rhythms or determine if a patient is experiencing a heart attack, or apps that turn smartphones into stethoscopes).

If the mobile app collects, creates, or shares consumer information, or if it diagnoses or treats a disease or health condition, then federal laws may apply. Examples of those laws include HIPAA and the Federal Food, Drug, and Cosmetic Act (FD&C Act). The FDA enforces the FD&C Act, which regulates the safety and effectiveness of medical devices, including certain mobile medical apps. The FDA focuses its regulatory oversight on a small subset of health apps that pose a higher risk if they do not work as intended.

Sharing Data for Research

There is a growing concern about health data being sold without patients' consent. Some organizations sell data on a regular basis. Doctors do have a legal and ethical responsibility to inform patients about using this system (Figure 10.8). They must give patients the opportunity to opt out of having their information included.

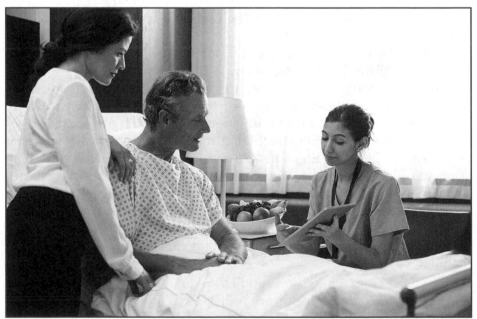

Monkey Business Images/Shutterstock.com

Figure 10.8   Doctors are legally obligated to inform patients when using a records system that collects de-identified health information.

An example is the exemption of health departments from complying with HIPAA regulations. For example, the Texas Department of State Health Services is required by law to collect hospital data from most hospitals in the state. The department shares that information. Between 1999 and 2008, the department shared the data regarding 27.7 million individual patient stays. Those files contained more than 200 data fields. The files are available to purchase in two forms—a research version and a de-identified version. In the research version, complete personal information, including birth dates and dates of care, are included. The de-identified version is free and does not include as much personal information.

While these practices are currently legal, there is much debate about whether they should continue, whether patients should sign informed consent forms prior to data sharing, and whether more regulations are needed.

Reporting a Security Breach

Information security laws, based on the constitutional concepts of privacy and ethical consideration for patient autonomy, are designed to protect individuals from unauthorized people obtaining access to their **protected health information** (PHI). If access does occur, it is referred to as a **breach**. A data breach occurs when there is a loss of, theft of, or other unauthorized access to data that contains sensitive personal information, resulting in the potential loss of confidentiality or integrity of the data.

In this context, a breach is the unauthorized acquisition, access, use, or disclosure of PHI, which compromises the security or privacy of such information. To help prevent this, national standards for securing data have been established (Figure 10.9). This includes **encryption** of data and certain guidelines that are to be followed. PHI is considered unsecured if it is not encrypted or destroyed.

When a breach does occur, state requirements for notification go into effect. These laws vary by state. Data breach notification laws typically cover PHI and require covered entities to implement a breach notification policy. These data breach notification laws include requirements for reporting incidents and notifying external entities.

No single federal law or regulation governs the security of all types of PHI. Determining which federal law, regulation, or guideline is applicable in a situation depends on the entity that collected the information and the type of information. Federal law includes obligations for protecting certain types of sensitive personal information. These obligations require certain facilities and organizations to implement information security programs and provide breach notification to people who are impacted by the breach.

protected health information
all individually identifiable information that is created or received by a healthcare provider or any other entity subject to HIPAA requirements; this information can be oral or written

breach   the unauthorized acquisition, access, use, or disclosure of protected health information that compromises the security or privacy of such information

encryption
the process of translating text into an unintelligible set of characters that can be transmitted with a high degree of security and then decrypted after reaching its secure destination

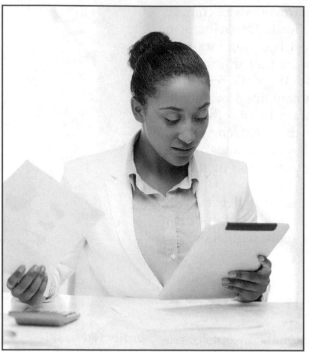

Syda Productions/Shutterstock.com

Figure 10.9 When using electronic health information, all healthcare workers must follow standards for keeping that data secure.

Data breach notification laws include both federal and state laws related to data breaches. The three laws discussed in this section are the Privacy Act, HIPAA, and the HITECH Act. Of course, other laws exist, including state laws and policies held by individual organizations.

The Privacy Act

The Privacy Act covers only federal agencies and records that are in the possession and control of federal agencies. This act, which was created in 1974, protects records that can be retrieved through personal information such as a name, address, or Social Security number. Under this act, an individual is entitled to access his or her records. A person can also request that changes be made to his or her record. The law prohibits disclosure of these records without the written consent of the individual to whom the records pertain. There are 12 disclosure exceptions outlined in the act, including law enforcement request, court order, and health and safety of an individual.

The Health Insurance Portability and Accountability Act (HIPAA)

HIPAA addressed the privacy of PHI and required adoption of a national privacy standard. This is the Standards for Privacy of Individually Identifiable Health Information, known as the *Privacy Rule*. The HIPAA Privacy Rule, effective as of April 2003, applies to health plans, healthcare clearinghouses, and healthcare providers who transfer financial and administrative information electronically.

The rule regulates PHI that is electronically transmitted or maintained, as well as documents on paper and in other formats. PHI does not include individually identifiable health information included in certain education and employment records that a covered entity keeps on file in its role as an employer.

The HIPAA Security Rule creates national standards that protect individuals' electronic PHI (e-PHI). Regulations in this rule include security standards for maintaining administrative, technical, and physical safeguards that ensure the confidentiality, integrity, and availability of e-PHI.

The rule also includes standards for protection against any threats or hazards to the security or integrity of PHI that an entity might reasonably expect. There are also specific standards for protection against any unauthorized uses or disclosures of PHI. The Centers for Medicare and Medicaid Services (CMS) has the authority to enforce the HIPAA Security Rule.

The Health Information Technology for Economic and Clinical Health (HITECH) Act

Before the HITECH Act was passed, the HIPAA Privacy and Security Rules were the only laws that covered PHI. These rules did not require covered entities or their business associates to notify individuals when the security or privacy of their PHI had been compromised. Health record companies were not required to make a breach notification either. The HITECH Act changed that. Now, covered entities, their business associates, and companies that sell health records are all required by law to notify affected individuals in the event of a breach.

A notice of Unauthorized Disclosure of Protected Health Information is included in Section 13402 of the HITECH Act. It requires covered entities to notify affected individuals when they discover that unsecured PHI has been, or is reasonably believed to have been, breached. The notification requirements are different depending on the number of individuals whose unsecured PHI was compromised. The notification requirements are explained in Figure 10.10.

Notification General Rule: HITECH Section 13402

Following a breach of unsecured protected health information, covered entities must provide notification of the breach to affected individuals, the Secretary, and, in certain circumstances, to the media. In addition, business associates must notify covered entities that a breach has occurred.

- **Individual Notice**

  Covered entities must notify affected individuals following the discovery of a breach of unsecured protected health information. Covered entities must provide this individual notice in written form by first-class mail, or alternatively, by email if the affected individual has agreed to receive such notices electronically. If the covered entity has insufficient or out-of-date contact information for 10 or more individuals, the covered entity must provide substitute individual notice by either posting the notice on the home page of its website or by providing the notice in major print or broadcast media where the affected individuals likely reside. If the

---

Figure 10.10   The HITECH Notification Rule.   *(Continued)*

Notification General Rule: HITECH Section 13402 (*Continued*)

covered entity has insufficient or out-of-date contact information for fewer than 10 individuals, the covered entity may provide substitute notice by an alternative form of written, telephone, or other means.

These individual notifications must be provided without unreasonable delay and in no case later than 60 days following the discovery of a breach and must include, to the extent possible, a description of the breach, a description of the types of information that were involved in the breach, the steps affected individuals should take to protect themselves from potential harm, a brief description of what the covered entity is doing to investigate the breach, mitigate the harm, and prevent further breaches, as well as contact information for the covered entity.

Additionally, for substitute notice provided via web posting or major print or broadcast media, the notification must include a toll-free number for individuals to contact the covered entity to determine if their protected health information was involved in the breach.

- **Media Notice**

Covered entities that experience a breach affecting more than 500 residents of a State or jurisdiction are, in addition to notifying the affected individuals, required to provide notice to prominent media outlets serving the State or jurisdiction. Covered entities will likely provide this notification in the form of a press release to appropriate media outlets serving the affected area. Like individual notice, this media notification must be provided without unreasonable delay and in no case later than 60 days following the discovery of a breach and must include the same information required for the individual notice.

- **Notice to the Secretary**

In addition to notifying affected individuals and the media (where appropriate), covered entities must notify the Secretary of breaches of unsecured protected health information. Covered entities will notify the Secretary by visiting the Health and Human Services website and filling out and electronically submitting a breach report form. If a breach affects 500 or more individuals, covered entities must notify the Secretary without unreasonable delay and in no case later than 60 days following a breach. If, however, a breach affects fewer than 500 individuals, the covered entity may notify the Secretary of such breaches on an annual basis. Reports of breaches affecting fewer than 500 individuals are due to the Secretary no later than 60 days after the end of the calendar year in which the breaches occurred.

(Continued)

Notification General Rule: HITECH Section 13402 *(Continued)*
• **Notification by a Business Associate** If a breach of unsecured protected health information occurs at or by a business associate, the business associate must notify the covered entity following the discovery of the breach. A business associate must provide notice to the covered entity without unreasonable delay and no later than 60 days from the discovery of the breach. To the extent possible, the business associate should provide the covered entity with the identification of each individual affected by the breach as well as any information required to be provided by the covered entity in its notification to affected individuals.

US Department of Health & Human Services.

Data Disposal Laws

Personal identifying information collected by businesses and government is stored in various formats, both digital and paper. Most states have enacted laws that require private or government entities, or both, to destroy, dispose, or otherwise make personal information unreadable or undecipherable after a certain amount of time and when they are no longer needed for care or other beneficial purposes. This is discussed further in Chapter 12.

The Federal Trade Commission's Disposal Rule also requires proper disposal of information in consumer reports and records to protect against unauthorized access to or use of the information. The rule applies to consumer reports or information derived from consumer reports. HIPAA also has disposal requirements for electronic protected health information.

The Computer Fraud and Abuse Act (CFAA) was passed in 1984 but has since been updated six times to create a computer security law that reflects the current technology environment. It is useful to refer to this law to find regulations on how to handle digital documents.

The Sarbanes Oxley Act of 2002 sets requirements for document retention times. This law could affect when you are allowed to shred sensitive records.

Chapter Summary

- The use of EMR and EHR has changed the way healthcare is delivered and the way information is retrieved, stored, and shared.

- Telemedicine and telehealth have required new laws to help prevent the loss of privacy and improve quality of care.

- Health information is often shared for research purposes, but patients should always be notified and be given an opportunity to opt out of this data sharing.

- Security breaches involving PHI are handled at the state level and involve several levels of notification.

- After a certain amount of time, or when it is no longer useful, personal identifying information should be disposed of according to state and federal law.

Vocabulary Matching

1. electronic record of health-related information about an individual that is created, managed, and consulted by authorized people within one healthcare organization

2. pretrial stage of litigation, in which both parties of a lawsuit identify information about the case

3. ability of systems to work and communicate with each other, usually by conforming to standards

4. use of technology to facilitate clinical care at a distance

5. unauthorized acquisition, access, use, or disclosure of protected health information that compromises its security

6. punishment for a criminal offense

7. term for healthcare-related applications that can be used on smartphones, tablets, and other devices

8. process of translating text into an unintelligible set of characters that can be transmitted with a high degree of security

9. electronic record of health-related information about an individual that is created, managed, and consulted by authorized people in more than one agency

10. use of a telecommunication system to deliver health-related services and information

11. individually identifiable information that is created or received by a healthcare provider or any other entity subject to HIPAA requirements

A. breach
B. discovery
C. electronic health record
D. electronic medical record
E. encryption
F. interoperability
G. mHealth
H. protected health information
I. sanction
J. telehealth
K. telemedicine

Multiple Choice

12. When using a(n) _____, an individual has control of what is entered into the system.
    A. electronic medical record
    B. electronic health record
    C. personal health record
    D. personal verification record

13. The term *PHI* means _____ health information.
    A. protected
    B. personal
    C. private
    D. portable

14. The _____ is a mutual recognition process by which states authorize a nurse licensed in one state to practice in other states without obtaining additional licensure.
    A. tele-nursing license
    B. nurse licensure compact
    C. nurse transference agreement
    D. cross-state nursing licensure

Completion

15. The Health Information Technology for Economic and Clinical Health (HITECH) Act was passed to increase the adoption of _____.

16. A(n) _____ is an electronic compilation of health information a person keeps about himself or herself.

17. The risks associated with use of an electronic health record system are highest during the _____ stage.

Discussion and Critical Thinking

18. What is the difference between electronic medical records, electronic health records, and personal health records?

19. What is the difference between telemedicine and telehealth? Provide examples of each.

20. How should an organization respond if a breach occurs? How can they prevent a breach?

21. How can the legal risks of changing from paper to electronic records be reduced?

22. Research data destruction laws. How do your state laws compare with those in other states? Do you think the laws in your state should be more or less strict? What would you like to have changed?

23. What legal issues are related to being in a Compact State? Why are these issues important for healthcare practitioners?

Activities

24. Review the scenario presented at the beginning of the chapter. After reading the chapter, has your response changed? What steps, other than encryption, should the healthcare organization have taken to protect the data? How should the organization notify the affected patients about the incident? Do they not need to notify them because the police are handling the theft investigation?

25. Watch the YouTube video called, "Peter Suderman Discusses the FDA Proposing to Regulate Medical Apps on Mobile Devices." Do you agree with the comments made in this video? Should the FDA regulate medical apps? If so, which ones?

Case Study

A company known as *RR* places physicians trained and licensed in the United States in time zones that are 8–10 hours ahead of or behind the United States. RR physicians in Australia, for example, work during the day in their time zone, which is during the evening in the United States. The organization charges hospitals a rate higher than the services provided in the United States to provide round-the-clock radiology coverage. This type of coverage helps hospitals in the United States remain compliant and meet guidelines for accreditation.

The primary liability issue in radiology occurs when the radiologist misses an obvious abnormality on an image. This error can lead to a delay in diagnosis or an incorrect diagnosis. Patients do not typically choose their radiologist. Instead, the hospital selects the service and/or radiologists for patients.

If a radiologist at RR misreads an image, he or she will usually be liable, but is the hospital liable? Would it matter if the hospital selected the services of RR but did not have control over what radiologist RR used? Is RR liable?

Chapter 11

Genetics and Drugs

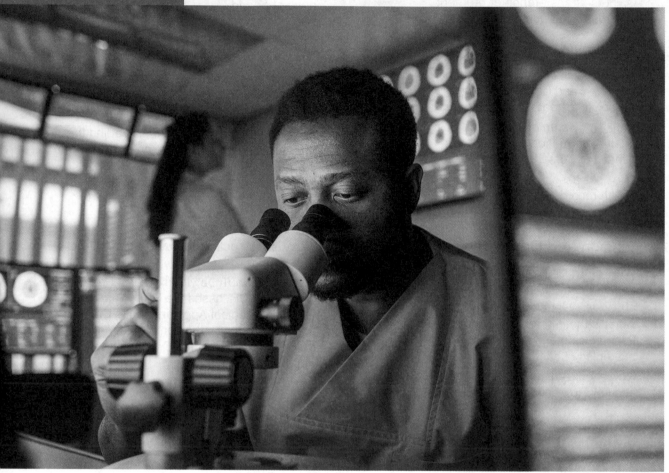

Gorodenkoff/Shutterstock.com

Chapter Outline

Genetics
    Genetic Technologies
    Genetic Research
    Genetic Testing
Drugs
    Drug Regulation
    Drug Approval Process
Medical Devices
Intellectual Property

Objectives

- Describe the laws and ethics related to genetic technologies, research, and testing.
- Explain the process and legal issues related to drug development and approval.
- Identify the agency responsible for regulating medical devices.
- Explain how innovations are protected through legal pathways.

Key Terms

clinical trials
cloning
gene therapy
genetic engineering
genetic mapping
genetics
human genome project
intellectual property
patent
stem cell
trademark

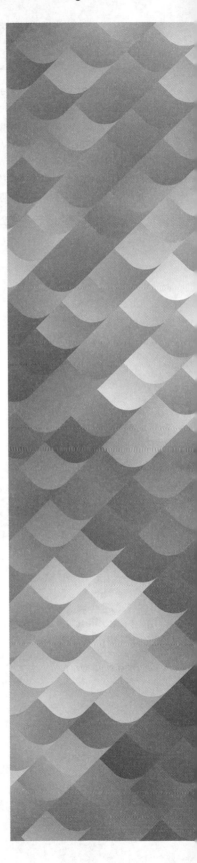

What Would You Do?

Imagine that you are a genetic counselor. A 38-year-old male patient is considering being tested for Huntington's disease. Huntington's disease is a progressive genetic disorder that can have devastating effects on a patient's quality of life. The patient's mother had the disease, so there is a good chance that the patient will have it as well. There is currently no cure for Huntington's disease. What would you recommend to the patient? If there is no cure, should tests be done for such diseases? Should insurance companies be required to pay for such testing? Would you be liable if you refused to conduct the test?

---

human genome project
international research program coordinated by the NIH and the US DOE that studied and identified all of the genes in the human body, collectively known as the *human genome*

Science, technology, and society are continuously changing, and these changes affect the health and safety of the public. As a result of these changes, laws may be created to promote further health and safety. For example, the technological advance of text messaging has led to laws prohibiting texting while driving to promote safety. The use of a substance found in an over-the-counter cold remedy to produce the illegal drug methamphetamine created the need for legal restrictions on the sale of specific cold medications. Telemedicine has expanded access to healthcare across state boundaries, which has required changes in cross-state provider licensure. These are just a few examples of how laws need to continuously evolve to keep pace with science and society.

While not all changes can be foreseen, advances in certain areas of healthcare are expected to contribute to the development of new laws and ethical guidelines. This chapter focuses on those evolving areas of the law. With the completion of the **human genome project** (the international, collaborative research program whose goal was the complete mapping and understanding of all the genes of human beings), changes related to genetic engineering, research, and testing are underway. Those topics are discussed in this chapter, as well as new medications and medical devices. Intellectual property is also addressed here. For innovations to occur, financial gain needs to exceed the costs, which is why intellectual property rights need to exist.

Genetics

genetics
a field of biology concerned with the study of heredity and gene variation

Genetics is a field of biology that is concerned with the study of heredity and gene variation. Genetic technologies, research, and testing all create new opportunities and risks. These opportunities can be revolutionary, such as the ability to prevent disease. But concerns about practices such as genetic testing are also an issue. As a result, laws are evolving along with the science of genetics.

Genetic Technologies

Genes are made up of deoxyribonucleic acid (DNA), an organism's genetic material inherited from one generation to the next. DNA holds many clues about human behavior, disease, and aging. As scientific advances lead to a better understanding of DNA, new DNA-based genetic technologies continue to emerge. Advances in genetic technology related to health include genetic engineering, cloning, and gene therapy. These advances can have positive effects on controlling human disease, but they come with legal and ethical challenges.

Genetic engineering is the process of manually adding new DNA to an organism or modifying an organism's DNA. The goal is to add one or more new traits that are not already found in that organism. Genetic engineering is also used to produce human chemicals (Figure 11.1). For example, human insulin DNA is placed into the DNA of a second organism, and that organism becomes an insulin-producing factory. Now, insulin and other chemicals, such as human growth hormone, are being mass-produced in bacteria. This process has reduced the cost and side effects of replacing missing human chemicals.

Cloning is the process of replicating the genes present within an organism's DNA molecule to make copies of that organism. Through this process, plants with desirable qualities can be rapidly produced from the cells of a single organism. Agricultural cloning can be used to increase the food supply to help alleviate starvation and to modify foods to help prevent nutritional deficiencies. However, concerns have been raised about the safety of genetically modified foods and the ethical implications of genetically modifying animals and plants.

Genetic mapping is the identification of the sequence and location of specific genes inside the chromosomes of cells. This was made possible by the human genome project. These blueprints for human beings make it possible to detect and, perhaps in the future, correct defective genes that may lead to poor health.

One of the most exciting potential applications of genetic mapping is the treatment of genetic disorders through the use of **gene therapy**. Gene therapy entails splicing a needed gene into the DNA of body cells that are still in their infancy. Some genetic disorders are quite serious or even fatal, and many are the result of relatively minor errors in DNA sequencing. Gene therapy can help solve those errors and treat genetic disorders.

The development of genetic technologies has raised issues. People have expressed concerns that organizations may use genetic

genetic engineering
any process by which genetic material is changed to make possible the production of new substances or new functions

cloning
the process of generating a genetically identical copy of a cell or an organism

genetic mapping
the creation of a graphic that shows how genes or DNA sequences are arranged on a chromosome

gene therapy
the use of genes to treat or prevent disease

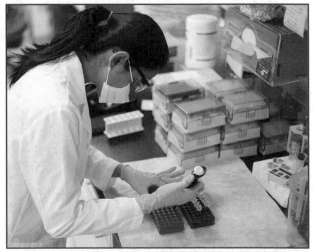

AshTproductions/Shutterstock.com

Figure 11.1 Genetic engineering can be used to create human chemicals, including hormones such as insulin and human growth hormone.

information learned in genetic testing against individuals through employment discrimination or restricting access to health insurance. The cloning of humans is a concern because of issues such as passing on defective genes, emotional risks, health risks from mutated genes, and the ability to control the creation of human beings. Concerns regarding gene therapy include using the process for genetic enhancement to create desired features such as a certain skin or hair color. Legal and ethical challenges also include the following questions:

- Who has the right to receive gene therapy?
- How much will the treatment cost?
- Are there limitations on what can be done?
- Is it ethical to alter a person's genes?
- Is it ethical to control the genes of the human population?

Ethical issues related to genetics have been raised for decades. The Nazis experimented with genetics to reduce the amount of Jewish blood in the human gene pool. They also encouraged breeding by Schutzstaffel (SS) soldiers (the notorious elite military unit of the Nazi party) with women who possessed Aryan genes to create a "master race."

In China, the national policy to limit population by restricting families to one child led to major ethical concerns in a society that prefers male children. If a woman gave birth to a female child, the child was sometimes killed so the family could try again to have a male child. In November 2013, China relaxed the one-child policy. Families now can have two children if one parent, rather than both parents, was an only child.

Genetic technologies can have positive effects on society as well. The recent development of DNA testing as a tool for identification has revolutionized some aspects of law enforcement and corrections (Figure 11.2). Rape cases are often solved with the help of a rape kit sample taken from the victim shortly after the crime. Furthermore, a number of prisoners who have served many years of incarceration are now being identified and freed based on DNA testing results from crime scene evidence that demonstrates that someone else committed the crime.

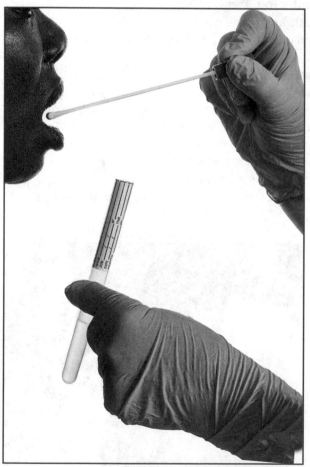

JPC-PROD/Shutterstock.com

Figure 11.2   DNA testing allows law enforcement to obtain important information from something as simple as a cheek swab.

Ethical Dilemma

Imagine that you are a genetic counselor. You meet with a couple who are having a baby. They tell you they are anxiously awaiting the news about the sex of the fetus, because they plan to have only one child, and they want a boy. If the fetus is a girl, they plan to abort the fetus and try again.

Some states have made sex selection abortions illegal. Do you agree with that law? Do you think it is ethical to abort a fetus based on its sex? Is it ethical to legally prohibit someone from choosing abortion due to the sex of the fetus? Can a genetic counselor in this situation refuse to conduct the test?

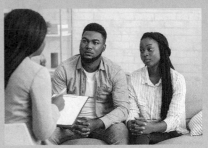

Prostock-studio/Shutterstock.com

Genetic Research

The World Medical Association's Declaration of Helsinki in 1964 first established an international code of ethics related to genetic research. The code prohibited most forms of genetic engineering. This was accepted by numerous professional medical organizations in the United States, including the American Medical Association (AMA). The international guidelines established by the Declaration of Helsinki have since been changed to allow certain forms of cell manipulation that develop therapeutic germ cells.

The topic of stem cell research has been very active and controversial in recent years. **Stem cells** are extracted from embryos and can grow into any cell or tissue in the body. As a result, limbs and organs can potentially be grown in a lab for transplants or the development of cures. Stem cells can provide the needed material to create every kind of human tissue (Figure 11.3). Through the use of these cells, scientists are working on the development of new treatments for a wide range of human diseases and conditions. Examples include diabetes, heart disease, spinal cord injuries, some forms of cancer, and Parkinson's disease.

Stem cells also provide material that is helping scientists better understand human development and the effect of certain substances on humans. A better understanding of normal human development may enable scientists to prevent or treat abnormal development. Stem cells also allow scientists to test millions of potential drugs and medicines without testing

stem cell
an unspecialized cell that can become one or more different types of specialized cells

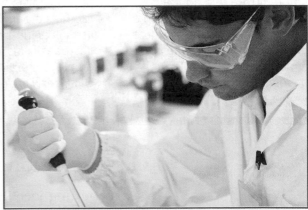

stefanolunardi/Shutterstock.com

Figure 11.3 Stem cells can be used to treat many diseases, but their use can be controversial.

on animals or humans. Scientists simulate the effect a drug has on a specific population of cells and determine whether the drug is useful.

One of the controversies surrounding stem cell research is related to the use of frozen embryos. After stem cells are removed, the embryos are destroyed. Some believe that the embryos are human beings and that destroying them is the same as killing a person. As a result, both federal and state laws related to stem cell research have been enacted.

In 2009, President Obama signed an executive order repealing a previous policy that limited federal tax dollars for embryonic stem cell research. In 2013, the Supreme Court rejected an appeal from two scientists to stop federal funding of research on human embryos, allowing federal funding for human embryonic stem cell research to continue. In 2016, the federal Cures Act helped expedite approval of stem cell and other genetic research, particularly that related to regenerative medicine.

Many states restrict research on aborted fetuses or embryos, but research is often permitted with consent of the patient. In addition, some states limit the use of state funds for cloning or stem cell research.

Career Corner

Clinical research associates (CRAs) supervise, monitor, and support the administration and progress of a clinical trial. A clinical trial is conducted for a *sponsor*, who wants to research pharmaceuticals, biological medical products, or devices. The sponsor may hire a CRA as an employee or a contractor.

CRAs can specialize in a specific area, such as asthma medications, or they may have a more general knowledge base and move from topic to topic. Growth potential for this career is strong, in part because personalized medicine is becoming more common. Clinical trials are needed to ensure that drugs and devices are effective and function properly.

A bachelor's degree in science, sociology, or psychology is a good foundation for this career. Experience in clinical trials or in health sciences is also helpful. Some employers prefer people with a CRA certification, such as the

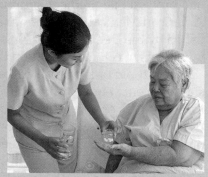

Pormezz/Shutterstock.com

one offered by the Association of Clinical Research Professionals.

Genetic Testing

Genetic testing identifies changes in chromosomes, genes, or proteins. The results of a genetic test can determine whether a person has a specific genetic condition. These tests also can help determine a person's chance of developing or passing on a genetic disorder. On May 21, 2008, President Bush signed the Genetic Information Nondiscrimination Act (GINA). Under this act, US employers and insurance companies are prohibited from discriminating against individuals based on the information found in genetic tests.

GINA prohibits insurance companies from giving people with certain genetic conditions reduced coverage or increased pricing. The law also prohibits employers from making hiring and firing decisions based on a person's genetic code (Figure 11.4). In addition, insurers and employers cannot request or demand a genetic test from their employees.

Yet genetic testing shows up regularly in court proceedings to prove paternity and to prove presence at crime scenes and involvement in crimes. This practice has been a burden on fathers trying to avoid paying child support, a benefit to coroners and others who must prove the identity of dead bodies, and a boon to wrongfully imprisoned people convicted due to faulty witness identification. This has led to the creation of DNA databanks, which are used by law enforcement to solve crimes.

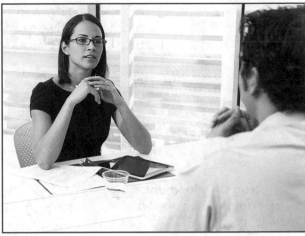

Monkey Business Images/Shutterstock.com

Figure 11.4 Under GINA, employers cannot refuse to hire someone based on his or her genetic information.

Drugs

Drugs are regulated and approved by the government. Laws related to drugs change over time as new drugs enter the market. The process of having drugs approved for sale and distribution is overseen by the government, and the approval process is lengthy and complex.

Drug Regulation

The Food and Drug Administration (FDA) is a regulatory agency within the Department of Health and Human Services. One of the FDA's key responsibilities is to regulate the safety and effectiveness of drugs sold in the United States. No drug can be sold in the United States without approval from the FDA. Once a drug has been approved, the FDA continues to monitor its safety and effectiveness as long as the drug is on the market. Beginning with the Food and Drugs Act of 1906, Congress has gradually refined and expanded the FDA's responsibilities in the drug approval and regulation process.

Drug Approval Process

Having a drug approved by the FDA is a lengthy process. The process begins with scientists developing the drug in a laboratory and testing it, often on animals. Next, a drug or biotechnology company develops a prototype drug from those initial plans. That company must seek and receive FDA approval to test the product on human subjects by submitting an investigational new drug (IND) application (Figure 11.5).

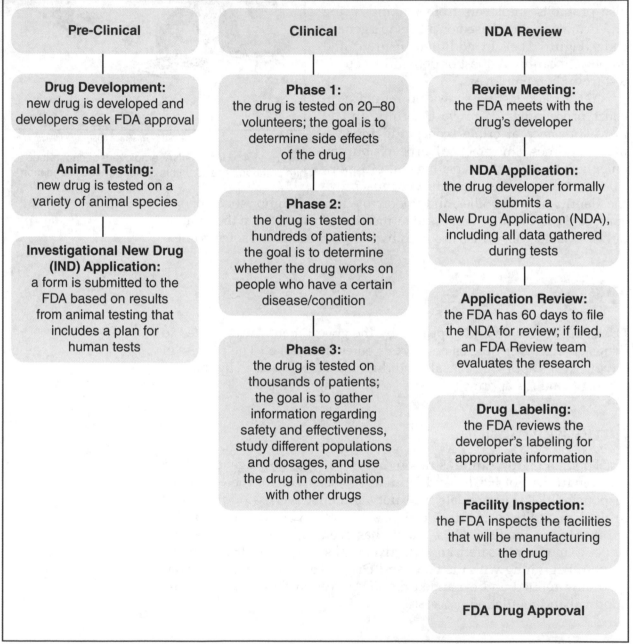

Figure 11.5   Although the FDA drug approval process is lengthy and complicated, it is important for ensuring the safety and effectiveness of drugs on the US market.

Tests performed on human subjects are called **clinical trials**. Clinical trials are conducted in three phases. At each phase, the number of subjects involved increases. After the tests are completed, the drug manufacturer compiles the resulting data and analysis in a new drug application (NDA). When the FDA reviews the NDA, it has three major concerns in mind. It evaluates the safety and effectiveness of the drug related to its proposed use; it ensures that the proposed labeling is appropriate; and it determines whether the drug lives up to the manufacturer's proposed strength, quality, and identity.

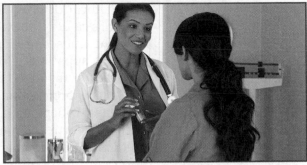

Rocketclips, Inc./Shutterstock.com

Figure 11.6 Under the FFDCA, drug companies must include accurate and appropriate information on their products' labels.

clinical trials
a series of research tests performed on human subjects to determine the effectiveness and safety of a new drug

At each step in this process, there are specific regulations and requirements to be followed. These requirements are detailed in the Federal Food, Drug, and Cosmetic Act (FFDCA). The FFDCA was passed to assure consumers that foods are pure and wholesome, safe to eat, and produced under sanitary conditions. The act also is intended to assure that drugs and devices are safe and effective for their intended uses; that cosmetics are safe and include appropriate ingredients; and that all labeling and packaging is truthful, informative, and not deceptive (Figure 11.6).

The main consumer watchdog in this system is the FDA's Center for Drug Evaluation and Research (CDER). CDER's best-known job is to evaluate new drugs before they can be sold. CDER ensures that drugs, both brand name and generic, work correctly and that their health benefits outweigh their known risks.

Medical Devices

The FDA's Center for Devices and Radiological Health (CDRH) regulates firms that manufacture, repackage, relabel, and/or import medical devices sold in the United States. In addition, CDRH regulates medical and non-medical electronic products that emit radiation, such as lasers, X-ray systems, and ultrasound equipment.

Medical devices are classified as Class I, II, and III. Class III devices receive more regulatory control than Class I devices. The basic regulatory requirements for manufacturers of medical devices distributed in the United States are related to labeling, registration, packaging, and reporting malfunctions.

Medical device law includes health technology, which is an evolving area. In addition to federal regulation, state laws related to product liability may also apply. The FDA regulates only those mobile apps that

intellectual property
creations of the intellect that are protected by the law, enabling people to earn recognition or financial benefit from what they invent or create

patent
a grant made by a government that gives the creator of an invention the sole right to make, use, and sell that invention for a specified period of time

trademark
a word, name, symbol, phrase, or other device used to identify and promote a product or service

are medical devices, the functionality of which could pose a risk to a patient's safety if they did not function as intended.

The subset of apps the FDA wants to regulate includes mobile medical apps that can be used as accessories to medical devices that are already regulated by the FDA. These might include apps that allow healthcare professionals to diagnose conditions after viewing an image on a smartphone or tablet (Figure 11.7). This subset also includes apps that transform a smartphone or other communications device into a medical device through attachments or sensors. This might include an app that turns a smartphone into a stethoscope.

Intellectual Property

The term **intellectual property** describes the area of law that involves protecting proprietary rights. Intellectual property includes patents, trademarks, copyrights, and other forms of exclusive rights to intangible property. Healthcare-related intellectual property includes **patents** on medications and **trademarks** on brand names for drugs.

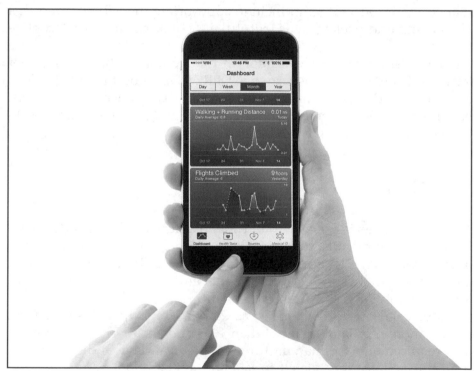

Denys Prykhodov/Shutterstock.com

Figure 11.7   The FDA regulates certain types of mobile medical apps.

Patent law is handled only at the federal level in the United States. Patents protect inventions from theft and apply to all sorts of inventions, not just those related to healthcare. A great deal of time and resources are required for the invention of new medications, healthcare software or devices, or other products. For this reason, patents are integral to organizations receiving a return on their investments. Patents generally provide exclusive use of a design for 14 or 15 years. If patents did not exist, private industries would not have the incentive or ability to conduct research and develop products to improve the delivery of healthcare. However, after an invention has been protected for the period defined in patent law, the right to use it becomes public, and the invention may be freely used by others.

Trademark law protects distinctive and non-functional terms, designs, and other methods of distinguishing goods or services from competitors. For example, eICU® is the trademark for a specific type of telemedicine equipment used in the intensive care unit. Trademarks do not protect the underlying goods or ideas themselves. Trademarks need to be registered and approved by the US Patent and Trademark Office. Importantly, trademarks are good for as long as the trademarked items are actually used in commerce. Registration and proof of use must be filed initially and then renewed after 5 years. Subsequently, it must be renewed every 10 years during actual use.

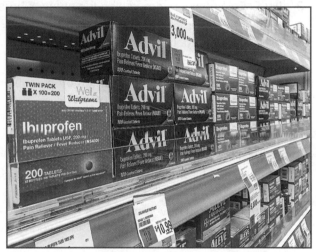

Roman Tirapolsky/Shutterstock.com

Patents and trademarks are intended to allow inventors and developers to make money on their new inventions and designs. The legal monopoly can, however, lead to an extended period of time when competition cannot bring down the price for the invention. In the case of medical trademarks, the cost of certain drugs may be higher even after the patent period ends due to long-term name recognition resulting from trademark protection (Figure 11.8). To reduce the costs of medical care, many insurance companies may provide incentives for drug distributors and patients to use non-brand name or generic drugs.

Figure 11.8 Trademark protection of brand names for over-the-counter pain relievers such as Advil® and Tylenol® has made these names much more recognizable by many people than their official US Pharmacopeia (generic) names of ibuprofen and acetaminophen, respectively.

Chapter 11 Review and Assessment

Chapter Summary

- Genetic research has been encouraged by federal and state law in efforts to advance medical science.
- The federal Food and Drug Administration (FDA) is responsible for approving drugs throughout the United States.
- The FDA regulates four classifications of medical devices, including certain smartphone apps.
- Federal patent and trademark protection is available to inventors and businesses who invest in and create new products and designs.

Vocabulary Matching

1. international research program that identified the genes in the human body
2. creations of the intellect that are protected by law, enabling people to earn recognition or financial benefit from the creations
3. field of biology concerned with the study of heredity and gene variation
4. word, name, symbol, phrase, or other device used to identify and promote a product or service
5. the use of genes to treat or prevent disease
6. series of research tests performed on human subjects to determine the effectiveness and safety of a new drug
7. creation of a graphic that shows how genes or DNA sequences are arranged on a chromosome
8. process of generating a genetically identical copy of a cell or organism
9. any process by which genetic material is changed to make possible the production of new substances or new functions
10. grant made by a government that gives the creator of an invention the sole right to make, use, and sell that invention for a specified period of time
11. unspecialized cell that can become one or more different types of specialized cells

A. clinical trials
B. cloning
C. gene therapy
D. genetic engineering
E. genetic mapping
F. genetics
G. human genome project
H. intellectual property
I. patent
J. stem cell
K. trademark

Multiple Choice

12. An organism's genetic material, known as _____, holds many clues to natural processes such as disease and aging.
    A. RNA
    B. stem cells
    C. DNA
    D. insulin

13. The _____ regulates firms who manufacture, repackage, relabel, and/or import medical devices sold in the United States.
    A. CRA
    B. HHS
    C. NIH
    D. FDA

14. Which act prohibits insurance companies and employers from discriminating against individuals based on information derived from genetic tests?
    A. DNA Information Act
    B. DNA Nondiscrimination Act
    C. DNA Restricted Use Act
    D. DNA HIPAA Act

15. Which of the following practices is commonly used in agriculture?
    A. cloning
    B. gene therapy
    C. stem cell research
    D. gene masking

16. Genetic _____ identifies the sequence and location of specific genes inside the chromosomes of a person's cells.
    A. therapy
    B. engineering
    C. treatment
    D. mapping

17. The Declaration of _____ first established an international code of ethics related to genetic research.
    A. Nuremburg
    B. China
    C. Sweden
    D. Helsinki

18. Genetic _____ can identify changes in chromosomes, genes, or proteins.
    A. therapy
    B. testing
    C. treatment
    D. engineering

19. Which of the following pieces of legislation prohibits insurance companies from discriminating against people based on genetic information?
    A. ACA
    B. OSHA
    C. FDA
    D. GINA

Completion

20. Genetic _____ is the process of manually adding new DNA to an organism or modifying an organism's DNA.

21. Patents on medications and trademarks on brand names are examples of _____.

22. Mobile medical _____ that are considered medical devices are regulated by the FDA.

23. Gene _____ entails splicing a required gene into the DNA of cells in their infancy.

Discussion and Critical Thinking

24. In the future, many more tests for genetic conditions will be available. Should screening for diseases or defects be allowed when there is no cure or treatment? Why or why not? Should insurance companies pay for genetic tests? Why or why not?

25. Supplements, such as vitamins and minerals, can be sold without FDA review and approval. These products are not classified as drugs. Do you think that supplements should be regulated by the FDA? Why or why not?

26. Why have international professional ethics rules been developed for genetic engineering?

27. Why is the drug approval process so thorough and complicated?

28. Why are patents approved for only a certain number of years?

Activities

29. Use the Internet to research genetically modified foods. Write a paper explaining how genetically modified foods affect human health. Describe the laws and regulations you think need to be in place, such as labels identifying genetically modified food. Explain your reasons with supporting research.

30. Research your state's laws on stem cell research. Write about your reaction to these laws. Do you agree with them? Why or why not?

Case Study

Visit the Thought Catalog website and find the article entitled "Man Does 30 Years in Prison Before Being Found Innocent By DNA Tests." Watch the accompanying video and read the information presented there. Discuss the role of DNA in the criminal justice system. How do you expect the use of DNA tests in criminal investigations to affect future laws and criminal investigations? Should laws be in place to review previous cases? How long should biological evidence be retained? How should states assist people who have been wrongfully convicted of crimes?

Chapter 12

Complexity of Facilities Administration

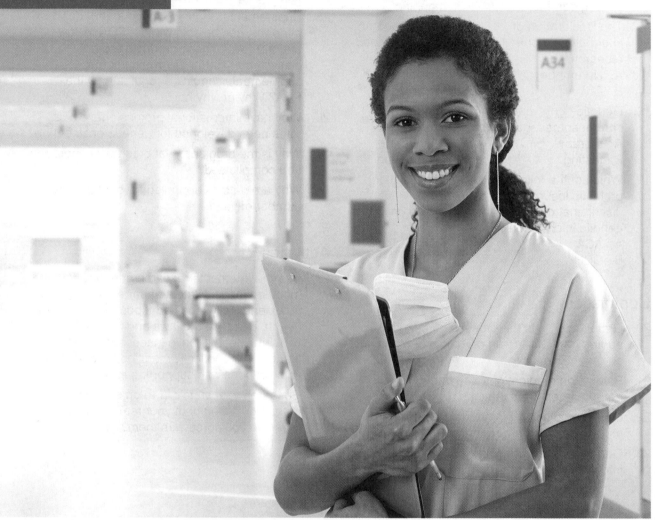

StockLite/Shutterstock.com

Chapter Outline

States and Healthcare Legislation

Patient Protection and Affordable Care Act

Medicaid

State Laws Related to Public Health

Healthcare Facilities and Departments

Medical Staff

Finance

Nursing Homes

Hospice Care

Medical Departments

Medical Records

Pharmacy

Clinical Laboratories

Critical Access Hospitals

Objectives

- Explain the legal responsibilities of states in carrying out federal healthcare legislation.
- Describe the legal and ethical responsibilities of various healthcare facilities and the departments within them.

Key Terms

accountable care organization (ACO)

Conditions of Participation (COP)

critical access hospital

Federal Medical Assistance Percentage (FMAP)

fee-for-service

health insurance exchanges

managed care

prospective payment system (PPS)

Sherman Antitrust Act

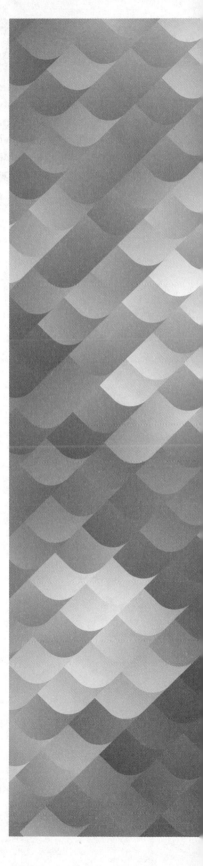

What Would You Do?

Imagine that you are a nurse in a residential care facility. The facility has a strict policy prohibiting staff from providing medical care for the residents. An 86-year-old resident begins to have breathing problems, so you call 911. The 911 operator says that help is on the way and instructs you to perform cardiopulmonary resuscitation (CPR) on the resident. Should you go against the residential care policy and perform CPR? Do you have a legal and/or ethical responsibility to do so?

Healthcare facilities and practitioners are licensed and regulated by federal, state, and local governments and laws. Voluntary methods of regulation, such as auditing by accredited organizations, also exist and can help healthcare facilities comply with the law. One example of a voluntary accreditation for hospitals and some ambulatory care centers is The Joint Commission accreditation. The Joint Commission is an independent, non-profit organization that accredits and certifies healthcare organizations and programs.

Laws related to states, healthcare facilities, and facility departments are shifting partly because of legislation at the federal level. The federal government influences healthcare delivery generally by providing funding or reimbursement tied to standards or qualifying conditions. State and local governments are much more involved in actual delivery of care. For example, states now have the ability to oversee health information exchanges, which includes many legal mandates, as a result of a federal law passed in 2010. In addition, facilities and their departments have to follow federal and state laws.

This chapter focuses on the responsibilities of states, healthcare facilities, and facility departments. These responsibilities are a result of both federal and state laws.

States and Healthcare Legislation

States have a long history of being involved in providing healthcare. Their roles have been expanded in many ways, but a recent driving force has been the passage of the Patient Protection and Affordable Care Act at the federal level. Other important laws passed by the federal government also can affect the states' roles in healthcare. Medicaid in particular contains several responsibilities for states. In addition, many states have laws pertaining to public health.

Patient Protection and Affordable Care Act

President Obama signed the Patient Protection and Affordable Care Act, also referred to as the *Affordable Care Act (ACA)*, into law in 2010. The ACA gives the states resources and power to build and run their own **health insurance exchanges**. These exchanges provide consumers with a variety of certified health plans and provide information and educational services to help patients understand the plans and options.

health insurance exchanges
state-run centers that provide and explain options for certified health insurance plans

Under the ACA, states have the option to establish one or more state or regional exchanges, partner with the federal government to run the exchange, or merge with other state exchanges. Every state was required to have a health insurance exchange by January 2014. If a state decided not to create an exchange, the federal government set up an exchange in the state. This gave the state the option of transitioning to a state exchange in the future.

The ACA includes two basic federal requirements for exchanges. These include: (1) minimum functions that exchanges must undertake directly or, in some cases, by contract; and (2) oversight responsibilities that exchanges must exercise in certifying and monitoring the performance of Qualified Health Plans. Plans that participate in the exchanges also must comply with state insurance laws and federal requirements in the Public Health Service Act.

Minimum functions that a healthcare exchange must provide, according to the ACA, include certification of plans, a toll-free hotline, website maintenance, and presentation of plan benefit options. All of this must follow a standardized format (Figure 12.1). An exchange's oversight responsibilities include developing regulatory standards in five areas that insurers must meet to earn certification under the ACA. These areas are marketing, network adequacy, accreditation for performance measures, quality improvement and reporting, and uniform enrollment procedures.

The ACA also states that exchanges must ensure that their plans comply with regulatory standards such as providing information on the availability of in- and out-of-network providers. Exchanges must also disclose plan data, including claims handling policies, financial disclosures, enrollment and disenrollment

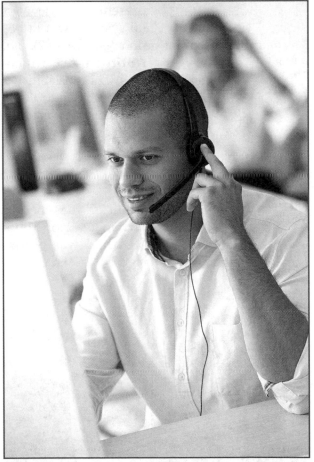

goodluz/Shutterstock.com

Figure 12.1 According to ACA specifications, healthcare exchanges must provide a toll-free hotline for users.

data, claims denials, rating practices, and cost sharing for out-of-network coverage.

Section 3022 of the ACA authorizes the Centers for Medicare and Medicaid Services (CMS) to create the Medicare Shared Savings Program (MSSP). An MSSP allows for the creation of an **accountable care organization (ACO)**. An ACO is a healthcare organization characterized by a payment and care delivery model in which provider reimbursements are linked to quality metrics and reductions in the total cost of care for an assigned population of patients.

A group of healthcare providers can coordinate to form an ACO, which then provides care to a group of patients. The ACO may use a range of payment models such as fee-for-service or capitation. The ACO is accountable to the patients and the third-party payer for the quality, appropriateness, and efficiency of the healthcare provided.

Some people have concerns about ACOs and antitrust issues. ACOs present a new legal problem because, through them, competing hospital systems would be able to come together and share pricing information (Figure 12.2). This may be considered illegal under the **Sherman Antitrust Act**, which prohibits certain anticompetitive business activities. The possibility that ACOs could allow hospitals to raise prices is contradictory to the basic concept of ACOs, which is to bring hospitals together to lower prices. Federal antitrust laws will likely have to change to accommodate ACOs.

accountable care organization (ACO)
a group of doctors, hospitals, and other healthcare providers who come together voluntarily to give coordinated, high-quality care to their Medicare patients

Sherman Antitrust Act
a federal statute that prohibits business activities that are anti-competitive, such as monopolies

Federal Medical Assistance Percentage (FMAP)
the percentage of Medicaid expenditures reimbursed to states by the federal government; varies by state

Medicaid

Medicaid has been discussed in previous chapters, but this section focuses on the state's legal responsibilities related to Medicaid. Medicaid was originally created in 1965 to enable states to provide medical assistance for certain low-income families. Assistance also can be extended to individuals who are old or disabled and whose income and resources are insufficient to meet the costs of medically necessary services.

The Medicaid program is funded by both the federal government and state governments. The federal government pays states for a specified percentage of expenditures from the program. This is called the **Federal Medical Assistance Percentage (FMAP)**. The FMAP varies by state based on criteria such as per capita income. On average, the FMAP is 57 percent. However, in wealthier states, the FMAP is only 50 percent. In poorer states, which might require more federal assistance, the FMAP may be as high as 75 percent. The maximum FMAP is 82 percent.

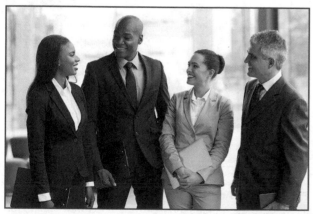

michaeljung/Shutterstock.com

Figure 12.2   Although ACOs offer some benefits, they might also create concerns regarding hospitals sharing pricing information.

FMAPs are adjusted in each state on a three-year cycle to account for economic changes. The federal government provides a matching dollar amount for state spending on Medicaid on an open-ended basis. States manage the Medicaid program on a day-to-day basis. Given the large amount of federal funds involved, the federal government oversees states' management of the program and shares responsibility with states to ensure program integrity.

States must fund their share of the Medicaid program that is provided by their state plan. This is a condition of federal financial participation. Before CMS approves an amendment to a state plan, they must verify that the state has sufficient funds to qualify for federal financial assistance for the covered services.

States can develop their own Medicaid provider payment rates, but they must adhere to federal requirements. States generally pay for services through fee-for-service or managed care payment methods. Under **fee-for-service** payment arrangements, states pay providers directly for services. States may develop their payment rates based on the costs of providing services, the average price for services in the private market, and a percentage of what Medicare pays for equivalent services.

Under **managed care** payment arrangements, states partner with organizations to deliver care through networks and pay providers. Approximately 70 percent of Medicaid participants are enrolled in a managed care delivery system that pays providers on a monthly rate. The methodologies for service rates are described in each state's Medicaid plan.

States must submit a State Plan Amendment for CMS to review and approve if they want to alter the way that providers are paid. Before the amendment goes into effect, states also must notify the public of the change. CMS reviews state plan amendment reimbursement methodologies for consistency with the Social Security Act and other federal statutes and regulations.

fee-for-service
in Medicaid, payment arrangement in which states pay providers directly for services

managed care
in Medicaid, payment arrangement in which states partner with organizations to deliver care and pay a set monthly rate to providers

State Laws Related to Public Health

States vary in their methods of establishing laws that are intended to protect the health of the public. These laws are extensive and cover everything from preventative healthcare to end-of-life care. Examples include laws related to smoking in parks, near buildings, and in bars and housing units with shared walls. Others include laws about texting while driving, wearing a helmet while riding a motorcycle, using marijuana, licensing medical professionals, and issuing penalties for driving while under the influence of alcohol and other drugs (Figure 12.3).

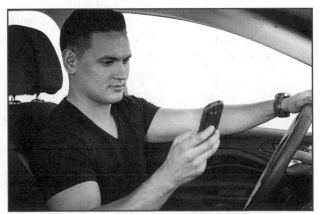

antoniodiaz/Shutterstock.com

Figure 12.3 Public health laws in the states cover topics such as texting while driving.

Healthcare Facilities and Departments

Many laws exist to regulate the operations of healthcare facilities and their specific departments. In addition to general employment laws, healthcare facilities must obey specific laws regarding their employees. A specific reimbursement system dictates the finances of healthcare facilities. Nursing homes and hospice care centers have specific laws addressing safety of residents and conditions for receiving federal funding. Each healthcare facility's departments also have important laws to follow, including medical records, the pharmacy, and clinical laboratories.

Medical Staff

Healthcare facilities have to abide by the same employment laws that other employers do. For example, they must follow laws related to providing breaks for employees, avoiding discrimination, and paying employees minimum wage. In addition to those laws, there are laws specific to employers of medical professionals and those that provide medical services. These include state laws related to criminal background checks, disaster management plans, appropriate licensure for operation, and medical licensures of employees. These healthcare-specific laws can be different in every state. The nursing-patient ratio laws, for example, vary greatly from state to state (Figure 12.4).

Finance

prospective payment system (PPS)
a method of reimbursement in which Medicare payments are made based on a predetermined, fixed amount

Most hospitals and many other healthcare facilities are required to use the **prospective payment system (PPS)** for billing. In a PPS, Medicare payments are made based on a predetermined, fixed amount. The payment amount for a particular service is determined by the service classification system (for example, diagnosis-related groups (DRGs) for inpatient hospital services). CMS uses a different PPS for different types of healthcare facilities, such as hospitals, hospices, and long-term care facilities.

Nursing Homes

Nursing homes are multi-residence housing facilities that provide intermediate residential care. There are numerous federal and state laws protecting residents in nursing homes and assisted-living facilities from low standards, abuse, and neglect. States issue licenses and inspect nursing homes and residential care facilities. If a nursing home is certified for Medicare or Medicaid participation, it must meet federal certification

Legislation and Staffing Ratios in the State of California
Some states have enacted laws that require minimum nursing-patient ratios. These laws mean that a specific number of nurses need to be present for a specific number of patients. California was the first state to enact such a law in 2004. Since then, other states and the District of Columbia have adopted legislation and/or regulations that address nurse staffing. Most of these states have legislation that is less strict than California's law. Under California's law, the Department of Health Services requires acute care hospitals to maintain minimum nurse-to-patient staffing ratios. Required ratios vary by unit, ranging from 1:1 in operating rooms to 1:6 (meaning one nurse to six patients) in psychiatric units. The minimum ratios vary by specialty and department. Examples of the required ratios include 1:2 in intensive care units (ICUs), neonatal ICUs, post-anesthesia recovery, and labor/delivery units; 1:4 in emergency departments and telemetry, antepartum, and postpartum units where nurses take care of both mother and child; 1:5 in medical and surgical units; and 1:6 in psychiatric units and in postpartum care units where nurses take care of only the mother. The legislation also requires hospitals to maintain a classification system to determine when additional staffing is necessary. This system also also assigns certain tasks only to licensed registered nurses, determines the competency of and provides appropriate training for nurses before assigning them to patient care, and maintains records of staffing levels.

Goodheart-Willcox, Inc.

Figure 12.4 California's staffing law.

standards in addition to state requirements. States also have nursing home abuse and injury laws.

Congress enacted the Nursing Home Reform Act in 1987. This act requires nursing homes that participate in Medicare and Medicaid to comply with certain rules for quality of care. These requirements mean that nursing homes must develop a written plan of care that includes services and activities that will help each resident reach his or her best possible physical, mental, and psychosocial well-being (Figure 12.5).

The Nursing Home Reform Act also established a certification process that requires states to conduct unannounced inspections of facilities, including resident interviews, at irregular intervals at least once every 15 months. These inspections generally focus on residents' rights, quality of care, quality of life, and the services provided. The Nursing Home Reform Act established certain rights for nursing home residents. To comply with the law, facilities must cater to and respect these rights. Inspections that are more specific can be conducted in response to complaints against nursing homes.

If an inspection reveals that a nursing home is not complying with the law, the Nursing Home Reform Act enforcement process begins.

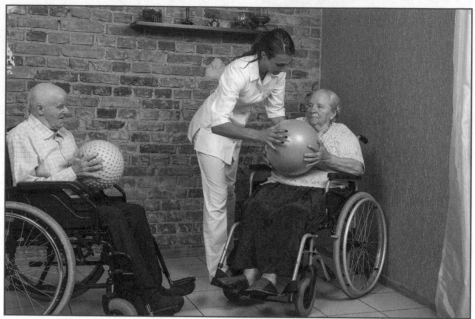

GBZero/Shutterstock.com

Figure 12.5 Nursing homes offer elderly people an opportunity to socialize and engage in activities that will improve their well-being.

The severity of this process depends on whether the issue of noncompliance puts a resident in immediate jeopardy, and whether it is an isolated incident, part of a pattern, or widespread throughout the facility. In the case of some violations, nursing homes have an opportunity to correct the problem before the process begins.

Hospice Care

There are federal and state regulations related to hospice care. Hospice care centers must meet the Medicare **Conditions of Participation (COP)** to become licensed and certified by state regulators. These conditions also must be met for CMS to allow a state to continue participating in the Medicare hospice program. Without certification, hospices cannot receive reimbursement for patients in their program. Obtaining certification does not necessarily mean that a hospice actually will comply with all the standards in any one patient's case. What it does mean is that regulators decided to certify the hospice as meeting the standards after their last inspection.

Medical Departments

Some departments within medical facilities have laws that are specific to those departments. For example, the medical records and pharmacy

Conditions of Participation (COP) conditions that healthcare organizations must meet to begin and continue participating in the Medicare and Medicaid programs

Ethical Dilemma

Imagine that you are the admissions representative at a nursing home. Your supervisor informs you that the organization is struggling financially and she needs you to improve the facility's admission rates of Medicare patients. She wants you to begin meeting with the discharge nurses at local hospitals and encourage them to send their patients to your nursing home instead of your main competitor. The supervisor states that she wants you to start taking them to lunch and, if the referrals increase, to take them to lunch on a quarterly basis.

You know that "kickbacks" are against the law, but you also know that your facility provides better care for the patients than the competing nursing home in the area. You want the patients to get the best care possible and need to keep your job. What would you do in this situation? Is lunch considered a kick-back

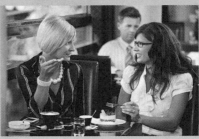

or a marketing meeting? What repercussions or consequences could you experience if you proceed?

departments of a hospital have laws that pertain to their processes. This section explains some of those department-specific requirements.

Medical Records

Healthcare organizations must establish appropriate retention and destruction schedules to ensure the availability of timely, relevant data and information for patient care purposes. The retention schedules must be designed to meet federal, state, and local legal requirements.

The responsibility to retain or destroy medical information has traditionally been given to health information management professionals. In the past, when health records were kept on paper, off-site storage was used as a method of maintaining records. Now that electronic health records (EHR) are required, healthcare facilities must determine which paper records should be entered into the EHR (Figure 12.6). For paper records that are not entered into the EHR, new methods of retention must be developed. Health information is now kept in multiple locations and in different types of storage. Because of this change, a clearly defined record retention and retrieval plan is required.

According to the American Health Information Management Association (AHIMA), a record retention schedule must help provide patient information in the case of legal requirements or other legitimate uses; include rules for what information is kept, how long it is kept, and the format in which it will be stored; and include clear rules that outline the format in which information should be maintained.

There is no single, standardized federal record retention schedule to which organizations and providers must adhere. However, there

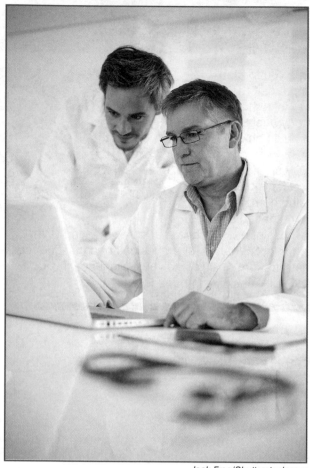

Figure 12.6   Deciding which paper medical records should be converted to electronic records, and entering the information accurately, is a major task for many healthcare organizations

are retention requirements that need to be reviewed when developing a compliant retention program. Healthcare organizations and providers should use federal record retention requirements found within the *Federal Register* and numerous acts, such as the Higher Education Act of 1965. These requirements must be compared with state-specific requirements to ensure that all records are maintained according to whichever presents the more restrictive timeline. Figure 12.7 contains a list of federal record retention requirements.

States also have requirements regarding record retention, which should be taken into account when an organization develops its own policy. If a state has no specific requirements, the healthcare organization should maintain health information as long as is specified by the state's statute of limitations, or long enough to comply with other laws and regulations.

In the case of a minor, a healthcare organization should retain the patient's information until he or she reaches the age of maturity, as defined by state law, plus the period of the statute of limitations. This longer period is recommended because the statute may not begin until the potential plaintiff realizes the relationship between an injury and care received. Healthcare organizations and providers should consider a state's retention requirements and statute of limitations to determine the best retention schedule.

As with retaining records, there is no singular federal or state requirement for destroying health information. Some states require the creation of a summary of destroyed information, the notification of patients when information is destroyed, or an explanation of the method used to destroy information. The process of destroying patient health information must follow any laws that do exist as well as an organization's written policy. Healthcare organizations must retain records that are involved in an open investigation, audit, or lawsuit until the case is closed.

Organizations should reassess their method of destruction each year. This reassessment should take into account current technology, accepted practices, and availability of timely and cost-effective destruction services. If no state law exists to the contrary, organizations must ensure that paper and electronic records are destroyed in a way that makes it impossible to reconstruct the information.

Federal Record Retention Requirements

Type of Documentation	Retention Period	Citation/Reference
abortions and related medical services documentation	three years	42 CFR 36.56 42 CFR 50.309
ambulatory surgical services	not specified	42 CFR 416.47
clinics, rehabilitation agencies, and public health agencies as providers of outpatient physical therapy and speech-language pathology services	determined by the respective state statute, or the statute of limitations in the state; in the absence of a state statute, five years after the date of discharge; in the case of a minor, three years after the patient becomes of age under state law or five years after the date of discharge, whichever is longer	42 CFR 485.721(d) 42 CFR 486.161(d)
clinics (rural health)	six years from date of last entry; longer if required by state statute	42 CFR 491.10(c)
comprehensive outpatient rehabilitation facilities (CORFs)	five years after patient discharge	42 CFR 485.60(c)
critical access hospitals (CAHs)	six years from date of last entry; longer if required by state statute, or if the records may be needed in any pending proceeding	42 CFR 485.638(c)
drug test results, students	not specified	34 CFR 99 Family Educational Rights and Privacy Act (20 USC §1232g)
home health agencies	five years after the month the cost report to which the records apply is filed with the intermediary, unless state law stipulates a longer period of time	42 CFR 484.48(a)
hospice care	retention periods are not specified	42 CFR 418.74
hospitals	five years	42 CFR 482.24(b)(1)
laboratory—all other records	two years	42 CFR 493.1777(d)(3) 42 CFR 493.1780(e)(4)
long-term care facilities	determined by state law; five years from the date of discharge when there is no requirement in state law; for a minor, three years after a resident reaches legal age under state law	42 CFR 483.75(l)(2)
psychiatric hospitals	five years	42 CFR 482.61

Figure 12.7 Federal record retention laws.

Career Corner

Health administrators are leaders in healthcare organizations such as hospitals, medical clinics, nursing homes, hospice centers, and home health agencies. In the public sector, they might work in county health departments, county hospitals, or national organizations. In the private sector, they might work at pharmaceutical companies, health insurance companies, or consulting firms.

These professionals direct the operations of the organization where they work. They are responsible for management functions such as facilities, services, programs, staff, budgets, and community and interagency relations. Health administrators may specialize in a specific area or have a more general skill set and background. Specialists lead specific clinical departments or services, while generalists manage or help to manage entire facilities or systems.

Health administrators are usually required to earn a bachelor's degree in health administration or a related field such as public health or public administration. In addition, some states require administrators to pass a licensing exam and complete a state-approved academic program.

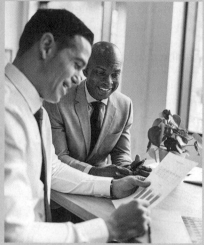

Flamingo Images/Shutterstock.com

Pharmacy

There are federal and state laws governing drug distribution and pharmaceutical care. These laws are related to drug purchasing, storage, record keeping, data protection, handling, labeling, administration, substitution, destruction, dispensing, and patient counseling. The drug distribution process is monitored to ensure the integrity of the drug product used in patient care and compliance with laws and regulations. These laws apply to pharmacies located within a healthcare facility as well as those that are not, such as a pharmacy in a grocery store.

There are three key federal laws related to drugs—the Pure Food and Drug Act (1906); the Federal Food, Drug, and Cosmetic Act (1938); and the Controlled Substance Act (1970). The Pure Food and Drug Act required all drugs marketed in the United States to meet minimum standards for strength, purity, and quality. The Federal Food, Drug, and Cosmetic Act established specific regulations for preventing people from tampering with drugs, foods, and cosmetics. The Controlled Substance Act created tighter regulations for groups of drugs that were being abused by society at the time (Figure 12.8).

Clinical Laboratories

States implement laboratory licensure laws, which apply to clinical laboratories. These laws include on-site inspections, proficiency assessment, and personnel training, which ensure that laboratories produce accurate and reliable results. The laws are related to personnel and administrative tasks as well as lab procedures. At the federal level, clinical labs are required to comply with the Clinical Laboratory Improvement Amendments (CLIA) of 1988. These state that all laboratories testing human specimens must be certified by the federal government to perform those tests.

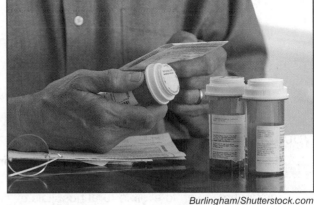

Burlingham/Shutterstock.com

Figure 12.8 There are several federal laws that regulate medication and drugs for safety.

Some states require laboratories to report notifiable diseases. For example, Maine's laws require laboratories and blood banks to report the recognition or strong suspicion of specific notifiable conditions. Definitions of notifiable diseases may vary by state. At the national level, the Centers for Disease Control and Prevention (CDC) has created the National Notifiable Diseases Surveillance System (NNDSS). This system enables public health officials to monitor the occurrence and spread of diseases.

State, local, territorial, and tribal health departments must notify the CDC of cases of specific diseases and conditions that they identify in their jurisdictions. Every year, the nation's epidemiologists determine which of these diseases and conditions should be notifiable and how to define a case.

Critical Access Hospitals

Critical access hospital (CAH) is a designation given to eligible rural hospitals by CMS. Congress created the CAH designation through the Balanced Budget Act of 1997 in response to numerous rural hospital closures during the 1980s and early 1990s. Since its creation, Congress has amended the CAH designation and related program requirements several times through additional legislation.

The CAH designation is designed to reduce the financial vulnerability of rural hospitals and improve access to healthcare by keeping essential services in rural communities. To accomplish this goal, CAHs receive certain benefits, such as cost-based reimbursement for Medicare services.

critical access hospital
designation given to eligible rural hospitals by CMS to help improve access to healthcare in rural communities

Chapter Summary

- Although states have much flexibility in overseeing health services in their state, federal laws have a profound impact on how the states carry out these services.

- The operations of all healthcare facilities, and various departments within these facilities, are highly regulated by law.

Vocabulary Matching

1. state-run centers that provide and explain options for certified health insurance plans

2. designation given to eligible rural hospitals by CMS to help improve access to healthcare in rural communities

3. payment arrangement in which states pay providers directly for Medicaid services

4. federal statute

5. method of reimbursement in which Medicare payments are made based on a predetermined, fixed amount

6. payment arrangement in which states partner with organizations to deliver care and pay a set monthly rate to providers for Medicaid services

7. group of doctors, hospitals, and other healthcare providers who come together voluntarily to give coordinated, high-quality care to Medicare patients

8. percentage of Medicaid expenditures reimbursed to states by the federal government

9. requirements that healthcare organizations must meet to begin and continue participating in Medicare and Medicaid programs

A. accountable care organization
B. Conditions of Participation
C. critical access hospital
D. Federal Medical Assistance Percentage
E. fee-for-service
F. health insurance exchanges
G. managed care
H. prospective payment system
I. Sherman Antitrust Act

Multiple Choice

10. Which of the following laws gives states the option of establishing health insurance exchanges?
    A. The Sherman Antitrust Act
    B. The Affordable Care Act
    C. The Public Health Act
    D. The Insurance Exchange Act

11. Which of the following requirements is *not* included in the minimum functions of a healthcare exchange laid out by the ACA?
    A. website maintenance
    B. certification of plans
    C. financial assistance
    D. toll-free hotline

12. Which of the following issues would *not* be covered by public health laws?
    A. wearing a helmet
    B. using medical marijuana
    C. Medicare reimbursement
    D. smoking in public places

13. The _____ Reform Act includes rules for quality of care and a certification process that requires unannounced inspections.
    A. Nursing Home
    B. Healthcare
    C. Home Health
    D. Hospice Care

14. Healthcare organizations are required to create schedules for _____ and destruction of information.
    A. filing
    B. creation
    C. definition
    D. retention

15. The _____ Act requires all drugs marketed in the United States to meet minimum standards for strength, purity, and quality.
    A. False Claims
    B. Controlled Substances
    C. Federal Register
    D. Pure Food and Drug

Completion

16. The _____ Act is a federal statute that prohibits certain anticompetitive business activities.

17. States must submit a State Plan _____ for CMS to review and approve before they alter the way healthcare providers are paid.

18. _____ care organizations come together to give coordinated, high-quality care to their Medicare patients.

19. Healthcare organizations must meet Medicare Conditions of _____ to receive funds in Medicare and Medicaid programs.

Discussion and Critical Thinking

20. Review the scenario presented at the beginning of the chapter. Can the nurse have his or her license suspended or revoked for not performing CPR? If the nurse does perform CPR, can he or she be fired from the retirement facility for not following the company's policy? Why do you think that facility had such a policy?

21. What is your opinion on the balance of federal and state regulations regarding healthcare facilities? Should more oversight control be shifted to the federal level or state level? Why or why not?

22. Explain the requirements for health insurance exchanges. Do you think that any requirements should be added or removed?

23. Do you think that the Sherman Antitrust Act is important? Explain your answer.

24. If someone were to ask you about destroying medical records, what advice would you give that person?

Activities

25. Use the Internet to research laws related to healthcare in the state of your choice. This might include regulations applied to nursing homes. Write a paper about the laws and include your opinion of them. Do you think they are too restrictive or not restrictive enough?

26. Create a timeline of the legal challenges the Affordable Care Act has faced and note the outcomes of each challenge.

Case Study

Decades ago, a religious organization purchased a hospital. Since that time, the organization has purchased dozens of other hospitals, all within the same area. Due to religious reasons, the organization has decided to discontinue performing abortions in their hospitals. The organization argues that it is against their religious beliefs to perform abortions because they believe that life begins at conception. They have the legal right to stop performing abortions for religious reasons.

There has been a public outcry because abortion is legal according to federal and state laws. The public also argues that they should have a choice of healthcare facilities and the hospital is there to serve the community. Because the religious organization owns so many hospitals in the region, women would now have to travel very far for an abortion.

What do you think? Should the hospitals be allowed to discontinue performing abortions? What laws, if any, support your opinion?

Unit 3 Healthcare, Law, and Ethics across the Lifespan

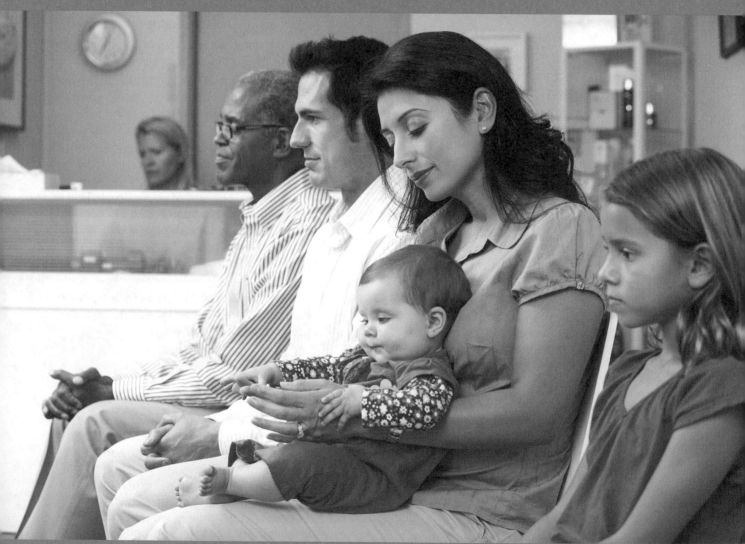

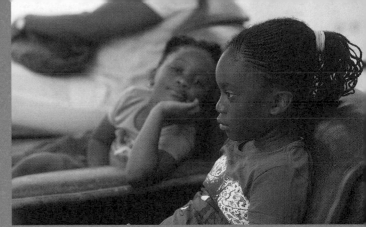

Chapter 10
Minors: Health Law and Ethics

Chapter 11
Adults: Health Law and Ethics

Chapter 12
Older Adults: Health Law and Ethics

Chapter 13

Minors: Health Law and Ethics

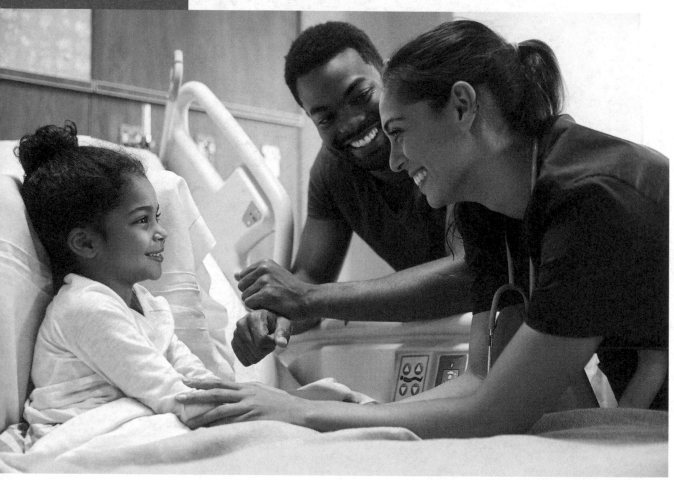

Monkey Business Images/Shutterstock.com

Chapter Outline

Healthcare and Minors
> The Rights and Responsibilities of Parents and Legal Guardians
> The Rights of Minors

Consent and Confidentiality

Reproductive Health
> Contraception
> Sexually Transmitted Infections
> Pregnancy
> Abortion

Mental Health

Cosmetic Surgery

Body Art

Child Labor Laws

Child Abuse

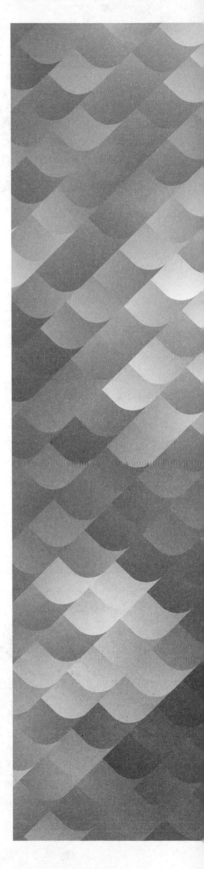

Objectives

- Describe the legal responsibilities of parents and the rights of children regarding healthcare.
- Describe the rules of confidentiality of medical records and under what circumstances a minor's information can be accessible to parents and others.
- Describe the rules for minors related to reproductive health.
- Discuss laws related to mental health.
- Describe the laws affecting minors related to cosmetic surgery.
- Explain the laws related to minors and body art.
- Explain labor laws related to the health of minors.
- Explain how federal and state laws address child abuse.

Key Terms

emancipated minor
emergency care doctrine
Fair Labor Standards Act
Federal Child Abuse Prevention and Treatment Act
judicial bypass
legal guardian
mature minor doctrine
minor

What Would You Do?

Imagine that you are a researcher working on a study about the health and well-being of children. A child tells you that her mother hits her and asks her to undress so she can take photos of her. What should you do? Are you required by law to report this to anyone? What are your ethical responsibilities? What if you do not tell anyone? Are there any legal actions that can be taken against you?

minor
a person younger than the age of full legal responsibility; any person younger than 18 years of age

A **minor** is typically defined as a person younger than 18 years of age or a person younger than the age of full legal responsibility. Most minors are considered not to have developed sufficient knowledge, judgment, and maturity to decide important and complex matters. As a result, minors are not permitted to vote, enter into enforceable contracts, consume alcohol, volunteer for the military, and, in most cases, consent to medical care (Figure 13.1). Laws regarding minors are intended to protect both the minor and society from harm. These laws generally permit minors to access medical care only with the consent of a parent or **legal guardian** in non-emergency situations.

As children mature, certain rights are granted to them, such as the right to work after they reach 16 years of age. One area of the law that has changed recently is the right of minors older than a given age to make certain healthcare-related decisions based on fundamental constitutional rights of privacy.

legal guardian
a person who has the legal authority (and the corresponding duty) to care for the personal and property interests of another person

Parents and guardians have a legal and ethical duty to care for and maintain custody of their children. The laws governing child custody differ from state to state. Each state allows for both child custody and guardianship over minors. Those rights can be taken from a parent only in exceptional situations, such as child neglect. Legal guardians are appointed by a court. Guardians have the right to make decisions about their children insofar as the terms of the guardianship allow, but those rights can be terminated by a court. In the situation of a divorce, one parent may have physical custody of the child, while both parents have joint legal custody. This means they share the authority and responsibility to provide for the minor's physical needs, living circumstances, and medical care.

In terms of providing protection, laws help prevent children from being subjected to abuse

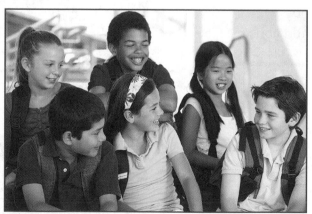

Monkey Business Images/Shutterstock.com

Figure 13.1   The rights of people less than 18 years of age are limited.

or being forced to work at young ages. Laws also help eliminate barriers to access to healthcare. More mature minors sometimes have reservations about seeking out healthcare services because of concerns about confidentiality, including having their parents or guardians notified.

Not seeking care when it is needed can have severe negative consequences. Laws have been established to allow minors to make some healthcare decisions on their own and obtain medical testing and treatment without anyone else being notified, in certain circumstances. Confidentiality and consent laws vary depending on the minor's age, the treatment needed, and the law of the state in which the person resides.

In this chapter, laws related to minors are discussed in general, but it is important to note that because these laws vary by state, healthcare providers are responsible for knowing their specific state laws.

Healthcare and Minors

Generally, minors have legal limitations on their decision-making capacity and healthcare-related rights. However, there are situations in which minors are able to make decisions on their own without parental consent or knowledge. This section explains the legal responsibilities of parents and guardians regarding the health of minors, as well as minors' rights with regard to their own care.

The Rights and Responsibilities of Parents and Legal Guardians

The law gives parents and legal guardians the power to make decisions for their minors' healthcare in most cases (Figure 13.2). For example, in non-emergency situations, minors typically require consent from a legally responsible adult to access medical care. However, this power is not absolute; there are some healthcare decisions that minors can make on their own. When the parent or guardian's healthcare decision conflicts with the desires of the minor, the minor may ask the courts to decide which decision is in the best interest of his or her health. Any minor may seek court action through an adult representative or *guardian ad litem*.

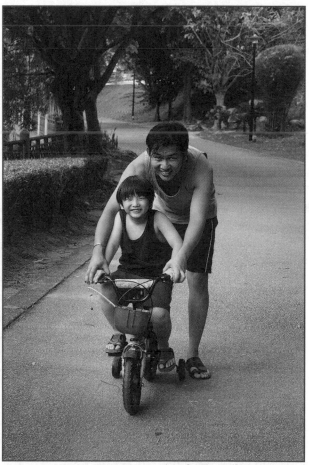

Figure 13.2 Parents and legal guardians have a responsibility to their children.

Obviously, younger children usually appear in court as a result of adults who have an interest in both the child and the subject matter.

A parent or guardian is not allowed to make medical decisions that would unnecessarily risk the life or health of the minor. For example, if a child needs a life-saving medication and the parents refuse to give it to the child, the child can be removed from the home. Along with the right to make healthcare decisions for their minor children, parents and guardians have a responsibility to pay for the care that children receive. Parents and guardians must pay for all of the healthcare treatment to which they give consent. Failure to pay for care may be considered neglect.

Career Corner

Pediatricians are physicians specializing in treatment for infants, children, and young adults. These physicians diagnose, treat, examine, and prevent diseases and injuries. They also monitor patients' development to ensure proper physical and mental health and development. Pediatricians also obtain and document patients' medical histories, discuss exam results with patients and guardians, and counsel patients on healthy eating, hygiene, and lifestyle.

Medical school takes four years to complete. The first two years are mostly spent in the classroom and laboratory. The third and fourth years involve clinical experience under the supervision of licensed physicians. After medical school, pediatricians must complete a three-year pediatric residency. Then they will be eligible to take the board examination for certification in general pediatrics.

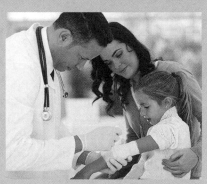

michaeljung/Shutterstock.com

The Rights of Minors

emancipated minor
a minor who is 16 years of age or older and has obtained legal independence from his or her parents or guardians

mature minor doctrine
a legal principle that allows minors to make decisions about their health and welfare, if they can show that they are mature enough to make a decision on their own

States have statutes that describe the types of healthcare minors can consent to and specifications for **emancipated minors**. The term *emancipated minors* describes anyone 16 years of age and older whom a court has determined can provide for themselves and are sufficiently mature to live on their own without the support of their families. These individuals are able to make their own healthcare decisions without consent from a parent or guardian.

Another type of minor, a *mature minor*, is also allowed by many states to make healthcare decisions on his or her own. The **mature minor doctrine** is a legal principle that states that an unemancipated minor may possess the maturity to choose or reject a particular healthcare treatment without the knowledge or agreement of parents or guardians. A mature minor must be able to demonstrate that he or she is able to make adult-like decisions. If this is the case, then the minor is permitted to make certain healthcare decisions. For example, a mature minor may be able to refuse a blood transfusion based on religious beliefs.

Statutes often indicate that if a minor is married or pregnant, he or she should be treated as an adult when it comes to healthcare decisions. In addition, many states permit minors to consent to birth control counseling as well as diagnosis and treatment for sexually transmitted infections and substance abuse without consent from or notification of a parent or guardian.

Each healthcare professional must understand the law in his or her state regarding treatment of and consent by minors. Minors should receive the same information that a parent or guardian would receive, but modified so that it is age-appropriate. Providers should document that the information was provided and why consent from the parent or guardian was not required. It is advisable for providers to seek a court order to accept consent from a minor if any doubt about the minor's maturity level exists. Of course, this is not always possible in an emergency situation.

Consent and Confidentiality

Unless otherwise specified by law, a medical provider may not reveal confidential information about a patient without the permission of the person who consented to the healthcare. There are some situations in which a healthcare provider may be required to disclose confidential information to someone other than the patient. Those exceptions, which

were described in Chapter 9, include duty to warn, suspected occurrence of abuse, and instances of notifiable diseases. In general, if a minor is able to legally give consent, then the rule of confidentiality applies.

If a minor is covered under his or her parent or guardian's health insurance plan, there is a chance that the minor's confidentiality may be compromised through billing information, itemized benefit statements, or other communication issued to the responsible adults (Figure 13.3). This may occur even if the provider agrees to keep the treatment confidential.

A minor who is seeking healthcare services under a parent or guardian's private insurance plan can contact the insurance company to determine whether all medical services will be reported to the insurance coverage holders. A minor also can potentially prevent medical information from being revealed by paying for care at the time of

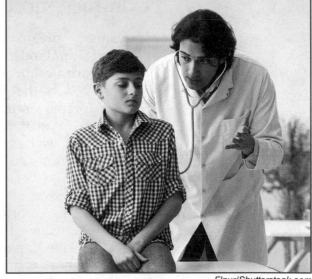

Elnur/Shutterstock.com

Figure 13.3 Minors being treated for drug addiction or other sensitive health problems may not want parents or guardians to know. It is important to know your state laws regarding these situations.

service and not using the insurance. With the increasing ability for patients to see their medical records, parents or guardians also may eventually see that a treatment has been provided by later reviewing the child's medical history.

In emergency situations, laws related to consent are different from those used in non-emergency situations. Medical treatment can be provided without getting parental or guardian consent if the time taken to obtain consent would delay treatment and increase the risk to a minor's life or health. For example, if the minor is involved in a car accident and sustains life-threatening injuries, treatment can be given without consent. Information about a minor's emergency treatment can be disclosed to the parents or guardians upon request, if their consent would have been necessary in a non-emergency situation. If the minor could have consented on his or her own, medical personnel may not be able to disclose treatment information to the parents or guardians. This is all covered in the **emergency care doctrine**, which protects healthcare providers from legal liability for medical battery.

emergency care doctrine
a legal process that assumes consent to a medical procedure during an emergency when the person is incapacitated and unable to give consent

Reproductive Health

Minors have unique rights when it comes to their reproductive health, such as the use of birth control. Situations involving sexually transmitted infections, pregnancy, and abortion also warrant special rights. These issues are addressed in this section.

Contraception

Unplanned pregnancies, sexually transmitted infections (STIs), acquired immunodeficiency syndrome (AIDS), and other health complications can occur when sexual intercourse takes place. Contraception can reduce the risk of developing these conditions. The United States Supreme Court has held that the federal constitutional right of privacy in matters relating to the use of contraception extends to minors as well as adults. For this reason, the government cannot restrict a minor's access to contraception without a compelling reason. The federal Title X family planning program provides funding to clinics that provide treatment regardless of age or marital status. As a result, Title X-supported clinics always provide confidential services to minors who request them.

Under Title X, family planning counseling and medical exams are part of a minor's confidential medical records. This information cannot be released without the minor's permission. This law also applies to any prescription for contraception that may be given. However, if the parents do not know about or consent to the treatment, they are not required to pay for it.

Sexually Transmitted Infections

A patient's treatment for a sexually transmitted infection (STI) is typically a confidential part of his or her medical record, but there are some cases in which another party or parties must be warned. For example, laws regarding notifiable diseases require that doctors and laboratories report some STIs and new cases of HIV/AIDS to the health department and/or the Centers for Disease Control and Prevention (CDC). These laws pertain to cases in minors as well as adults.

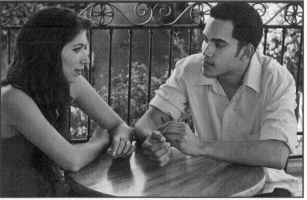

photomatz/Shutterstock.com

Figure 13.4   Some states have laws requiring individuals with STIs to inform their partners of the diagnosis. This includes young adult couples, who might still be minors.

In addition, some states require a person who is infected with an STI to warn sexual partners of the disease or risk criminal sanctions (Figure 13.4). This requirement includes minors. The STIs included in the partner notification law are typically HIV/AIDS, syphilis, gonorrhea, and chlamydia. The patient also can have the health department or a doctor notify the partner(s). Partner notification typically occurs within 2 to 3 working days of identification, unless there is an indication of potential partner violence.

Some states require doctors to ask patients who are infected with HIV/AIDS about others who may have been exposed to the infection through sex or needle sharing. The health department or physician can then notify people who are at risk about where to get counseling, testing, and treatment if they are infected.

Laws related to HIV testing vary in different states. For example, in New York, consent for HIV testing is not determined by age. Instead,

 ## Ethical Dilemma

Imagine that you are a licensed vocational nurse working at a high school. A 17-year-old student who tested positive for HIV a few months ago visits the health office to discuss some symptoms he is having. He informs you that he is having unprotected sex with his girlfriend. He is afraid that she will leave him if he tells her he is HIV-positive. The student also is fearful that his girlfriend will tell other students about his condition, and that he will be abandoned and teased by his friends. What is your legal responsibility in this situation? Do you need to inform the parents or guardians? Do you need to inform the girlfriend? What ethical considerations exist?

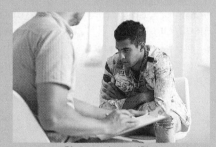

Photographee.eu/Shutterstock.com

consent is determined by factors such as if they have the capacity to understand the consequences of the test, if the child is married, if a female minor is pregnant, and if the child is in foster care.

Pregnancy

There is no law specifically addressing the rights of pregnant minors. Prenatal care, delivery, and postnatal care are very expensive, so it is unlikely that a hospital or doctor would agree to treat a minor without first receiving the consent of her parents or guardians. If a parent or guardian refuses to consent to prenatal care, the pregnant minor may be able to turn to the courts for help.

In terms of delivery, the only circumstance in which the consent of the minor would definitely be accepted is if she came to the emergency room already in labor. This would qualify as an emergency case and the hospital staff could deliver the baby without parental or guardian consent because of the emergency care doctrine.

Abortion

In the United States, abortion is legal. However, for minors, the laws regarding abortion differ from state to state. For example, in some states, minors do not need parental permission (consent) to have an abortion. In other states, parental notification is required, but parental permission is not. In these cases, consent is not needed, but the parent or guardian must be notified that the procedure is going to take place. In some states, the law requires that one parent or adult family member (such as an adult sibling, aunt, or uncle) give permission for an abortion, while other states' laws specifically require that one parent give permission.

judicial bypass
a legal provision that allows a minor to circumvent the necessity of obtaining parental consent by obtaining consent from a court instead

In states with laws that require notification or permission, a **judicial bypass** may be used by a girl younger than 18 years of age who wishes to have an abortion. Through this process, a judge can excuse the minor from the legal requirement to tell her parents or legal guardian about the procedure. All states are required to provide the judicial bypass option to minors who want to have an abortion without notifying their parents. In some states, there may be a 24- or 48-hour waiting period from the time the minor speaks to a counselor in a clinic or doctor's office until the time of the procedure.

Mental Health

Mental health professionals, such as counselors and psychiatrists, can provide minors with some services without having to notify anyone. This includes treatment for substance abuse, self-injury, depression, and eating disorders. A minor 14 years of age or older can request outpatient care without notifying a parent if the treatment does not include medication. This applies only if the medical care is limited to 6 sessions or 30 days, whichever comes first. After that, care must be discontinued or a parent or guardian must be informed and give consent for treatment to continue (Figure 13.5).

During those first 6 sessions or 30 days, the parent or guardian will not be informed of the treatment unless the minor consents or the professional feels the minor is likely to harm someone, including himself or herself. The right to treatment is predicated on the condition that action must be taken to ensure that a minor does not harm anyone, including himself or herself. Even in this situation, however, the healthcare provider must first tell the minor that the parent or guardian will be notified.

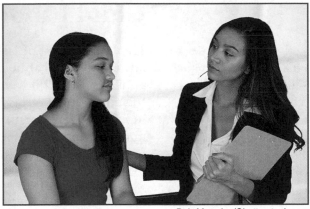

Rob Marmion/Shutterstock.com

Figure 13.5 Minors can receive mental health treatment for 6 sessions or 30 days without having to notify a parent or guardian.

Cosmetic Surgery

Consent from a parent or legal guardian is required for all cosmetic surgery procedures performed on minors. In addition, the patient must have matured physically and have the intellectual and emotional capacity to handle the surgery. In 2000, the federal government passed a new regulation stating that no person younger than 18 years of age may undergo a breast augmentation procedure, even with parental consent, except for some rare occasions in which that breast augmentation is truly a reconstructive procedure.

Body Art

Skin painting and piercing have health risks. The use of unclean needles may transfer bloodborne diseases such as HIV/AIDS or hepatitis and can cause infections. Certain body art also can be related to gangs, and those affiliations can contribute to violence. Therefore, there are state laws that restrict minors from obtaining certain body art. In states that require consent of a parent or guardian, the parent or guardian must accompany the minor to the business where the procedure will be performed and sign a document that describes the tattoo or body piercing.

Child Labor Laws

**Fair Labor
Standards Act**
law that contains
regulations related to
employment of minors,
including restricting
the hours that children
younger than 16 years
of age can work
and forbidding the
employment of children
younger than 18 years
of age in certain jobs
that are deemed too
dangerous

The Department of Labor monitors child labor and enforces child labor laws. The **Fair Labor Standards Act** (FLSA) addresses the employment and abuse of child workers. This law includes provisions that protect the educational opportunities of minors and prohibit their employment in jobs that are harmful to their health and safety. For example, minors may not work manufacturing or storing explosives, mining coal, fighting forest fires, or operating power-driven meat processing machines. The FLSA also restricts the hours that minors younger than 16 years of age can work.

Child Abuse

**Federal Child Abuse
Prevention and
Treatment Act**
key federal legislation
that addresses child
abuse and neglect;
provides federal
funding to states in
support of prevention,
assessment,
investigation,
prosecution, and
treatment activities;
and provides grants to
public agencies and
nonprofit organizations
for demonstration
programs and projects

The **Federal Child Abuse Prevention and Treatment Act** (CAPTA) is federal legislation that provides minimum standards and funding for states to support prevention, assessment, investigation, prosecution, and treatment related to child abuse. Since being amended by the CAPTA Reauthorization Act of 2010, this law defines child abuse and neglect as any action or inaction that results in death, serious physical or emotional harm, sexual abuse, or exploitation; or an action or inaction that presents a risk of serious harm.

CAPTA requires that states include a list of minimum actions or behaviors into their legal definitions of child abuse and neglect. This legislation provides grants for states to create demonstration programs and projects. Additionally, CAPTA identifies the federal government's role in supporting research, evaluation, technical assistance, and data collection activities. It also established the Office on Child Abuse and Neglect and the National Clearinghouse on Child Abuse and Neglect Information.

All states have laws related to child abuse, but each state's law is different. Most states have civil definitions for child abuse and neglect that determine when an intervention by state child protective agencies should occur. In most states, certain individuals are required by law to report suspected child abuse (see Chapter 6 for further discussion of mandatory reporting laws).

It can be difficult to balance laws created to protect children while simultaneously permitting parents and legal guardians to raise their families without government intrusion. One example of this is some families' preference to use spanking for discipline. At what point does spanking become abuse?

Another example is cultural healing practices such as *cupping* and *coining*. Cupping is a cultural healing practice in which evacuated glass cups are applied to the skin to draw blood toward or through the surface. Cupping leaves burns and bruises on the child's skin. In the practice of coining, a coin is used to scrape the skin, and this often leaves marks (Figure 13.6). Is this a cultural norm or child abuse?

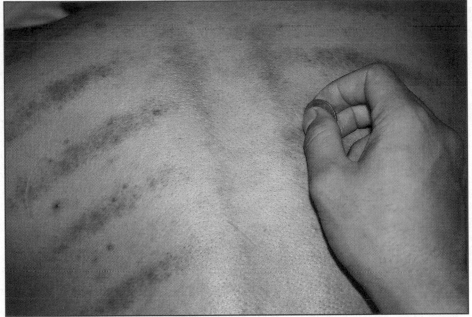

Figure 13.6   Coining is an old Asian practice that some may consider abuse.

The marks left by coining and cupping do not constitute child abuse. However, uninformed individuals may see these marks, misidentify them as child abuse injuries, and misreport minority parents as child abusers. In an article for *The Journal of Law in Society*, W.Y. Chin referred to the following incident:

> "A Vietnamese father brought his feverish son to the emergency room. The doctors saw marks on the boy's skin and mistakenly believed the father abused the boy. Law enforcement officials arrested the father who tried to explain that the marks were caused by 'coining,' a benign folk remedy that treats various ailments by using the edge of a coin or similar object to scrape or 'scratch' the skin. The humiliated father later committed suicide."

Laws about mandatory reporting are controversial. People have concerns about the loss of privacy and how broad the definition of what constitutes abuse is (as illustrated in the previous example about coining). The main concern is that the government is interfering with the rights of parents and legal guardians to raise and discipline their children as they desire. However, no one wants children's lives to be put at a greater risk if they are not removed from an abusive home, so these laws remain in place despite privacy concerns.

Chapter Summary

- Parents and guardians have a legal duty to provide appropriate healthcare to a minor under their care.
- Children have limited rights to consent to care independently under certain circumstances.
- Minors have special rights related to reproductive health.
- Mental health services to minors may be provided without parental consent if medication is not involved.
- Cosmetic surgery is not permitted on minors except in cases of needed reconstruction.
- Some states have limited the application of body art to minors, and some states that allow it require written parental consent.
- Labor laws have been established, in part, to protect the health and safety of minors.
- Federal and state laws attempt to protect minors from child abuse while honoring parental rights to childrearing.

Vocabulary Matching

1. legal provision that allows a minor to circumvent the need to obtain parental consent by obtaining consent from a court instead
2. law that contains regulations related to employment of minors, including restricting the hours that children can work and forbidding certain types of employment
3. legal principle that allows minors to make decisions about their health and welfare if they can show that they are mature enough to make a decision on their own
4. minor who is 16 years of age or older and has obtained legal independence from his or her parents or guardians
5. person who has the legal authority (and the corresponding duty) to care for the personal and property interests of another person
6. legal process that assumes consent to a medical procedure during an emergency when the person is incapacitated and unable to give consent
7. person younger than the age of full legal responsibility; any person younger than 18 years of age
8. federal legislation that provides funding to states to support prevention, assessment, investigation, prosecution, and treatment activities related to child abuse

A. emancipated minor
B. emergency care doctrine
C. Fair Labor Standards Act
D. Federal Child Abuse Prevention and Treatment Act
E. judicial bypass
F. legal guardian
G. mature minor doctrine
H. minor

Multiple Choice

9. Generally, minors must obtain consent from a(n) _____ before gaining access to medical care.
   A. physician
   B. teacher
   C. legal guardian
   D. counselor

10. The legal term for an adult representative sought through court action is _____.
    A. police power
    B. *respondeat superior*
    C. habeas corpus
    D. *guardian ad litem*

11. _____ minors can provide for themselves, and the court has determined that these minors are mature enough to live on their own.
    A. Emancipated
    B. Surrogate
    C. Conditional
    D. Independent

12. The _____ doctrine legally allows minors who are mature enough to reject a healthcare decision made by their parents.
    A. minor privacy
    B. surrogate
    C. temporary maturity
    D. mature minor

13. Which of the following laws provides funding and requires standards for states to protect children from abuse?
    A. Sex Offender Registration and Notification Act
    B. CAPTA
    C. Mature Minor Doctrine
    D. Emergency Care Doctrine

Completion

14. If a minor is in a life-threatening situation and there is not time to obtain consent from a parent or legal guardian to provide medical care, the provider can assume consent under the _____ doctrine.

15. The _____ Act enforces child labor laws.

16. The _____ doctrine states that unemancipated minors may possess the maturity to choose healthcare treatments for themselves.

17. Minors can be treated for _____ sessions or 30 days without notifying a parent or guardian.

Discussion and Critical Thinking

18. Review the scenario presented at the beginning of this chapter. How would you respond in this situation? Explain your answer.

19. Do you disagree with any of the laws mentioned in this chapter? If so, please explain which laws and why you disagree with them.

20. If you were a parent, what healthcare decisions would you want your minor children to decide for themselves without speaking to you? Explain your answer.

21. List at least three reasons for parents having control over most healthcare decisions related to minors.

22. Why might a minor seek mental health services without obtaining parental permission?

23. How might a minor's intended confidential medical treatment be disclosed to a parent?

Activities

24. Review at least two healthcare-related laws in your state that affect minors. Write a paper describing why you do or do not support these laws. Discuss any changes that you would recommend.

25. Watch the YouTube video called "Childhood Obesity Deemed Child Abuse In Controversial...," and then write a reaction paper. Should parents or legal guardians with morbidly obese children be charged with child abuse? Why or why not?

26. Search the Internet for three child labor laws that exist in your state. Create a table identifying the differences in these three laws. Then write a reaction paper about the differences that you identified.

Case Study

Sharon, a 16-year-old who lives with her mother, is HIV-positive. Sharon has never told her mother that she is HIV-positive, and now she has developed an AIDS-related illness. Sharon is in need of medical attention, but she does not want to tell her mother. She will not seek out medical care if she is required to inform her mother of her HIV status. Can a physician treat Sharon without parental consent? Explain the laws related to this situation.

Chapter 14

Adults: Health Law and Ethics

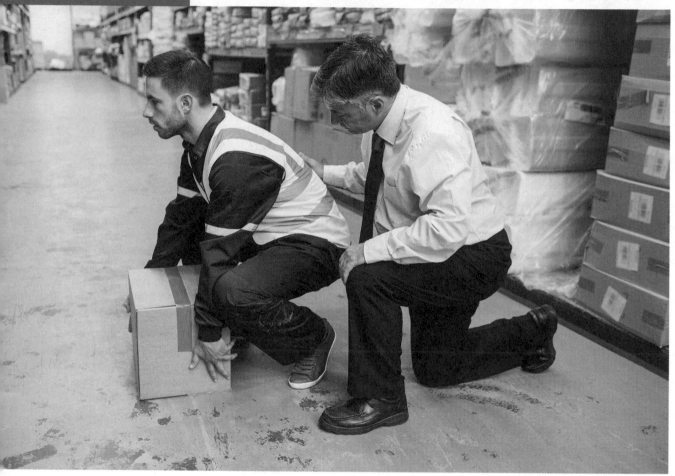

wavebreakmedia/Shutterstock.com

Chapter Outline

Government Programs That Enhance Health

Language, Culture, and Healthcare

    Language

    Culture

Occupational Laws

Public Health Laws

    Driving

    Medical Marijuana

    Domestic and Intimate-Partner Violence

    Assisted Conception and Reproduction

    HIV Testing

    Mental Health

Public Policy Support of Autonomy

    Advance Directives

    Powers of Attorney

    Conservatorships

Drug Testing

Opioid Prescribing Laws

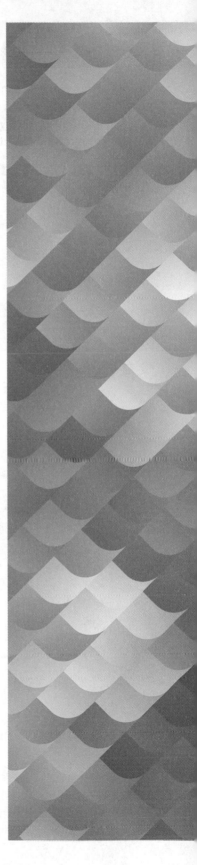

Objectives

- Identify government programs that enhance the health of various members of society.
- Explain the legal responsibilities of medical providers regarding non-English speakers and situations in which culture affects healthcare decisions.
- Describe the laws that mandate health and safety in the workplace.
- Discuss public health laws that affect adults.
- Explain provisions that help patients maintain their autonomy when they cannot communicate their preferences.
- Describe laws related to testing for drugs.
- Explain why new laws have been established to control the use of opioid drugs.

Key Terms

advance directive

Civil Rights Act of 1964

competence

conservatorship

culture

durable power of attorney for
    healthcare

fiduciary duty

Occupational Safety and Health
    Administration (OSHA)

What Would You Do?

Imagine that you are a nurse practitioner in New York. You have just informed your 30-year-old patient that he is HIV-positive. What is your responsibility in this situation? Can you require that he tell you who his previous sexual partners were? If so, are you allowed to contact them? What can you tell them?

Adults (people 18 years of age and older) typically have the ability to direct their own healthcare decisions. There are laws in place to guide professionals and organizations in providing care to adults that respects their autonomy, protects the public, and enables healthcare providers or a surrogate decision maker to make healthcare-related decisions for adults who are not able to make decisions for themselves. Yet there are times when laws take precedence over personal decision making. This chapter focuses on key laws that affect the health and safety of adults between 18 and 64 years of age.

Government Programs That Enhance Health

Government programs are available to assist residents. Some of these programs legally must be offered to citizens and therefore are referred to as *entitlement programs*. These entitlement programs include Social Security, Medicare, and Medicaid. There are additional health-related programs that the federal and state governments provide, which are also described in this section. The criteria for qualifying for these programs vary by program.

Medicare is a health insurance program for the elderly and disabled. Medicaid is a health insurance program for low-income individuals and families. Medicare was created by the Social Security Act, and Medicaid was created by the Social Security Amendments of 1965. Health insurance through Medicare is generally offered to people 65 years of age and older. However, some disabled adults, kidney transplant recipients, and kidney failure patients on dialysis are also eligible for Medicare, which is why it is included in this chapter.

Numerous states offer Children Health Insurance Programs (CHIP) for low-income families. Federal employees receive insurance coverage through the Federal Employees Health Program (FEHP).

Active members of the military, their families and beneficiaries, and veterans are entitled to healthcare benefits via the US Department of

Veteran Affairs (Figure 14.1). The Indian Health Services program provides healthcare services for Native Americans and Alaska Natives. This program was made available by the 1988 Indian Healthcare Improvement Act.

In addition to health insurance programs, there are many other programs that can support the health of individuals and families, such as government housing programs. Many federal housing grants or loans, such as the Section 8 Housing Program, help people find affordable living arrangements. Food assistance programs are designed to help low-income families combat hunger. Food stamps, which came about as a result of the Federal Food Stamp Act of 1964, are one example of these programs. This program provides low-income individuals with food stamps that can be exchanged like money at authorized stores. The federal government pays for the benefit that is received, while states pay to determine eligibility for the program, distribute the stamps, and run the program.

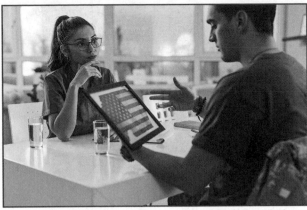

Drazen Zigic/Shutterstock.com

Figure 14.1   Veterans of all ages are eligible for healthcare services through the US Department of Veteran Affairs.

Language, Culture, and Healthcare

What do language and culture have to do with providing medical care? As described in previous chapters, proper healthcare depends on good communication, understanding patient instructions, and honoring the patient's right to autonomy. All of these aspects of healthcare can be negatively affected if differences in language and culture are not understood.

Language barriers can create unequal access to healthcare and health information. **Culture** influences how people access and utilize the healthcare system; their health behaviors; and how they express, prevent, and treat health issues. There can be differences between the Western medical system and the system used by people with different cultural perspectives.

culture
the sum of attitudes, customs, and beliefs that distinguishes one group of people from another

For example, blood transfusions are against the cultural beliefs of some people. Others refuse vaccinations for religious reasons. In some cultures, people are often put in a trance to hallucinate and communicate with gods or spirits, which may be viewed as a psychiatric illness in the dominant culture. Laws are designed to respect patients' autonomy when cultural beliefs vary from dominant beliefs, but there are times when laws need to override cultural and religious preferences to protect the safety of children and the general public.

While language and culture affect the healthcare provided for people of all ages, it tends to have a strong impact on adults, as they are

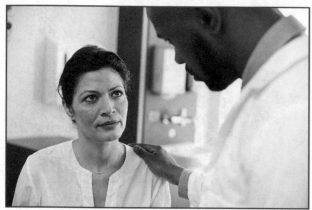

Monkey Business Images/Shutterstock.com

Figure 14.2 Adults are generally responsible for making their own healthcare decisions, so information must always be presented in a way they can understand.

legally able to make their own healthcare decisions in most cases (Figure 14.2). Therefore, this topic is included in this chapter on adults and health law and not the other chapters. That does not mean, however, that minors and older adults are not impacted by language and cultural differences.

Language

As a healthcare worker, you will likely encounter patients whose primary language is not English, and healthcare has a language of its own. Therefore, people who have limited English skills can be particularly confused when it comes to healthcare. As a provider of care, you have a legal and ethical responsibility to help ensure equal treatment for limited English speakers. There are federal mandates and state laws that healthcare facilities and clinicians must obey to provide this equal treatment.

Civil Rights Act of 1964
federal legislation that outlawed discrimination based on race, color, religion, sex, or national origin

The **Civil Rights Act of 1964** continues to be the single most important piece of federal legislation for providing Limited English Proficiency (LEP) individuals with a legal right to language assistance services. The legal foundation for language assistance is contained in Title VI of the Civil Rights Act, which states the following:

"No person in the United States shall, on the ground of race, color, or national origin, be excluded from participation in, be denied the benefits of, or be subjected to discrimination under any program or activity receiving federal financial assistance."

The Civil Rights Act was passed by Congress to ensure that federal funds were not used to support discriminatory programs or activities. The Supreme Court interpreted this law to equate discrimination based on language with national origin discrimination. Title VI applies to all federal agencies.

In healthcare, federal financial assistance includes money from federal agencies such as Medicaid, Medicare, the Health Resources and Services Administration, and the National Institutes of Health. The US Department of Health & Human Services (DHHS) Office for Civil Rights is responsible for enforcing the Civil Rights Act along with the Americans with Disabilities Act, the Age Discrimination Act, and the Hill-Burton Act.

Any organization or individual that receives funding through DHHS is subject to oversight from the Office for Civil Rights (OCR). The OCR has the authority to investigate complaints about language barriers, to initiate its own reviews, and to withhold federal funds for noncompliance. In 1946, Congress passed a law that gave hospitals, nursing homes, and other healthcare facilities grants and loans for construction and modernization. In return, they agreed to provide a reasonable volume of services to people who were unable to pay and to make their services available to everyone residing in the facility's area. The program stopped providing funds in 1997, but about 170 healthcare facilities nationwide are still obligated to provide free or reduced-cost care because they received federal funds.

The Executive Order (EO) 13166, *Improving Access to Services for Persons with Limited English Proficiency*, was signed by President Clinton in 2000. This EO requires federal agencies to examine the services they offer and determine where they might add services for LEP individuals. Once they have done that, federal agencies must develop and establish a system to provide those services to LEP people. The EO also requires federal agencies to ensure that facilities receiving federal financial assistance provide access to their LEP applicants and beneficiaries.

The US Department of Justice issued a Policy Guidance Document entitled "Enforcement of Title VI of the Civil Rights Act of 1964—National Origin Discrimination Against Persons With Limited English Proficiency (LEP Guidance)" to assist federal agencies with meeting the requirements laid out in the EO.

This LEP Guidance document sets forth the compliance standards that recipients of federal financial assistance must follow to ensure that their programs and activities normally provided in English are accessible to LEP individuals. This is intended to prevent discrimination based on national origin, which would violate Title VI's prohibition against national origin discrimination.

These laws mean that all healthcare facilities should be providing language assistance services, especially after receiving federal funds. Several states also require some forms of health information to be distributed to LEP patients. The topics and languages included in this information vary by state. If you are involved in providing healthcare information, you should be aware of the rules in a particular location (Figure 14.3).

Some states have laws requiring language assistance services to be available at specific types of facilities or as a condition of licensure. Massachusetts, for example, requires all emergency departments and acute psychiatric facilities to provide access to trained interpreters for their patients on a 24-hour, 7-day basis. Illinois requires interpreters to be provided in state mental health facilities during the intake and evaluation process. States such as Colorado, New Jersey, and Rhode Island have established laws that require language services as a condition of licensure.

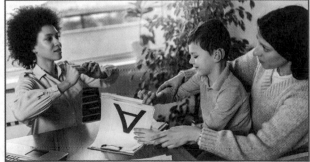

adriaticfoto/Shutterstock.com

Figure 14.3 In many states, language assistance requirements are not limited to speech. Assistance must also be available for people with hearing and vision impairments.

Culture

The social norms and behaviors of groups, known as *culture*, affect people's health-related decisions and practices. Therefore, laws have been established to respect both cultural and religious autonomy. While this is the intent, there are times when the law must override cultural and religious preferences. For example, as stated previously, some religious groups do not agree to blood transfusions. In life-threatening situations, adults can refuse a blood transfusion, but they cannot prevent their children from getting a blood transfusion.

In some instances, laws cede to religious freedom. For example, all states have legislation requiring students to receive specified vaccines. Some states grant religious exemptions for people who have religious beliefs against immunizations (Figure 14.4). At other times, laws, culture, and religion do not coexist so easily. As described in the previous chapter, the practice of coining has clashed with laws related to child abuse.

Deciding whether a practice is cultural or considered child abuse may relate to the proximate cause of harm. This means an event is so related to a harm that has occurred that it must be considered a cause of the harm. Not getting a child vaccinated may contribute to him or her becoming ill sometime, while an injury caused by coining is immediate and a direct cause of harm.

Sometimes laws developed to respect one culture can be considered discriminatory for others. The laws surrounding the use of peyote are a good example of this. For millennia, Native Americans have used peyote, a cactus plant, as part of their spiritual and healing practices. These practices are used in their culture to induce spiritual experiences, treat physical illnesses such as asthma and diabetes, cure infections, and reduce pain.

The issue of concern is that peyote contains mescaline, a powerful psychoactive drug that causes hallucinations. The United States Drug Enforcement Association (DEA), a division of the US Department of Justice, classifies peyote as a "Schedule I" drug (a category of drugs not considered legitimate for medical use). It is illegal to possess, sell, or use peyote in the United States. However, there are exceptions to the DEA classification of peyote cacti as a controlled substance. It is legal for Native Americans who belong to federally recognized tribes to use peyote for religious purposes.

Many states offer limited exceptions to the peyote laws for religious use by non-Native Americans, but the laws vary. Some non-Native Americans claim that making it legal for only Native Americans to use peyote is discriminating against others.

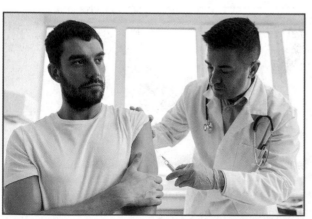

Syda Productions/Shutterstock.com

Figure 14.4 Some patients' cultures or beliefs mean they are opposed to vaccination.

Occupational Laws

Most adults are employed, and there are several federal and state laws that protect employees and the general public while working. These include laws related to safety, sexual harassment, discrimination, noise levels, exposure to smoke, drug testing, and family medical leave. The United States Department of Labor's **Occupational Safety and Health Administration (OSHA)** is the federal agency that enforces these types of laws.

The OSHA Act of 1970 sought to prevent death and serious injuries in the workplace. The law requires employers to create working conditions that are free of known dangers. The Act also created OSHA, which is an organization that creates and mandates protective workplace safety and health standards. These standards are designed to make work environments and practices safer for workers in the United States.

OSHA provides workers with information, training, and assistance. Workers may file a complaint to OSHA if they believe their employer is not following certain standards, and someone from the organization will inspect their workplace. Examples of OSHA regulations include protecting workers in nail salons from infectious diseases, protecting workers in medical facilities from needlesticks, and managing ergonomic safety.

Occupational Safety and Health Administration (OSHA)
a federal agency that regulates workplace safety and health

Public Health Laws

There are numerous health-related laws at the community level. Examples include laws related to smoking, advertising, the sale of alcohol and cigarettes, wearing seat belts, texting while driving, prostitution, and public intoxication.

Driving

Each state has its own licensing and license renewal criteria for drivers of commercial and private motor vehicles. In addition, certain states require physicians to report unsafe drivers or drivers with specific medical conditions to the driver licensing agency. Examples of reportable medical conditions include seizures and vision problems.

Marijuana

Currently, the use of both medical and recreational marijuana is illegal at the federal level, although legislation to legalize it is being considered by Congress. However, the District of Columbia and several states—including Alaska, California, Colorado, Florida, Illinois, Maine, Massachusetts, Michigan, Nevada, Oregon, Vermont and Washington—have adopted expansive laws legalizing marijuana for recreational use. Most recently,

Illinois became the second most-populous state to legalize recreational marijuana. Vermont was the first state to legalize marijuana for recreational use through the legislative process, rather than via a ballot measure. Vermont's law allows adults age 21 and over to grow and possess small amounts of cannabis. However, it does not permit the sale of non-medical cannabis. Some other state laws similarly decriminalized marijuana, but did not initially legalize retail sales.

Most other states allow for limited use of medical marijuana under certain circumstances. Some medical marijuana laws are broader than others, with types of medical conditions that allow for treatment varying from state to state. Louisiana, West Virginia, and a few other states allow only for cannabis-infused products, such as oils or pills.

Domestic and Intimate-Partner Violence

Most states have enacted mandatory reporting laws that require certain healthcare professionals to report specified injuries and wounds and suspected abuse or domestic violence (Figure 14.5). These laws are different from laws that cover reporting for elder abuse, vulnerable adult abuse, and child abuse. The difference lies in the fact that these laws do not specify a protected group. Instead, these broader laws include all individuals to whom specific healthcare professionals provide treatment or medical care.

These reporting laws vary from state to state but generally fall into four categories. The categories include required reporting of injuries caused by weapons; required reporting of injuries that occur during a crime, in violent circumstances, or by any non-accidental means; specific required reporting of domestic violence; and a lack of general mandatory reporting laws.

Assisted Conception and Reproduction

Artificial insemination is the process by which a woman is medically impregnated using semen from her husband, male partner, or a third-party donor. When donors utilize sperm donation clinics, legislation states that legally the donor is not liable for children born via artificial insemination with his donation. The donor has no legal responsibility for his offspring and cannot sue for parental rights at a later time.

The Food and Drug Administration regulates sperm donation clinics. These clinics offer donor screenings and quality checks, and they have specific rules regarding record keeping. The FDA requires that all sperm donors be tested for HIV and hepatitis. The state of California considers it a felony for someone who knows he has HIV/AIDS to donate sperm.

Examples of Mandatory Reporting Laws for Domestic Violence and Intimate-Partner Violence for Selected States	
State	**Example Mandatory Reporting Laws**
California	California Penal Code §§11160 and 11161 require any healthcare practitioner employed in a health facility, clinic, physician's office, or local or state public health department or clinic to report suspected abuse to local law enforcement. This law applies when a health practitioner treats a physical condition that the practitioner knows or reasonably suspects is the result of assaultive or abusive behavior, as defined by state law. This law also applies if a healthcare practitioner provides treatment for a self-inflicted wound or any wound inflicted by a firearm. California Penal Code § 13823.11 states that, at a minimum, suspected sexual assault or suspected attempted sexual assault should be reported to law enforcement authorities.
Colorado	Colorado Revised Statute § 12-36-135 requires physicians, nurses, and other healthcare practitioners to report treating any wounds that he or she believes are intentionally inflicted. Healthcare practitioners must also report injuries that he or she believes were inflicted as a result of a crime or domestic violence.
Florida	Florida Statute § 790.24 requires any physician, nurse, or other employee of a hospital, sanitarium, clinic, or nursing home to report treating a gunshot wound or life-threatening injury resulting from violence to the sheriff's department. Knowingly avoiding reporting such an incident is considered a misdemeanor. Florida Statute § 877.155 requires any person to report treating second- or third-degree burns affecting 10% or more of the body to the sheriff's department if the burns are determined to be caused by a flammable substance and if they suspect the injury is a result of violence or other crime.
North Dakota	North Dakota Century Code § 43-17-41 requires a physician, physician assistant, or any other specified healthcare professional to report diagnosis or treatment of a wound, injury, or other physical trauma that is self-inflicted or inflicted via a knife or gun, and which the healthcare professional suspects is the result of a crime. If the healthcare professional reports suspected domestic or sexual abuse, he or she must provide the patient with information about a relevant support organization or assistance program.
Tennessee	Tennessee Code Annotated § 38-1-101 requires all hospitals, clinics, sanitariums, doctors, physicians, surgeons, nurses, pharmacists, undertakers, embalmers, or others to report treating injuries caused by a knife, firearm, or other deadly weapon. Injuries caused by other means of violence, suffocation, or poisoning must also be reported to law enforcement officials. Tennessee Code Annotated § 36-3-621(C)(1) requires any healthcare practitioner licensed or certified under Title 63 (excluding veterinarians) to report known or suspected injuries that are the result of domestic violence or domestic abuse to the department of health, office of health statistics, on a monthly basis. Identifying information shall not be disclosed.

Goodheart-Willcox Publisher

Figure 14.5 Examples of State Mandatory Reporting Laws.

Certain states have regulations requiring that artificial insemination be done with a licensed physician supervising the process. Most states have set a standard that determines the legal parents of a child conceived through artificial insemination. This standard considers a married woman's husband to be the legal father of that child.

Career Corner

Genetic counselors help individuals and couples considering genetic testing identify their risks for certain genetic disorders, such as breast cancer. These professionals have a background in counseling and medicine. They assist patients in understanding hereditary genetic conditions and the probability of passing on such genetic traits to their offspring. Genetic counselors work in clinical settings, education, research, public health, public policy, private practice,

administrative positions, and as consultants.

Prior to qualifying for employment as a genetic counselor, an individual must attain a bachelor's degree in public health, social work, biology, nursing, or psychology. Then he or she must earn a master's degree in genetics. Courses in subjects such as clinical genetics, cytogenetics, molecular genetics, social theory, population genetics, and ethics are taken while earning this master's degree.

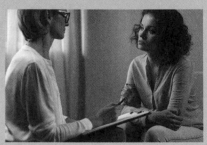

Motortion Films/Shutterstock.com

Certification for this profession may be obtained from the American Board of Genetics Counseling. Applicants must have earned a degree from an accredited genetics program and pass an exam to be certified.

HIV Testing

There are situations in which people are required by law to take an HIV test. These laws vary from state to state and are related to topics such as joining the military or arriving in prison. In some states, healthcare providers are required to obtain informed consent specifically for the HIV test. In other states, the general consent for medical treatment is sufficient for the provider or facility to conduct the test.

Pre- and post-test counseling is covered in certain state laws. This counseling includes personalized help with understanding the test, HIV/AIDS, and prevention and treatment strategies. Typically, pre-test counseling is either required for everyone or only those at high risk. In some states, post-test counseling is required only if you test positive. In many states, doctors, nurses, and other healthcare professionals can provide this counseling. In other states, counselors are required to have special education and certification.

Most states only let certain people administer the test, such as doctors, nurses, emergency medical technicians, and employees of the state department of health or corrections. Many states require the use of a specific type of test and specify where it needs to be analyzed. State laws usually determine when and if a second test is needed to confirm the results. A second test is generally done only if the test is positive, but some states always run tests twice.

Some states require the test results to be delivered face-to-face by healthcare providers or specially trained HIV counselors. In other states, these results can be delivered in the same way as any other medical test, such as by mail or over the telephone.

In some states, a patient's spouse, sexual partners, and anyone the patient shared hypodermic needles with or who could have contracted HIV from the patient may be told the results of the test without identifying the patient. Identification is voluntary and partner notification can be done by the patient or the health department personnel. The health department will not reveal the name of the patient who has tested positive.

Mental Health

Mental health laws reflect the complex balance of personal rights and government interests in protecting the public. You can exhibit symptoms of mental illness without losing your ethical rights to autonomy and your constitutional rights to privacy and freedom. Courts have determined that there must be evidence that you are a danger to yourself and others before you can be compelled to undertake mental health treatment or be incarcerated "for your own good."

There are situations in which an adult needs to be involuntarily admitted to a medical facility for mental illness. Of course, these adults also need to be protected from being wrongfully held against their will. Individual states have laws related to involuntary commitment.

There are special considerations to take into account when handling medical records for patients who have received psychiatric care (Figure 14.6). Patients generally have the right to review their records at any reasonable time within three working days of the request, and they can obtain copies of the records. However, notes on psychiatric care are different.

Access to psychotherapy notes may be restricted prior to litigation or if allowing someone to access the information may cause harm to someone. Information in the record may also have restricted access if it was obtained from someone other than a healthcare provider under a promise of confidentiality and allowing access would reveal the source of the information.

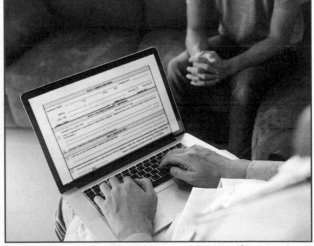

wutzkohphoto/Shutterstock.com

Figure 14.6 Special rules apply to the medical records of psychiatric patients.

Generally, providers must obtain specific statutory authorization, written client authorization, or a court order before sharing confidential patient information with another provider. Providers are allowed to release mental health records to ensure continuity, accountability, and coordination of service delivery. During a psychiatric crisis, providers must allow access to community support services records for continuity of care.

Providers also can release mental health records for psychiatric hospitals to admit, diagnose, care for, and treat involuntary patients. These records also can be released in dangerous situations. HIPAA includes exceptions for law enforcement purposes in relation to subpoenas, court orders, and other requirements of law.

Public Policy Support of Autonomy

There are laws in place to help patients maintain their autonomy when they may not be able to communicate their preferences. The three primary forms are advance directives, powers of attorney, and conservatorships. While many people tend to think of them when they are elderly, these forms may be necessary at any time in life. For example, adults of any age may not be able to communicate their healthcare treatment preferences if they are in a coma due to an auto accident, or if they experience cognitive impairment due to a traumatic brain injury.

Advance Directives

advance directive
a legal document that allows people to communicate decisions about their end-of-life care ahead of time

Once an attending physician determines that a patient lacks decision-making capacity, the medical community looks to advance directives and surrogate decision makers to help make medical decisions for the patient. **Advance directives** are statements made by the patient, when he or she was competent, that indicate to the appointed surrogate decision maker which medical interventions the patient accepts or refuses (Figure 14.7).

When a patient is no longer competent to make informed decisions, advance directives help to uphold his or her autonomy. These directives provide guidance and help ease the pressure on family members who have to make choices for the patient.

However, four primary problems can occur with advance directives:

- the patient may change his or her mind, particularly regarding life-sustaining treatments, and fail to update the advance directive to reflect the desired change

- the directive may conflict with the patient's best interests, given that the situation may not be identical to what is stated in the directive

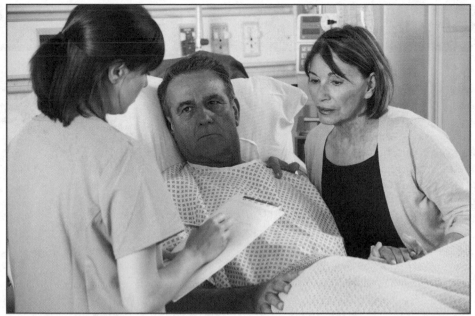

Monkey Business Images/Shutterstock.com

Figure 14.7 Advance directives are best created while a patient is still competent and can appoint a surrogate decision maker.

- the patient may not have fully understood certain emergency life-sustaining treatments; thus advance directives were not made with informed decision-making capacity
- the advance directive is too vague and fails to describe individual preferences for the specific case

Despite these complications, advance directives allow a patient to express his or her values and beliefs regarding medical care. Discussing advance directives encourages physicians, patients, and the patients' family members to determine which life-sustaining treatments should be undergone before it is too late. This will help all parties avoid a great deal of stress in the future.

Advance directives are state-specific, and so are the laws related to providers not adhering to them. Overall, states require medical providers to follow advance directives and have procedures for physicians to follow if they choose not to carry out requests outlined in advance directives.

Powers of Attorney

There are two forms of legal documents that are more legally binding than advance directives and that transfer the legal powers of one person to another person. These are the power of attorney and the durable power of attorney for healthcare.

Ethical Dilemma

Diana, a 28-year-old woman, experienced complications after surgery and is now in a coma. Prior to surgery, Diana signed a living will indicating that she did not want to be kept on life support systems if she went into a coma. The physician caring for Diana believes that she may not remain in this condition and does not want to remove her life support.

Diana's parents want the life support removed, as that is what their daughter wanted. They are suing the hospital for malpractice and asking for $36 million for their daughter's pain and suffering and for ongoing medical expenses. The parents claim that the hospital is overriding Diana's wishes so that they can make more money from her care.

What is the family's role in end-of-life decisions? How are advance directives involved in rationing healthcare as resources dwindle? Should a living will be mandatory?

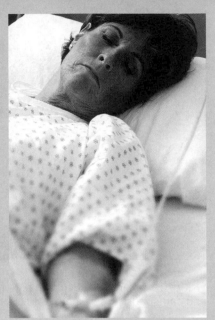

GWImages/Shutterstock.com

The *power of attorney* empowers another person to act in your absence or during periods of incapacity. These documents are usually notarized statements that specify that one or more people have full binding legal authority on issues related to property and business affairs. The power of attorney is commonly used by adults of any age but can be effectively used by older adults to ensure continuity of ability, that payments are made for care, or that contracts for services can be created.

Another form of legal document that applies to personal care is known as a **durable power of attorney for healthcare** (Figure 14.8). These documents must often be witnessed or notarized but are readily available at most hospitals, doctors' offices, and law offices. The medical field encourages the use of these documents because they reduce the burden on caregivers who want to avoid guessing a person's wishes.

A durable power of attorney for healthcare is seen as a way to not only recognize the continuing dignity and autonomy of the patient, but also to avoid malpractice claims. In many cases, these documents also help avoid unwanted and expensive care that might otherwise be provided as a result of pressure on the caregiver to practice defensive medicine.

durable power of attorney for healthcare
a legal authorization for somebody other than yourself to make decisions regarding your health and medical care

---

POWER OF ATTORNEY FOR HEALTHCARE

Designation of Agent: I designate the following individual as my agent to make healthcare decisions for me:

Name of agent: _____

Address: _____

Telephone: _____

Agent's Authority: My agent is authorized to make all healthcare decisions for me, including decisions to provide, withhold, or withdraw artificial nutrition and hydration and all other forms of healthcare to keep me alive, except as I state here: _____

_____

_____

When Agent's Authority Becomes Effective:

My agent's authority becomes effective when my primary physician determines that I am unable to make my own healthcare decisions. _____
(initial)

My agent's authority to make healthcare decisions for me takes effect immediately. _____
(initial)

Agent's Obligation: My agent shall make healthcare decisions for me in accordance with the power of attorney for healthcare, any instructions I give in Part 2 of this form, and my other wishes to the extent known to my agent. To the extent my wishes are unknown, my agent shall make healthcare decisions for me in accordance with what my agent determines to be in my best interest. In determining my best interest, my agent shall consider my personal values to the extent known my agent.

Agent's Postdeath Authority: My agent is authorized to make anatomical gifts, authorize an autopsy, and direct disposition of my remains, excepts as I state here or in Part 3 of this form:

_____

_____

_____

Goodheart-Willcox Publisher

Figure 14.8   The durable power of attorney for healthcare authorizes someone else to speak on behalf of a patient.

Both types of powers of attorney may be created to provide power while a patient still has capacity. These documents also may be limited to "speak" only after a patient has been declared incapable of making decisions by the doctor.

Conservatorships

If advance directives or powers of attorney are not in place when incapacity occurs, formal court action is required to grant others the power to speak on the patient's behalf. This process creates a **conservatorship**. Under conservatorship, the court actually takes away power from the

conservatorship
a legal relationship that gives one or more individuals or agencies the responsibility of the personal affairs of the protected person

fiduciary duty
duty to act in a person's
best interest

patient and gives it to another person to act in the patient's best interest. This establishes a **fiduciary duty**, which means that the conservator must act in the best interest of the patient, or *conservatee*. Actions taken by conservators are typically subject to review, which can involve special accountings and reports to the court.

If the patient has an advance directive, then his or her agent will make those decisions that the patient can no longer make. Determining whether the patient has the capacity to make decisions and when the conservator should take over is not always an easy decision for providers. To be deemed capable, the patient must be able to understand the nature and consequences of his or her decisions. Specifically, a patient must be able to understand and communicate, to reason and deliberate, and possess a set of values and goals.

competence
the capacity of a
person to understand
a situation and to act
reasonably

However, there is no single clinically accepted standard of decision-making capacity. Note that **competence** and decision-making capacity are not the same. Competence and incompetence are legal designations determined by courts and judges. Decision-making capacity is clinically determined by physician assessment.

What happens if the patient does not have an advance directive? The physician and one person from a specified list may decide to withhold treatment if there is no legal guardian or power of attorney. The list, in order of priority, includes (1) the patient's spouse, (2) the patient's reasonably available adult children, (3) the patient's parents, and (4) the patient's closest living relative.

Drug Testing

Drug testing can be required as a pre-employment screening or performed at random for employees, athletes, people who are on probation or incarcerated, and people with certain occupations (Figure 14.9). Employees in occupations such as law enforcement, truck driving, and healthcare may be required to undergo drug tests. Some states or municipalities mandate testing for additional occupations, such as food processing workers, people working in security, and heavy equipment operators.

The Drug-Free Workplace Act of 1988 requires *some* federal contractors and *all* federal grantees to agree that they will provide drug-free workplaces as a condition of receiving a contract or grant from a

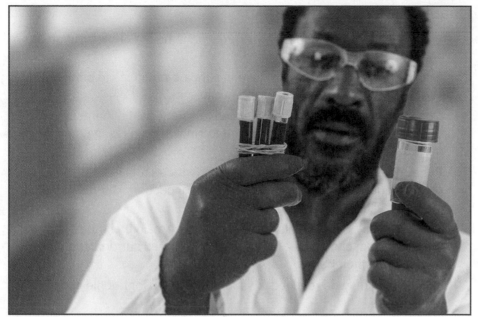

Figure 14.9   Drug tests are important to protect the general public as well as maintain workplace safety.

federal agency. Employers not covered by the federal Drug-Free Workplace Act of 1988 may be covered by the laws of their particular states. When there is both a federal and state law in existence, employers must comply with both.

Opioid Prescribing Laws

Opioid overdose is a continuing public health crisis, and states have taken steps attempting to reduce overuse of these medications. These attempts include imposing strict limitations on the amount of the drugs or the duration for which opioids may be prescribed to patients with acute pain, as well as who may prescribe them.

Mid-level practitioners (MLPs) can usually prescribe controlled substances, but their ability to prescribe opioids varies from state to state. Of all the MLPs, nurse practitioners, physician assistants, and optometrists have the highest authority among states to prescribe opioids.

Chapter Summary

- Various laws exist to enhance and protect the health of different groups in society.
- Both federal and state laws require healthcare practices to provide interpreters for non-English-speaking citizens.
- Occupational laws include laws related to safety, sexual harassment, discrimination, noise levels, exposure to smoke, drug testing, and family medical leave.
- Public health laws that affect adults include those related to driving, use of marijuana, domestic violence, assisted conception, HIV testing, and mental health.
- Several types of documents can help patients retain their autonomy while they are incapacitated by allowing their designated surrogate to make decisions on their behalf.
- Drug testing may be required in various situations for people in certain occupations.
- Opioid prescribing laws have recently changed in an attempt to reduce the overuse of opioid medications.

Vocabulary Matching

1. duty to act in a person's best interest
2. legal authorization for someone other than yourself to make decisions regarding your health and medical care
3. federal legislation that outlawed discrimination based on race, color, religion, sex, or national origin
4. federal agency that regulates workplace safety and health
5. legal relationship that gives one or more people responsibility for the personal affairs of the protected person
6. legal document that allows people to communicate decisions about end-of-life care ahead of time
7. the sum of attitudes, customs, and beliefs that distinguishes one group of people from another
8. person's capacity to understand a situation and to act reasonably

A. advance directive
B. Civil Rights Act of 1964
C. competence
D. conservatorship
E. culture
F. durable power of attorney for healthcare
G. fiduciary duty
H. OSHA

Multiple Choice

9. Programs such as Medicare, Medicaid, and Social Security must legally be offered to citizens, and so are called _____ programs.
   A. federal
   B. entitlement
   C. local
   D. healthcare

10. The _____ Act provides important rights for Limited English Proficiency (LEP) individuals.
    A. Social Security
    B. Affordable Care
    C. Language Rights
    D. Civil Rights

11. "Schedule _____" is a category of drugs that are not considered legitimate for medical use.
    A. I
    B. II
    C. III
    D. IV

12. Which of the following abbreviations describes the federal agency that enforces national workplace safety regulations?
    A. OCR
    B. DEA
    C. OSHA
    D. DOJ

13. State laws related to prescribing opioids are related to _____.
    A. the patient's diagnosis
    B. the patient's age
    C. who can prescribe them
    D. the type of facility the provider works in

14. In some states, pre- and post-test counseling are required for _____ tests.
    A. cancer
    B. HIV/AIDS
    C. mental health
    D. genetic

Completion

15. A durable power of _____ for healthcare legally authorizes someone to make decisions regarding your health and medical care.

16. _____ is a federally run health insurance system for people 65 years of age and older, some disabled adults, and patients with kidney failure or who have had kidney transplants.

17. Compentence and incompetence are legal designations determined by courts and judges, while decision-making _____ is clinically determined by a physician.

18. Laws have been established to respect both cultural and _____ autonomy.

Discussion and Critical Thinking

19. Public health laws are designed to maintain the safety and well-being of the public. Some people believe that this is too much government intervention and that the people should be able to make their own decisions. For example, if someone does not want to wear a seat belt or helmet, he or she should not be forced to wear one. What are your thoughts on public health laws? Do we have too many or too few? Why?

20. Should healthcare providers be required by law to have regular HIV tests? Why or why not?

21. Explain the Civil Rights Act requirement related to the use of medical interpreters.

22. Explain how culture and language affect the delivery of quality healthcare.

23. Describe the agency that enforces laws that protect people in the workplace.

24. Who is a mandatory reporter?

25. Describe how a durable power of attorney benefits both patients and caregivers.

Activities

26. There are different views on the mandatory reporting of adult domestic and intimate-partner violence. Search the Internet to learn about these different views. Then write a paper on the different perspectives. Include your opinion of mandatory reporting laws.

27. Research the domestic violence laws in your state. Write a paper summarizing these laws and include your thoughts on them. Are they too lenient? Are they too strict?

Case Study

Imagine that you are a medical assistant in a medical practice. A patient comes in with her husband two weeks after a visit to the emergency room. Her initial visit was for a fall. She presented with a broken arm and some bruises on the side of her face from hitting the ground. The husband insists on being in the room when she is seen by the physician.

When the physician enters the examination room, the husband explains the fall and the patient remains silent. When the physician states that she wants the patient to answer her questions, the husband says that she does not speak English well.

You and the physician leave the room. You saw from the patient's chart that she has been in the emergency room many times for falls. You state that you are concerned this is a situation of domestic violence. The physician says that she cannot be certain and that you should just focus on the injuries. What should you do? Will your actions depend on the state that you live in?

Chapter 15

Older Adults: Health Law and Ethics

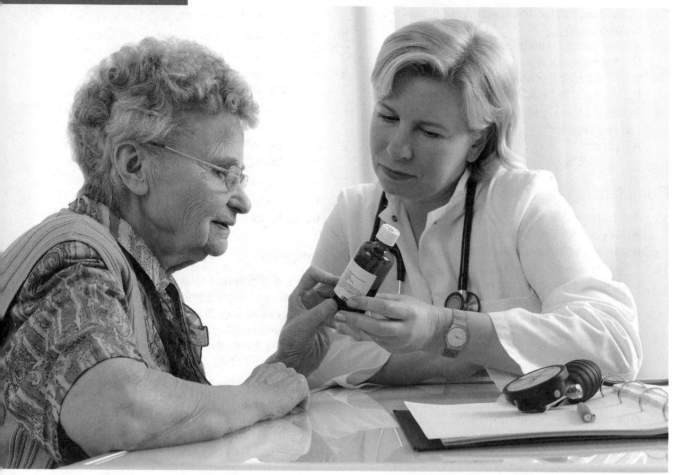

Alexander Raths/Shutterstock.com

Chapter Outline

Competency and Decision Making

Public Policy Supporting Patient Autonomy and Safety

    Restraints

    Do Not Resuscitate Orders

    Organ Donation

    Physician-Assisted Suicide

Elder Abuse

Healthcare Facilities and Services

    Senior Centers

    Adult Day Care Centers

    Home Health Care Service Agencies

    Assisted-Living Facilities

    Nursing Homes

    Hospice Care

End-of-Life Issues

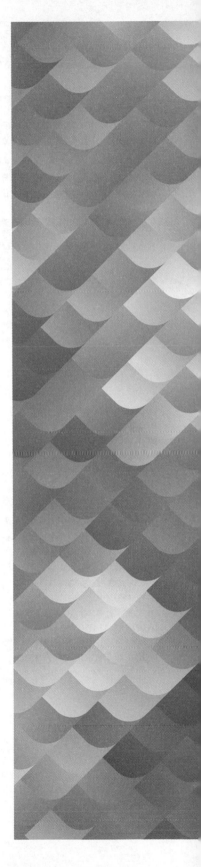

Objectives

- Recognize the effects of age on competency and decision-making capacity.
- Understand how public policy addresses autonomy and safety for the senior population.
- Describe the laws regarding elder abuse.
- Understand the differing types of senior-focused healthcare facilities and services.
- Explain issues that may arise with end-of-life care.

Key Terms

do not resuscitate orders

elder law

hospice care

institutional abuse laws

Older Americans Act

physician-assisted suicide

restraints

What Would You Do?

Imagine that you are a physician working in the emergency room at a rural hospital. It is 2:34 a.m. when Mr. Harris, who is 84 years of age, arrives. His daughter, who cares for him, has brought him in because he is experiencing difficulty breathing, chest pain, and intense coughing and wheezing. He also has a history of severe depression. You diagnose Mr. Harris with acute pneumonia and he refuses treatment. His daughter insists that he receive treatment. Does the patient have the ability to make his own decisions? If not, how should you proceed? What if you agree with the daughter?

In 2019, approximately 52 million people in the United States were 65 years of age or older. The number constituted 16 percent of the US population of 328,239,523. By 2030, the over-65 population will constitute about 20 percent of the entire population. By 2034, there will be 77.0 million people 65 years or older, compared to 76.5 million under the age of 18. By 2060, the US Census Bureau predicts that the senior population will be about 95 million.

Elder law encompasses all legal issues related to aging. The **Older Americans Act** (OAA), enacted in 1965 by President Lyndon B. Johnson, is considered the most important legislation for older adults in the United States. The original OAA created the Administration on Aging (AOA), which acts as the primary advocate for issues concerning the elderly. The OAA also granted money to states to develop research and programs in the field of aging. Later, the OAA was amended to include funding for various services and programs designed to assist senior citizens and their families.

The OAA was amended again in 2006 to help older individuals avoid institutional care; improve state health and nutrition programs for seniors; and increase coordination of federal, state, and local services for elders. Key issues in elder law include regulation of federal benefits, estate and financial planning, and elder abuse. This chapter focuses on elder law related to health, including topics such as competency, independence, end-of-life decisions, and elder abuse.

elder law
the area of legal practice that focuses on issues that affect the growing population of older adults

Older Americans Act
legislation that provided states with funding for community planning and social services, research and development projects, and personnel training in the field of aging; established the Administration on Aging

Competency and Decision Making

People are generally considered to be senior citizens at 65 years of age, when they are still perfectly competent. They become eligible for special privileges and programs simply because of their numeric age. Special privileges include everything from discounted prices for pancakes at restaurants to eligibility for Medicare hospital services.

Despite the best innovations of modern science, the aging process cannot be stopped, and individuals who live long enough may gradually lose both physical and mental capacity. Informed adults understand that this normal process will likely happen to them, so they make plans in anticipation of future needs while they are still capable (Figure 15.1). Many, however, ignore the inevitable, wait for disability to occur, and let other family members, friends, or the government step forward and provide care through a variety of means. Capacity to act autonomously in your own interest is assumed for adults, and lack of capacity must be demonstrated before others become involved with an older adult's care.

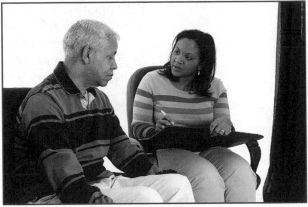

Ron Marmion/Shutterstock.com

Figure 15.1 Older adults who plan ahead might assign a surrogate decision maker and write living wills.

Older adults can suffer from dementia, delirium, depression, stroke, and other conditions that impair their cognitive ability and their ability to make decisions. The elderly may lack the ability to comprehend and remember information or experience impaired brain functions that affect judgment and planning. At what point do you determine that a patient is no longer capable of making health decisions for himself or herself? In those situations, who makes the decisions? The law provides a number of methods to help answer these questions, including advance directives, powers of attorney, and conservatorships (see Chapter 14).

Public Policy Supporting Patient Autonomy and Safety

As noted in Chapter 14, public policy encourages individuals to communicate authority and instructions to others. This is consistent with the ethical doctrine of autonomy. It also reduces risk of liability and malpractice claims for healthcare workers and medical facilities. The following situations can apply to patients of any age but are often associated with the elderly because of their increasing chance of declining health.

Restraints

Restraints on older adults can be misused and lead to patient harm or death. Restraints can include human actions, physical devices, or drugs that restrict a person's freedom of movement. They are used sometimes with older adults to prevent injuries to people who are at risk of accidents due to physical or mental illness. However, restraints are sometimes used improperly, such as for coercion, staff convenience, or punishment.

restraints
methods used to stop or limit a patient's movement

Patients have the right to refuse to be restrained unless they may cause harm to themselves or others.

There are legal and ethical issues to consider when using restraints. In certain situations, it is legally justifiable for an individual or group of individuals to restrain a person. The restraint of an individual outside such situations, or the use of excessive force, is not justifiable. It is important, from a legal and ethical perspective, to ensure that a provider does not unjustifiably restrain patients.

Do Not Resuscitate Orders

do not resuscitate order
a medical order written by a doctor that instructs healthcare providers not to use cardiopulmonary resuscitation (CPR) if breathing stops or the heart stops beating

Do not resuscitate orders, also known as *DNRs*, are used in hospital systems to honor the wishes of patients. These documents are more limited in scope than advance directives. If a properly executed DNR is in a patient's medical file and an emergency event occurs, such as respiratory failure or cardiac arrest, the staff will not resuscitate the patient.

Some states have begun to implement the Out-of-Hospital Do Not Resuscitate Declaration and Order (Figure 15.2). This law allows a qualified person to communicate that he or she does not want to be resuscitated if the heart or lungs stop working in a location that is not a hospital or other healthcare facility. If other advanced directives exist, an out-of-hospital DNR may override them.

An out-of-hospital DNR may be canceled by the individual at any time. This is done through a signed and dated document, by destroying or canceling the document, or by communicating to healthcare providers at the scene the desire to cancel the order. Emergency Medical Services (EMS) may have procedures in place for marking a person's home so they know such an order is in place.

Organ Donation

The Health Resources and Services Administration (HRSA) is the federal agency responsible for overseeing the transplant system in the United States. However, state laws facilitate organ and tissue donation commitments and transplants.

All 50 states allow people to legally consent to be a designated donor. According to the Administration on Aging, 13 states require donor education in school and 17 states require driver's education programs to include information about organ and tissue donor awareness. Organ donations can be made by executing a document that is part of a valid driver's license, by completing an organ donation card, or through requests made in a will or durable power of attorney.

Physicians are legally bound to execute a patient's organ donation request. State laws may specify when they are exempt from this requirement.

Medical Society of New Jersey

MSNJ

DO NOT RESUSCITATE

ALL FIRST RESPONDERS AND EMERGENCY MEDICAL SERVICES PERSONNEL ARE AUTHORIZED TO COMPLY WITH THIS OUT-OF-HOSPITAL DNR ORDER.

This request for no resuscitative attempts in the event of a cardiac and/or respiratory arrest for:
_____,has been ordered by the physician whose signature
PLEASE PRINT NAME
appears below. This order is in compliance with the patient's/surrogate's wishes and it has been determined and documented by the physician below that resuscitation attempts for this patient would be medically inappropriate.

It is expected that this DNR order shall be honored by all **Emergency Medical Services (EMS)** personnel, **First Responders**, and other healthcare providers who may have contact with this patient during a medical emergency.

PATIENT/SURROGATE SIGNATURE:_____

PATIENT ADDRESS: _____

THE ABOVE NAMED PATIENT IS UNDER THE CARE OF:

PHYSICIAN NAME:_____
PLEASE PRINT NAME

PHYSICIAN ADDRESS:_____

TELEPHONE NUMBER:(   ) _____ - _____

MEDICAL FACILITY AFFILIATION:_____

PHYSICIAN SIGNATURE:_____   DATE:_____

THIS DOCUMENT SHOULD BE PROMINENTLY DISPLAYED
AND READILY AVAILABLE TO EMS PERSONNEL
(see reverse for instructions)

INSTRUCTIONS FOR FIRST RESPONDERS/EMS

2015 © Medical Society of New Jersey

Figure 15.2   This out-of-hospital DNR used in New Jersey clearly states a patient's wishes.

Ethical Dilemma

Mr. Young is 85 years of age and has been hospitalized following a severe stroke. He has been married for 31 years. His wife visits him at the hospital regularly. She hand-feeds him his lunch and dinner and is a very devoted wife. In Mr. Young's durable power of attorney for healthcare, his wife is listed as his surrogate decision maker in case he loses decision-making capacity.

After completing the durable power of attorney, Mr. Young spoke to his doctor and requested that no cardiopulmonary resuscitation be attempted if he suffers cardiac arrest. The DNR order was completed and filed in his medical chart. Later, Mr. Young informed his primary nurse that he did not want a feeding tube. The nurse informed Mr. Young's physician of this statement.

The physician discussed the matter the following day with both Mr. Young and his wife. This time Mr. Young said nothing. His wife made the comment, "His mind is not always clear. I know that he wouldn't want to die without food or water."

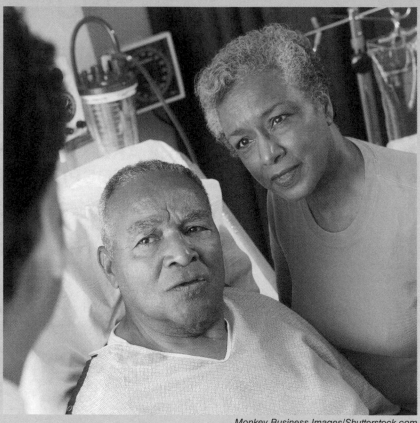

Monkey Business Images/Shutterstock.com

Later, outside the patient's room, Mrs. Young told the nurse and doctor, "He doesn't understand what he's saying. He doesn't want to die that way. If he does have another stroke, I will become the decision maker, so what he says doesn't matter anyway."

What are some ethical issues involved in this situation? Who could assist in this situation? How should the physician handle the situation?

Physician-Assisted Suicide

physician-assisted suicide
suicide committed with the aid of a physician

Physician-assisted suicide is facilitated by means or information, such as a drug prescription or indication of a lethal dosage, provided by a doctor who knows how the patient intends to use such means or information. The majority of states have statutes explicitly criminalizing assisted suicide. Oregon and Washington are examples of states that permit physician-assisted suicide. These laws are called the *Death with Dignity Acts.*

In 1997, Oregon enacted its Death with Dignity Act, which allows terminally ill Oregonians to end their lives through the voluntary self-administration of lethal medications, expressly prescribed by a physician for that purpose. Washington's Death with Dignity Act, which went into effect in 2009, allows terminally ill adults to request lethal doses of medication from medical and osteopathic physicians to end their lives. This act applies only to Washington residents who have less than six months to live.

Elder Abuse

Abuse of elders is a criminal offense in all 50 states and the District of Columbia. Many states also have mandatory reporting laws. These laws require specified professionals to report suspected elder abuse to law enforcement officials or state social service agencies for investigation and potential prosecution (Figure 15.3). Different laws define elder abuse differently and specify various professionals as mandatory reporters.

All 50 states, the District of Columbia, Guam, Puerto Rico, and the Virgin Islands have laws that authorize the use of adult protective services (APS) when elder abuse occurs. Generally, these APS laws create a system for reporting and investigating elder abuse. The laws also establish provisions for social services to help the victim and stop the abuse. In most states, these laws apply to abused adults who have a disability, vulnerability, or impairment as defined by state law, not just to the elderly. Some states, however, have specific elder protective services laws or programs.

institutional abuse laws
laws that protect against abuse found in institutional settings, including systemic forms of abuse

Some state laws regarding APS only relate to individuals who reside in the community, while other APS laws also include individuals who reside in long-term care facilities. These laws are known as **institutional abuse laws**.

As mentioned previously, certain professionals are required by law to report suspected elder abuse. For example, Illinois has a law that requires some professionals to report suspected abuse of older adults who are unable to report the abuse themselves due to a medical condition. This law specifies healthcare professionals providing care for older individuals in areas such as adult care, education, state service to seniors, and social work environments.

Healthcare Facilities and Services

Certain types of healthcare facilities and agencies are used primarily by the elderly. These include senior centers, adult day care centers, home health care service agencies,

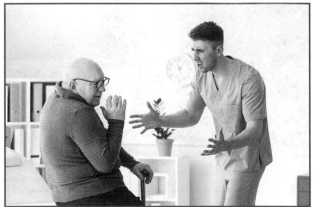

Pixel-Shot/Shutterstock.com

Figure 15.3 Elder abuse can be verbal or psychological as well as physical.

assisted-living facilities, nursing homes, and hospice care. Administrators and healthcare providers need to be aware of the federal and state laws related to these settings and services. Those laws are highlighted in this section.

Senior Centers

In 1965, Congress passed the Older Americans Act (OAA) because policymakers had concerns about a lack of community social services for older adults. The original legislation authorized grants to states for community planning and social services, research and development projects, and personnel training on the topic of aging. The OAA also established the Administration on Aging, which administers the newly created grant programs and address matters concerning older adults.

Title III of the OAA addresses grants for state and community programs on aging. Senior centers fall into this category. They are places where people, usually 55 or 60 years of age and older, can gather to share meals, exercise, participate in social activities, and receive support services. Under Title III, the federal government gives states funds to distribute grant money. Those who receive grant money from the state are required to follow certain regulations. The states have designated responsibilities to ensure that senior centers adhere to those regulations.

Adult Day Care Centers

Adult day care centers are designed to provide care and companionship to seniors who need assistance or supervision during the day (Figure 15.4). These centers can be public or private, nonprofit or for-profit. The majority of states require adult day care service facilities to obtain licensure or certification in accordance with each state's standards. This means that some require licensure, others require certification, and some require both.

Nearly all states require some kind of training for day care employees. Most states also have minimal requirements regarding initial and ongoing training. Some requirements are general, while others are more specific, mandating a certain type of training and number of hours. Training might be required for skills such as medication administration, handling medical crises, infection control, and patient rights.

Many states have specific requirements for adult day care providers who serve people with dementia. Most of these requirements relate to staffing and training. There are many

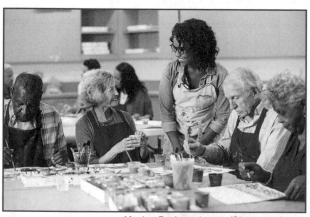
Monkey Business Images/Shutterstock.com

Figure 15.4 Older adults may benefit from companionship, which can be found at adult day care centers.

other regulations with which administrators and providers in these areas should become familiar. Examples include mandatory versus optional services, the administration of medications, staffing requirements (including staffing ratios), and inspections.

Home Health Agencies

Home health agencies provide services to patients who need post-hospital and ongoing care at home. While home health nurses and rehabilitation therapists may be needed for patients of all ages, the elderly population has a particularly frequent need for home care. Medicare pays for home health services for patients who meet its qualifications. Agencies that participate in Medicare have to follow many rules and regulations.

In fact, Medicare has hundreds, if not thousands, of conditions and rules. For example, a home health agency must be in compliance with all state and local regulations. These agencies need to be licensed and in good standing with their state health departments as well as duly licensed for business with their cities and counties.

Healthcare professionals who work for an agency must keep their licenses current and in good standing. If an agency is out of compliance with any state or local requirements, the Centers for Medicare and Medicaid Services (CMS) can demand their reimbursements back for all services given while the agency is out of compliance. CMS may also terminate a non-compliant agency from Medicare participation.

 ## Career Corner

Home health aides work with people who are sick, disabled, and elderly. These professionals assist people with activities of daily living such as dressing, bathing, and light housekeeping. Home health aides provide services that enable people to stay in their homes instead of having to live in a higher level of care facility. Therefore, home health aides help patients maintain their independence. While many home health aides do work in people's homes, they also work in residential care facilities, transitional housing, and assisted-living facilities.

There is no standardized educational requirement for home health aides. In some states, a high school diploma or equivalent is required. In other states, preparation classes are required prior to working in this field. These preparation classes are typically offered at community colleges or vocational and technical schools. Many aides receive on-the-job training. Some

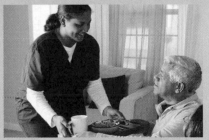
Rob Marmion/Shutterstock.com

employers prefer aides to be certified. The certification process requires passing an exam after 75 hours of training and skills testing.

Assisted-Living Facilities

Assisted-living facilities are primarily regulated at the state level. There are also a variety of legislative and regulatory initiatives at the federal level that are important to senior living providers and the residents they serve. At the state level, regulations are related to protecting the patient's autonomy as well as safety. In this case, autonomy means allowing residents to decorate their rooms as they please and select meals that they would like to eat (Figure 15.5). State assisted-living regulations can be found on the Assisted Living Federation of America website.

Nursing Homes

Certain federal and state laws exist to protect the residents of nursing homes. Under these laws and regulations, residents are entitled to security, privacy, and optimal health. The Nursing Home Reform Act of 1987 is the primary piece of federal nursing home regulation. This act includes guidelines for every federally funded nursing home facility. The Nursing Home Reform Act, as well as other laws, sets forth guidelines related to basic rights, health, and safety. In addition, the act specifies that nursing homes receiving funds from Medicare and Medicaid must pass minimum regulations set out by the government.

State nursing home laws can vary. Some states require more from facilities to earn state approval and outline stricter guidelines than other states. Nursing homes should always be aware of their states' regulations, which can be found through each state's health department.

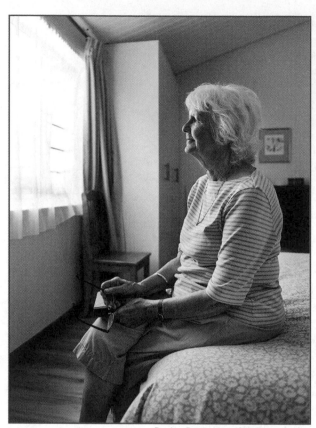

Daxiao Productions/Shutterstock.com

Figure 15.5   The autonomy of older adults is protected in assisted-living facilities.

hospice care
medical care that focuses on patient comfort and quality of life rather than curing the patient's disease; generally appropriate for someone with a terminal illness and life expectancy of six months or less

Hospice Care

Hospice care provides medical services, emotional support, and spiritual resources for people who are terminally ill and in the final stages of life. Hospice care may be provided in the community, at home, or in a facility. In the United States, federally recognized hospice care began with implementation of parts of the Social Security Act.

Regulations governing the conditions for Medicare participation for hospice agencies are explained in the US Code of Federal Regulations.

If they want to become licensed and certified by state regulators, hospices must meet these "Conditions of Participation." Continued participation in the Medicare hospice program is dependent on meeting these conditions. Compliance with these standards is required for hospices to receive reimbursement for enrolling Medicare patients in their program.

The federal laws regarding hospice care are extensive and include regulations for restraints, staffing requirements, reporting a death, and core services that must be provided. State regulations are also extensive and cover a variety of topics including laundry service, equipment maintenance, bereavement care for the family, and pharmaceutical services.

End-of-Life Issues

Optimally, patients will have established advance healthcare directives as described in Chapter 10. These formal, written documents express the patients' wishes and empower others to make critical medical care judgments However, end-of-life conditions may not be as straightforward as hoped for those who have made advance plans.

Although laws and professional ethical rules protect people who hold power to authorize care for an elderly person, it may be difficult to implement the patient's intent. For instance, the person holding the healthcare power through the advance directive may or may not have the courage to withhold life-sustaining treatment. That person's personal morals or emotions may come into play. While earlier agreement with the patient may have seemed comfortable, actually making a decision to provide or not provide care, holding life in the balance, may create a conflict between the patient's intent and the person who actually has to authorize action. In such cases, there may be several options.

If a successor agent is identified in the healthcare directive, the first person may resign or defer to the second and withdraw from the position of conflict. This, of course, requires that the successor agent be willing to make the decisions. Alternatively, if time permits, the authorized agent may apply to a court to authorize care.

End-of-life situations may also require healthcare providers themselves to refresh their knowledge of laws and rules for end-of-life care. It is essential that they understand the laws and professional rules of conduct affecting the local area. This includes an understanding of federal, state, and local laws, as well as the applicable professional rules.

In addition, healthcare facilities and programs may have established social work or professional hospice services to assist in the end-of-life process. These services may be provided directly by the facility or through contract services that may be funded in part by Medicare.

Chapter Summary

- Competency may decline as a person ages, and law provides for creating advance directives to guide medical care in times of incapacity.

- Laws provide for maximizing autonomy through, for example, rules regarding use of restraints, do not resuscitate orders, and organ donation.

- Elder abuse is a crime in all 50 states; some states also have elderly abuse laws for institutional care.

- Facilities and services for elderly patients range from activity and care centers for generally healthy seniors to residential facilities that provide degrees of medical care ranging from light assistance to end-of-life services in hospices.

- Laws exist to help with end-of-life situations when an issue arises with carrying out the patient's wishes.

Vocabulary Matching

1. ending one's own life using information or medication provided by a physician

2. medical care that focuses on patient comfort and quality of life, generally provided for patients with a life expectancy of six months or less

3. legislation that provided state funding for various projects for aging citizens and established the Administration on Aging

4. medical order written by a physician that instructs healthcare providers not to use CPR if a person's breathing stops or the heart stops beating

5. methods used to stop or limit a patient's movement

6. laws that protect against abuse in institutional settings

7. area of legal practice that focuses on issues that affect the growing population of older adults

A. do not resuscitate order
B. elder law
C. hospice care
D. institutional abuse laws
E. Older Americans Act
F. physician-assisted suicide
G. restraints

Multiple Choice

8. If a(n) _____ order is on file, the medical staff will not resuscitate the patient.
   A. DNCPR
   B. DPA
   C. EMR
   D. DNR

9. Oregon and Washington have _____ Acts that permit physician-assisted suicides.
   A. Respectful Death
   B. Death with Dignity
   C. Death with Integrity
   D. Death with Pride

10. Abuse of elders is a criminal offense in _____ of the states and the District of Columbia.
    A. half
    B. some
    C. all
    D. ten

11. Which of the following facilities provides care and companionship to seniors who need assistance or supervision during the day?
    A. hospitals
    B. nursing homes
    C. adult day care
    D. hospice care

12. Which of the following healthcare facilities provides care to patients who need post-hospital and ongoing care at home?
    A. home health care agency
    B. home clinic services
    C. home hospital care
    D. home therapy care

13. The _____ Act created guidelines for basic rights, health, and safety for the elderly in certain healthcare facilities.
    A. Older Americans
    B. Elderly Assistance
    C. Elderly Protection
    D. Nursing Home Reform

Completion

14. _____ are pharmacological or physical methods used to protect older adults, but which are sometimes misused.

15. _____ can be made by executing a document that is part of a valid driver's license.

16. Hospice care is focused on patient comfort and _____ of life rather than curing a patient's disease.

17. _____ agencies provide services to patients who need post-hospital and ongoing care at home.

18. The _____ capacity of older adults may be affected by conditions such as dementia, delirium, and stroke.

Discussion and Critical Thinking

19. What would you include in your advance directive? Under what circumstances would you want to complete a do not resuscitate order?

20. Explain the purpose of a do not resuscitate order. What are some relevant laws that apply to this document?

21. Why are advance directives for healthcare particularly important for older adults?

22. Cite examples of when applying physical restraints is appropriate and authorized.

23. What is the difference between a senior center and an adult day care center?

Activities

24. Visit the government website for the Oregon Death with Dignity Act. Read about the requirements of the law and any recent reports, and then write a reaction paper. Include any information that surprised you. Do you believe that the act is comprehensive? What is your opinion of the act?

25. Use the Internet to research Dr. Kevorkian and his mercy killings. Write a paper summarizing the case and your reaction to it.

26. Use the Internet to find and research the hospice laws in your state. Write a paper summarizing the key laws and your reaction to them.

Case Study

Ms. Hoffman is a 69-year-old widow. She was driving home from the grocery store and was badly injured in a car accident. As a result, she has been in a coma and on life support for two days. According to Ms. Hoffman's durable power of attorney for healthcare, her son is designated as her agent.

The son wants to take his mother off life support, but the physician believes that Ms. Hoffman has a chance of coming out of the coma, as she exhibits brain activity. How should the physician handle the situation?

References

Chapter 1

American Bar Association, Center for Professional Responsibility (2015). Rule 1.15: *Safekeeping Property*. http://www.americanbar.org/groups/professional_responsibility/publications/model_rules_of_professional_conduct/rule_1_15_ safekeeping_property.html

Centers for Medicare and Medicaid Services (2019). *Historical, National Health Expenditure Data*. https://www.cms.gov/research-statistics-data-and-systems/statistics-trends-and-reports/nationalhealthexpenddata/nationalhealthaccountshistorical

Clark, M. and Crawford, C. (1994). *Legal Medicine in History*. http://ebooks.cambridge.org/ebook.jsf?bid=CBO9780511599668

NEJM Catalyst (2017). *What Is Value-Based Healthcare?* https://catalyst.nejm.org/doi/full/10.1056/CAT.17.0558

Porter, Michael E., PhD. (2010). What Is Value in Health Care? *N Engl J Med* 2010; 363:2477–2481. https://www.nejm.org/doi/full/10.1056/NEJMp1011024

Zalta, E. (2014). *Kant's Moral Philosophy*. http://plato.stanford.edu/entries/kant-moral

Health Sciences Institutional Review Boards, University of Wisconsin KnowledgeBase. *Brief Overview of Regulatory Basis of IRB Authority and Review Responsibilities*. https://kb.wisc.edu/hsirbs/page.php?id=19228

Josephson, M. (n.d.). *Making Ethical Decisions*. http://josephsoninstitute.org/MED/

Kaiser Permanente (n.d.) *Ethics Committee*. http://mydoctor.kaiserpermanente.org/ncal/facilities/region/gsaa/area_master/departments/ethicscommittee/

Lasagna, L. *Modern Physicians' Oath*. http://www.hospicepatients.org/modern-physicians-oath-louis-lasagna.html

McCormick, T.R. (2008). *The Principle of Nonmaleficence*. http://depts.washington.edu/bioethx/tools/princpl.html#prin2

National Library of Medicine, History of Medicine Division (2002). *Hippocratic Oath*. http://www.nlm.nih.gov/hmd/greek/greek_oath.htm.

Thompson, E. (December 5, 1987). Fundamental ethical principles in healthcare. *British Medical Journal* (Clinical research ed.), 295(6611), 1461–1465.

Chapter 2

Abbott, A.D. (1988). *The System of Professions: Essay on the Division of Expert Labor*. Chicago: University of Chicago Press.

American Medical Association (2001). *Principles of Medical Ethics*. http://www. ama-assn.org/ama/pub/physician-resources/medical-ethics/code-medical-ethics/principles-medical-ethics.page?

Chapter 3

Centers for Medicare and Medicaid Services. *National Health Expenditure Data*. https://www.cms.gov/research-statistics-data-and-systems/statistics-trends-and-reports/nationalhealthexpenddata/nationalhealthaccountshistorical

Congressional Constitution Caucus (n.d.). *U.S. Constitution*. http://congressionalconstitutioncaucus-garrett.house.gov/ resources/us-constitution

Massachusetts Court System (2015). *Massachusetts Law about Health Insurance.* http://www.mass.gov/courts/case-legal-res/law-lib/laws-by-subj/about/healthinsurance.html

Miller, R.D. (2006). *Problems in Health Care Law.* Sudbury, MA: Jones & Bartlett Publishers.

National Center for Complementary and Integrative Health (June 2013). *Ephedra.* https://nccih.nih.gov/health/ephedra

United States Court of Appeals (2011). *Thomas More Law Center, et al. v President Barack Obama, et al.* http://www.ca6.uscourts.gov/opinions.pdf/11a0168p-06.pdf

US History (2013). *Bill of Rights and Later Amendments.* http://www.ushistory.org/documents/amendments.htm

US National Archives and Records Administration (n.d.). *Transcription of the 1789 Joint Resolution of Congress Proposing 12 Amendments to the U.S. Constitution.* http://www.archives.gov/exhibits/charters/bill_of_rights_transcript.html

Chapter 4

American Association of Naturopathic Physicians (2015). *Licensed States & Licensing Authorities.* http://www.naturopathic.org/content.asp?pl=16&sl=57&contented=57

American Board of Neurological Surgery (2015). *Training Requirements.* http://www.abns.org/Board%20Certification/Training%20Requirements/July%20202013.aspx/

American Nurses Association. *Advocacy.* https://www.nursingworld.org/practice-policy/health-policy/health-system-reform/quality/advocacy/

National Healthcareer Association. (n.d.). *Certified Billing and Coding Specialist.* http://www.nhanow.com/billing-coding.aspx

Oregon.gov (n.d.). *Midwifery: How to Get Licensed.* http://www.oregon.gov/OHLA/DEM/Pages/Midwifery_How_to_Get_Licensed.aspx

United States Bureau of Labor Statistics. (January 8, 2014). *Home Health Aides.* http://www.bls.gov/ooh/healthcare/home-health-aides.htm

United States Department of Health and Human Services (August 2011). *Community Health Workers Evidence-Based Models Toolbox.* http://www.hrsa.gov/ruralhealth/pdf/chwtoolkit.pdf

University of Maryland Medical Center (2011). *Naturopathy.* http://www.umm.edu/altmed/articles/naturopathy-000356.htm

Wise Law Group, LLC. (2012). *Pharmacy Laws.* http://www.resource4pharmacymalpractice.com/laws.html

Chapter 5

American Law Institute (1977). *Restatement of the Law, Second, Torts.* http://lexinter.net/LOTWVers4/restatement_(second)_of_torts.htm

American Law Institute (1981). *The Restatement (Second) of Contracts.* http://www.lexinter.net/LOTWVers4/restatement_(second)_of_contracts.htm

American Law Institute and the National Conference of Commissioners on Uniform State Laws (n.d.). *Uniform Commercial Code.* http://www.law.cornell.edu/ucc

Official California Legislative Information (n.d.). *California Uniform Commercial Code.* http://www.leginfo.ca.gov/cgi-bin/calawquery?codesection=com

Chapter 6

Child Welfare Information Gateway (2019). *Penalties for failure to report and false reporting of child abuse and neglect.* Washington, DC: U.S. Department of Health and Human Services, Children's Bureau)

United States Bureau of Labor Statistics (January 8, 2014). *Forensic Science Technicians.* http://www.bls.gov/ooh/life-physical-and-social-science/forensic-science-technicians.htm

US Department of Health & Human Services. *HHS FY 2018 Budget in Brief.* https://www.hhs.gov/about/budget/fy2018/budget-in-brief/cms/medicare/index.html

US Department of Justice, Southern District of Florida. *Owner of Numerous Miami-Area Home Health Agencies Sentenced to 20 Years in Prison for Role in $66 Million Medicare Fraud Conspiracy.* https://www.justice.gov/usao-sdfl/pr/owner-numerous-miami-area-home-health-agencies-sentenced-20-years-prison-role-66

United States Department of Health and Human Services (2014). *Annual Report of the Departments of Health and Human Services and Justice.* https://oig.hhs.gov/publications/docs/hcfac/FY2014-hcfac.pdf

Chapter 7

Cleverley, William O.; Song, Paula H.; and Cleverley, James O. (2010). *Essentials of Healthcare Finance.* Sudbury, MA: Jones & Bartlett Publishing.

Medicaid.gov (n.d.). *Eligibility.* http://www.medicaid.gov/affordablecareact/Provisions/Eligibility.html

Syracuse University (2015). *Speech-Language Pathology.* http://csd.syr.edu/about/index.html

United States Bureau of Labor Statistics (January 8, 2014). *Speech-Language Pathologists.* http://www.bls.gov/ooh/Healthcare/Speech-language-pathologists.htm

United States Department of Health and Human Services (n.d.). *Comparison of the Anti-Kickback Statute and Stark Law.* https://oig.hhs.gov/compliance/provider-compliance-training/files/starkandakscharthandout508.pdf

Chapter 8

Agency for Healthcare Research and Quality (June 2015). *National Healthcare Quality and Disparities Reports.* http://www.ahrq.gov/research/findings/nhqrdr/index.html

Carrier, E., Reschovsky, James D., Katz, David A., Mello, Michelle M. (2013). High physician concern about malpractice risk predicts more aggressive diagnostic testing in office-based practice. *Health Affairs*, 32(8). http://content.healthaffairs.org/content/32/8/1383.abstract

Healthcare Finance. *List: 769 hospitals fined for medical errors, infections, by CMS.* https://www.healthcarefinancenews.com/news/list-769-hospitals-fined-medical-errors-infections-cms

Johns Hopkins Medicine News and Publications (2016). *Study Suggests Medical Errors Now Third Leading Cause of Death in the U.S.* https://www.hopkinsmedicine.org/news/media/releases/study_suggests_medical_errors_now_third_leading_ cause_of_death_in_the_us

LaFountain, R.C. and Lee, C.G. (2011). *Medical Malpractice Litigation in State Courts.* http://www.ncsconline.org/d_research/csp/Highlights/CH_Medical_Malpractice_April_2011.pdf

Levinson, Daniel R. (2010). Adverse Events in Hospitals: *National Incidence Among Medicare Beneficiaries.* http://oig.hhs.gov/oei/reports/oei-06-09-00090.pdf

United States Department of Health and Human Services (n.d.) *Quality Improvement.* http://www.hrsa.gov/quality/toolbox/methodology/qualityimprovement/part2.html

Chapter 9

American Medical Association (n.d.) *Informed Consent.* http://www.ama-assn.org/ama/pub/physician-resources/legal-topics/litigation-center/case-summaries-topic/informed-consent.page

Cooper, S. (June 2010). *Taking no for an answer—refusal of life-sustaining treatment. Virtual Mentor*, 12. http://virtualmentor.ama-assn.org/2010/06/ccas2-1006.html

Derse, A.R. (2005). What part of "no" don't you understand? Patient refusal of recommended treatment in the emergency department. *Mount Sinai Journal of Medicine*, 72(4), 221–227

Jaworska, A. (2009). *Advanced Directives and Substitute Decision-Making*. http://plato.standford.edu/entries/advance-directives/

Kohls, L. Robert (April 1984). *The Values Americans Live By*. http://www.claremontmckenna.edu/pages/faculty/ alee/extra/American_values.html

Pantilat, S. (2008). *Ethics Fast Fact: Decision-Making Capacity*. http://missinglink.ucsf.edu/lm/ethics/Content%20Pages/fast_ fact_competence.htm

Richards, E. (2009). *Battery—No Consent*. http://biotech.law.lsu.edu/map/BatteryNoConsent.html

Savulescu, J., & Momeyer, R.W. (1997). Should informed consent be based on rational beliefs? *Journal of Medical Ethics*, 23, 282–288. JSTOR database

Supreme Court of North Carolina (1956). *Kennedy v Parrott*. https://scholar.google.com/scholar_case?case=13899581076859360328&hl=en&as_sdt=6&as_vis=1&oi=scholar

The Law, Science, and Public Health Law Site (1993). *Good Samaritan Laws*. http://biotech.law.lsu.edu/Books/lbb/x894.htm

Tunzi, M. (July 15, 2001). Can the Patient Decide? Evaluating Patient Capacity in Practice. *American Family Physician*, 64(2). http://www.aafp.org/afp/2001/0715/p299.html#afp20010715p299-f2

University of Virginia (2013). *Extension Doctrine*. http://www.med-ed.virginia.edu/courses/rad/consent/2/extension_doctrine.html

Chapter 10

Mangalmurti, S.S., Murtagh, L., Mello, M. (November 18, 2010). Medical malpractice liability in the age of electronic health records. *New England Journal of Medicine*, 363. http://www.nejm.org/doi/full/10.1056/NEJMhle1005210

National Council of State Boards of Nursing (November 10, 2014). *Compact State Nurse Licensure: An Overview*. https://www.ncsbn.org/6694.htm

Rodwin, M.A. (2010). Patient data: property, privacy & the public interest. *American Journal of Law & Medicine*, 36(2010), 586–618

Stevens, G. (January 28, 2010). *Federal Information Security and Data Breach Notification Laws*. http://www.fas.org/sgp/crs/secrecy/RL34120.pdf

United States Department of Health and Human Services, Health Resources and Services Administration (2006). *The Critical Care Workforce: A Study of the Supply and Demand for Critical Care Physicians*. http://bhpr.hrsa.gov/healthworkforce/reports/studycriticalcarephys.pdf

United States Department of Health and Human Services (2015). *The Privacy Act*. http://www.hhs.gov/foia/privacy/index.html

Vigoda, M., Callahan, Dennis J., and Dougherty, M. (October 2008). E-record, e-liability: addressing medico-legal issues in electronic records. *Journal of AHIMA*, 79(10). http://library.ahima.org/xpedio/groups/public/documents/ahima/bok1_040399.hcsp?dDocName=bok1_040399

Chapter 11

Bulloch, Marilyn, PharmD, BCPS, FCCM. Opioid Prescribing Limits Across the States. *Pharmacy Times* (2019-02-05). https://www.governing.com/gov-data/safety-justice/state-marijuana-laws-map-medical-recreational.html

Human Genome Project Information Archive (2013). *Genetics Legislation*. http://www.ornl.gov/sci/techresources/Human_Genome/elsi/legislat.shtml

State Marijuana Laws in 2019 Map. *Governing* (2020). https://www.governing.com/gov-data/safety-justice/state-marijuana-laws-map-medical-recreational.html

United States Food and Drug Administration (October 27, 2014). *Development & Approval Process (Drugs)*. http://www.fda.gov/drugs/developmentapprovalprocess/default.htm

Yin, S. (July 20, 2011). *FDA Proposes Guidance for Certain Mobile Medical Apps.* http://www.medscape.com/viewarticle/746673

Chapter 12

Agency for Healthcare Research and Quality (August 13, 2014). *State-Mandated Nurse Staffing Levels Alleviate Workloads, Leading to Lower Patient Mortality and Higher Nurse Satisfaction.* http://innovations.ahrq.gov/content.aspx?id=3708

American Association of Naturopathic Physicians (2012). *Licensed States & Licensing Authorities.* http://www.naturopathic.org/content.asp?pl=16&sl=57&contented=57

American Health Information Management Association (August 2011). *Retention and Destruction of Health Information.* http://library.ahima.org/xpedio/groups/public/documents/ahima/bok1_049252.hcsp?dDocName=bok1_049252

American Society of Transplantation. *United States Resources.* https://www.myast.org/education/specialty-resources/organ-donation-education-tools/united-states-resources

Centers for Medicare and Medicaid Services (n.d.) *State Marketplace Resources.* https://www.cms.gov/CCIIO/Programs-and-Initiatives/Health-Insurance-Marketplaces/State-Marketplace-Resources.html

Cornell University Law School (November 30, 2001). *42 CFR 419.20 - Hospitals subject to the hospital outpatient prospective payment system.* http://www.law.cornell.edu/cfr/text/42/419.20

Medicaid.gov (n.d.) *Financing & Reimbursement.* http://www.medicaid.gov/Medicaid-CHIP-Program-Information/By-Topics/Financing-and-Reimbursement/Financing-and-Reimbursement.html

National Conference of State Legislatures (2015). *Health Insurance Exchanges or Marketplaces: State Profiles and Actions.* http://www.ncsl.org/portals/1/documents/health/health_insurance_exchanges_state_profiles.pdf

Page, L. and Fields, R. (2012). *13 Legal Issues for Hospitals and Health Systems.* http://www.beckershospitalreview.com/hospital-management-administration/13-legal issues-for-hospitals-and-health-systems.html

Rural Assistance Center (2013). *FQHC Frequently Asked Questions.* http://www.raconline.org/topics/clinics/fqhcfaq.php

United States Census Bureau. *Older People Projected to Outnumber Children for First Time in U.S. History.* https://www.census.gov/newsroom/press-releases/2018/cb18-41-population-projections.html

United States Department of Health and Human Services (n.d.). *What are Federally qualified health centers (FQHCs)?* http://www.hrsa.gov/healthit/toolbox/RuralHealth1Toolbox/Introduction/qualified.html

University of Maryland Medical Center (2011). *Naturopathy.* http://www.umm.edu/altmed/articles/naturopathy-000356.htm

Chapter 13

Becker, Christian D, MD, PhD, et al. Legal Perspectives on Telemedicine Part 1: Legal and Regulatory Issues. *Perm J* 2019; 23:18–293. https://www.thepermanentejournal.org/issues/2019/summer/7170-telemedicine.html

Chin, W.Y. (2005). Blue spots, coining, and cupping: How ethnic minority parents can be misreported as child abusers. *The Journal of Law in Society, 88,* 88–115.

Cornell University Law School (1990). *42 U.S. Code § 13031 - Child abuse reporting.* http://www.law.cornel.edu/uscode/text/42/13031

Chapter 14

Chen, A.H., Youdelman, M.K., & Brooks J. (2007). The legal framework for language access in healthcare settings: title VI and beyond. *Journal of General Internal Medicine, 22,* 362–367. http://dx.doi.org/10.1007%2Fs11606-007-0366-2

Cornell University Law School (n.d.). *42 U.S. Code § 1996a - Traditional Indian religious use of peyote*. http://www.law.cornell.edu/uscode/text/42/1996a

Family Violence Prevention Fund (2010). *Compendium of State Statutes and Policies on Domestic Violence and Healthcare*. http://www.futureswithoutviolence.org/userfiles/file/HealthCare/Compendium%20Final.pdf

Hudson, Kathy L, Ph.D., and Francis S. Collins, M.D., Ph.D. The 21st Century Cures Act—A View from the NIH. *N Engl J Med* 2017; 376:111–113. https://www.nejm.org/doi/10.1056/NEJMp1615745

Michigan Department of Community Health (January 2006). *It's the Law*. http://www.michigan.gov/documents/Its-The-Law-Michigan-01-06_147015_7.pdf

National Conference of State Legislatures (July 6, 2015). *States with Religious and Philosophical Exemptions from School Immunization Requirements*. http://www. ncsl.org/issues-research/health/school-immunization-exemption-state-laws.aspx

National Conference of State Legislatures (October 15, 2015). *State Medical Marijuana Laws*. http://www.ncsl.org/issues-research/health/state-medical-marijuana-laws.aspx

Voth, E.A. (November 2001). Guidelines for prescribing medical marijuana. *The Western Journal of Medicine*, 175. http://www.ncbi. nlm.nih.gov/pmc/articular/PMC1071601/

Chapter 15

Administration on Aging (2011). *Aging Statistics*. http://www.aoa.acl.gov/Aging_Statistics/index.aspx

Hospice Patients Alliance (n.d.). *Hospice Law & Regulations (Federal & State Laws On Hospice: The Uniform Standards of Care)*. http://www.hospicepatients.org/hospic38.html

Illinois Department on Aging (2015). Report Abuse. http://www.illinois.gov/aging/ProtectionAdvocacy/Pages/abuse_ reporting.aspx

Jones, R.C. & Holden, T. (2004). A guide to assessing decision-making capacity. *Cleveland Clinic Journal of Medicine*, 71. http://ccjm.org/content/71/12/971. full.pdf

National Association of State Units on Aging (2008). *Senior Center Practices*. http://www.nasuad.org/documentation/nasuad_materials/SeniorCenterPractices.pdf

Glossary

A

abandonment termination of the patient-professional relationship in a manner that denies the patient necessary medical care (9)

accountable care organization (ACO) a group of doctors, hospitals, and other healthcare providers who come together voluntarily to give coordinated, high-quality care to their Medicare patients (12)

accreditation the process for authorizing or approving a facility, program, or person that conforms to formal standards (4)

advance directive a legal document that allows people to communicate decisions about their end-of-life care ahead of time (14)

allied health professionals healthcare workers who deliver services involving the identification, evaluation, and prevention of diseases and disorders; dietary and nutrition services; and rehabilitation and health systems management (4)

amendments additions to the US Constitution that address topics not covered in the original Constitution (3)

Americans with Disabilities Act (ADA) law that prohibits discrimination against people with disabilities in employment, transportation, public accommodation, communications, and governmental activities; also establishes requirements for telecommunications relay services (7)

Anti-Kickback Statute a criminal statute that prohibits the exchange (or offer to exchange) of anything of value in an effort to receive the reward of federal healthcare program business (7)

articles sections of the US Constitution (3)

assault an intentional attempt to injure or harm another person; no physical contact is necessary for an assault to occur (5)

autonomy an individual's right to self-determination that is free from undue interference from others (2)

B

battery the intentional offensive or harmful touching of another person without that person's consent (5)

beneficence the act of performing goodness, kindness, or charity, including all actions intended to benefit others based on a moral obligation to do so (2)

Bill of Rights the first ten amendments to the US Constitution, which protect the individual rights of citizens (3)

bioethics the study of the ethical and moral implications of new biological discoveries and biomedical advances (2)

breach the unauthorized acquisition, access, use, and disclosure of protected health information that compromises the security or privacy of such information (10)

breach of duty a failure to perform some obligation or promise; the neglect or failure to fulfill the standard of care when one person or company has an obligation toward another person or company (5)

business disparagement false and injurious statements related to a business; requires proof of a specific economic loss (5)

C

Cabinet the advisory body to the President of the United States, which is made up of the heads of various federal agencies (3)

case law law that is made by courts as they resolve issues presented to them (3)

causation the relationship between an action or condition and its effect or result (5)

certification a document that formally recognizes the recipient as having successfully achieved a specific level of training or demonstrated a specific level of competence (4)

checks and balances the limitations of each branch of government and the coordination among the branches required to operate the government (3)

civil law noncriminal law; typically addresses nonviolent circumstances and events that are perceived as wrongs suffered (5)

civil liability the legal obligation to pay damages or perform another court-enforced action as a result of private wrongs (noncriminal acts) or breach of contract (5)

civil litigation a formal legal procedure or action in court that determines legal rights and responsibilities (5)

Civil Rights Act of 1964 federal legislation that outlawed discrimination based on race, color, religion, sex, or national origin (14)

clinical trials a series of research tests performed on human subjects to determine the effectiveness and safety of a new drug (11)

cloning the process of generating a genetically identical copy of a cell or an organism (11)

code of ethics a set of rules established to guide the conduct of members of a profession (4)

Commerce Clause a clause in the US Constitution that grants Congress extensive power to regulate the economy, particularly the flow of items and information between the states (3)

common law rules derived from English law (French law in Louisiana) and tradition that have often been formally adopted into state laws or used to determine decisions in American courts (3)

Common Rule the common name for 45 CFR Part 46, Subpart A, which outlines the authority of IRBs and helps protect fetuses, neonates, pregnant women, prisoners, and children involved in research studies (2)

competence the capacity of a person to understand a situation and to act reasonably (14)

Conditions of Participation (COP) conditions that healthcare organizations must meet to begin and continue participating in the Medicare and Medicaid programs (12)

conservatorship a legal relationship that gives one or more individuals or agencies the responsibility of the personal affairs of the protected person (14)

conspiracy an agreement made by two or more people to perform an illegal or harmful act (6)

contract law rules-based statutes and case law related to enforcing promises (5)

crime an act, or failure to act, that is deemed injurious of public welfare or morals and for which someone can be punished by the government (6)

criminal law a system of law consisting of a body of rules and statutes that define conduct prohibited by the government because such conduct is an offense against the state and threatens and harms public safety and welfare (6)

criminal negligence the failure to use reasonable care to avoid consequences that threaten or harm the safety of the public and that have a foreseeable outcome (6)

critical access hospital designation given to eligible rural hospitals by CMS to help improve access to healthcare in rural communities (12)

culture the sum of attitudes, customs, and beliefs that distinguishes one group of people from another (14)

D

decision-making capacity the patient's ability to make a specific decision at a point in time (9)

defamation any intentionally false communication, either written (libel) or spoken (slander), that harms a person's reputation; decreases the respect toward the person; or induces disparaging, hostile, or disagreeable opinions or feelings against a person (5)

defendant a person against whom an action or claim is brought in a court of law; may also be called a *respondent* (5)

defensive medicine patient care that involves conducting more tests or treatment than would be called for if litigation or malpractice was not of particular concern (8)

discovery the pretrial stage of litigation in which both parties of the lawsuit identify information about the case (10)

do not resuscitate order a medical order written by a doctor that instructs healthcare providers not to use cardiopulmonary resuscitation (CPR) if breathing stops or the heart stops beating (15)

due process the legal requirement that the government provide fair treatment through the normal judicial system (6)

Due Process Clause a clause in the Fourteenth Amendment that has been interpreted to mean that citizens cannot be deprived of life or liberty without notice and a right to be heard (3)

durable power of attorney for healthcare a legal authorization for somebody other than yourself to make decisions regarding your health and medical care (14)

E

e-discovery a process in which electronic data is searched for, located, and secured for the purpose of using as evidence in a civil or criminal legal case (10)

elder law the area of legal practice that focuses on issues that affect the growing population of older adults (15)

electronic health record an electronic record of health-related information about an individual that conforms to nationally recognized interoperability standards and that is created, managed, and consulted by authorized clinicians and staff in more than one agency (10)

electronic medical record an electronic record of health-related information about an individual that is created, managed, and consulted by authorized clinicians and staff within one healthcare organization (10)

emancipated minor a minor who is 16 years of age or older and has obtained legal independence from his or her parents or guardians (13)

emergency care doctrine a legal process that assumes consent to a medical procedure during an emergency when the person is incapacitated and unable to give consent (13)

Emergency Medical Treatment and Active Labor Act (EMTALA) a law created to ensure public access to emergency services regardless of ability to pay (7)

encryption the process of translating text into an unintelligible set of characters that can be transmitted with a high degree of security and then decrypted after reaching its secure destination (10)

Equal Protection Clause a clause in the Fourteenth Amendment that is intended to end all remaining discrimination resulting from slavery and requires state laws to protect each citizen equally (3)

ethics a set of principles of right and wrong conduct; a system of values that guides behavior in relationships with people in accordance with social roles (1)

executive branch the portion of the government that is empowered to implement the laws established by the legislative branch (3)

express consent the verbal or written authorization of care (9)

extension doctrine statute that allows a healthcare professional to extend a patient's original consent to a procedure in an extenuating circumstance when further issues occur during the original procedure (9)

F

Fair Labor Standards Act law that contains regulations related to employment of minors, including restricting the hours that children younger than 16 years of age can work and forbidding the employment of children younger than 18 years of age in certain jobs that are deemed too dangerous (13)

False Claims Act law that prohibits any individual or business from submitting, or causing someone else to submit, a false or fraudulent claim for payment to the government; allows individuals to sue on behalf of the government on knowledge of past or present fraud against the federal government (7)

false imprisonment the restraint of a person in a bounded area without justification or consent (5)

Federal Child Abuse Prevention and Treatment Act key federal legislation that addresses child abuse and neglect; provides federal funding to states in support of prevention, assessment, investigation, prosecution, and treatment activities; and provides grants to public agencies and nonprofit organizations for demonstration programs and projects (13)

Federal Medical Assistance Percentage (FMAP) the percentage of Medicaid expenditures reimbursed to states by the federal government; varies by state (12)

fee-for-service In Medicaid, payment arrangement in which states pay providers directly for services (12)

fee-for-service model payment model in which healthcare providers are compensated according to volume of hours or other measures of care (1)

felony a serious crime that typically involves violence and is usually punishable by at least one year in a state prison, or death (6)

fiduciary duty duty to act in a person's best interest (14)

fraud the intentionally false representation of a material fact that is calculated to deceive and does deceive another person to legal detriment or loss (5)

full faith and credit the Constitution's requirement that each state recognize the equal powers of each state to establish its own law; has been used to ensure that barriers to commerce and rights of citizenship do not interfere with the nation functioning as a single entity (3)

G

gene therapy the use of genes to treat or prevent disease (11)

general intent a mental plan to do something that is against the law, whether the specific results that eventually occur were meant to happen or not (6)

general liability insurance insurance that protects against injuries and property damage resulting from general risk associated with business or property ownership, such as "slip-and-fall" accidents (8)

genetic engineering any process by which genetic material is changed to make possible the production of new substances or new functions (11)

genetic mapping the creation of a graphic that shows how genes or DNA sequences are arranged on a chromosome (11)

genetics a field of biology concerned with the study of heredity and gene variation (11)

H

Health Information Technology for Economic and Clinical Health (HITECH) Act a federal law established to promote the adoption of health information technology while protecting patient privacy (3)

health insurance exchanges state-run centers that provide and explain options for certified health insurance plans (12)

Health Insurance Portability and Accountability Act (HIPAA) law that aims to protect the confidentiality and security of healthcare information and help control administrative costs (7)

Hippocratic Oath an oath attributed to the ancient Greek known as Hippocrates that requires a new physician to swear upon a number of healing gods to uphold professional ethical standards; strongly binds the student to the teacher and the greater community of physicians (2)

hospice care medical care that focuses on patient comfort and quality of life rather than curing the patient's disease; generally appropriate for someone with a terminal illness and life expectancy of six months or less (15)

human genome project international research program coordinated by the NIH and the US DOE that studied and identified all of the genes in the human body, collectively known as the *human genome* (11)

I

implied consent a patient action that leads to the presumption that medical care has been authorized (9)

implied contract an enforceable promise or agreement created by the action of the involved parties without a specific written or spoken agreement (5)

informed consent written or verbal agreement to a healthcare procedure that is given after a person understands the accompanying benefits and risks (9)

institutional abuse laws laws that protect against abuse found in institutional settings, including systemic forms of abuse (15)

Institutional Review Boards groups of experts convened to review proposed research activities at an institution with the focus of protecting the rights and welfare of human subjects recruited to participate in those research activities (2)

insurance a contract that states that one party (the insurance company) will pay for certain types of monetary loss in the event of loss or damages occurring from some predefined categories of risk in return for the payment of money in advance, called a *premium* (8)

intellectual property creations of the intellect that are protected by the law, enabling people to earn recognition or financial benefit from what they invent or create (11)

intentional infliction of emotional distress a tort that involves purposeful misconduct that is so extreme that it causes the victim severe emotional trauma (5)

intentional torts deliberate civil wrongs (5)

interoperability the ability of systems to work and communicate with each other, usually achieved by conforming to standards (10)

invasion of privacy intrusion into the personal life of another person without just cause (5)

J

judicial branch the portion of the government made up of judges and courts that resolve issues involving the application of laws (3)

judicial bypass a legal provision that allows a minor to circumvent the necessity of obtaining parental consent by obtaining consent from a court instead (13)

justice the principle that requires giving others what is due to them, including the fair distribution of benefits, risks, and costs (2)

L

law a rule or action that is prescribed by a governmental authority and has a binding legal force (1)

legal guardian a person who has the legal authority (and the corresponding duty) to care for the personal and property interests of another person (13)

legislative branch the portion of the government made up of lawmakers elected by the people; includes the House of Representatives and the Senate (3)

libel defamation that occurs in a written format (5)

license a legally authorized permit to work in a given field (4)

M

managed care In Medicaid, payment arrangement in which states partner with organizations to deliver care and pay a set monthly rate to providers (12)

mandatory reporter a person who has a legal requirement to report an event or issue to someone else; might include reporting child or elder abuse (6)

mature minor doctrine a legal principle that allows minors to make decisions about their health and welfare, if they can show that they are mature enough to make a decision on their own (13)

medical ethics committee a group of knowledgeable healthcare-related experts who are convened to provide advice and assistance in resolving unusual, complicated ethical problems that involve issues affecting the care and treatment of patients (2)

medical malpractice the improper, unskilled, or negligent treatment of a patient by a healthcare professional (5)

mHealth healthcare-related applications that can be used on smartphones, tablets, and other wireless devices (10)

minor a person younger than the age of full legal responsibility; any person younger than 18 years of age (13)

misdemeanor a minor crime; maximum punishment includes fines and up to one year in jail (6)

money damages payments awarded by the court in a liability suit (5)

morality the quality of practicing the right conduct; defines correct conduct according to an individual's ideals and principles (1)

N

negligence the failure to act as a reasonable person of ordinary prudence would act in a certain situation (5)

negligence per se negligence in which the duty is presumed if the act violated a law intended to protect the public; unlike ordinary negligence, the conduct is automatically considered negligent, and the focus of the suit will be whether the conduct proximately caused damage to the plaintiff (5)

non-malfeasance the principle that requires a practitioner to do no harm to a patient by not performing up to professional standards, such as through ineffective, careless, or intentional wrongful acts (2)

notifiable diseases conditions that are required by law to be reported to government authorities (9)

O

Occupational Safety and Health Administration (OSHA) a federal agency that regulates workplace safety and health (14)

Older Americans Act legislation that provided states with funding for community planning and social services, research and development projects, and personnel training in the field of aging; established the Administration on Aging (15)

P

patent a grant made by a government that gives the creator of an invention the sole right to make, use, and sell that invention for a specified period of time (11)

Patient Protection and Affordable Care Act (ACA) law that was passed to help decrease the number of Americans who do not have health insurance and help reduce the overall cost of healthcare (7)

personal health record an electronic record of health-related information about an individual that conforms to nationally recognized interoperability standards and is controlled by the individual (10)

philosophy the study of the truths and principles of existence, reality, knowledge, values, or conduct that guide behavior (1)

physician-assisted suicide suicide committed with the aid of a physician (15)

plaintiff a person or group who is accusing another person or group of wrongdoing (5)

police power the basic right of state and local governments to make laws and regulations for the benefit of their communities (3)

privileged communication information exchanged between people who are in certain recognized relationships, such as a physician-patient relationship, that cannot be disclosed without the consent of the protected party (6)

profession a calling that requires specialized training and membership in a group that establishes and enforces codes of conduct or codes of ethics, including requirements for continuing education and payment of periodic membership fees (2)

professional malpractice insurance a contract between an insurance company and a healthcare professional under which the company will pay for certain types of monetary liability created if the professional makes errors when treating a patient (8)

professional organization a group that consists of individuals who are subject to specific standards regarding training and experience as well as ethical rules (4)

prosecutor a representative of the government who brings charges and leads government efforts to prove the guilt of a defendant in court (6)

prospective payment system (PPS) a method of reimbursement in which Medicare payments are made based on a predetermined, fixed amount (12)

protected health information all individually identifiable information that is created or received by a healthcare provider or any other entity subject to HIPAA requirements; this information can be oral or written (10)

Public Health Service Act law that structured the United States Public Health Service as the primary division of the United States Department of Health, Education, and Welfare, which later became the United States Department of Health and Human Services (7)

punitive damages a type of award that is designed to punish a defendant and deter bad conduct (5)

R

regulation a rule made and maintained by an authority (1)

Rehabilitation Act law that prohibits discrimination based on disability in programs run by federal agencies, programs that receive federal financial assistance, federal employment, and the employment practices of federal contractors (7)

restraining order a court order intended to protect an individual from further harm from someone who has hurt him or her (5)

restraints methods used to stop or limit a patient's movement (15)

revocation an official government act that permanently takes away all rights afforded by a license (4)

risk the possibility of loss or injury (8)

risk management a program or practice to examine causes of loss and to design or implement preventive actions or methods to reduce loss once a cause is identified (8)

rule an explicit or understood regulation or principle that governs conduct within a specific activity or situation (1)

S

sanctions in criminal law, describes the punishment for a criminal offense (10)

scope of practice the range of procedures and actions an individual is permitted to perform; based on education, experience, competence, and formal training (8)

separation of powers a purposeful structuring of the government to avoid one person or group of people wielding uncontrolled centralized power (3)

Sherman Antitrust Act a federal statute that prohibits business activities that are anti-competitive, such as monopolies (12)

slander defamation that occurs in a verbal manner (5)

specific intent a conscious intention and premeditation to do something that is prohibited by law and which will cause a specific harm or result (6)

standard of care the degree of caution or actions expected of a person, such as a healthcare practitioner, in the course of professional duties (5)

Stark Anti-Referral Law law that prohibits physician referrals of designated health services for Medicare and Medicaid patients if the physician (or an immediate family member) has a financial relationship with that entity (7)

statute of limitations a written law that limits the period of time during which a person can assert his or her right to bring a claim, or forever lose the right to bring a claim (5)

statutes laws established by a legislative body (3)

statutory law the body of law established by legislatures, as opposed to common law that has been developed over time by case law (3)

stem cell an unspecialized cell that can become one or more different types of specialized cells (11)

strict liability the imposition of liability that makes a person or company responsible for actions or products that cause damages, regardless of any intent, caution, or preventive acts (5)

Supremacy Clause a clause in Article VI of the US Constitution that establishes that all federal laws and all treaties made under the authority of the United States are the "supreme law of the land" (3)

surrogate decision maker a person who has been entrusted by a once competent patient to make decisions on the patient's behalf when he or she is unable to make those decisions (9)

suspension a temporary negation of the rights and privileges granted by a license (4)

T

telehealth the use of a telecommunications system to deliver health-related services and information (10)

telemedicine the use of technology to facilitate clinical care at a distance (10)

tort an act of wrongdoing that results in injury to another person or damage to another's property (5)

trademark a word, name, symbol, phrase, or other device used to identify and promote a product or service (11)

21st Century Cures Act act that promotes and funds research into preventing and curing serious illnesses, including mental illnesses (7)

U

Uniform Commercial Code set of laws and regulations that govern all commercial transactions in the United States (5)

United States Constitution the formal charter of the United States, which defines the powers and limitations of the national government and the rights of the people (3)

V

value-based healthcare delivery model payment model in which healthcare providers are compensated based on patient health outcomes (1)

vicarious liability liability for loss or damages of one person or entity attributable to another person based on their relationship, even if the second person or entity was not directly involved in causing the loss (8)

Index

Note: Page numbers followed by *f* indicate figures.

I

J

K

L

M